Borders

ELDER MISTREATMENT

Abuse, Neglect, and Exploitation in an Aging America

Panel to Review Risk and Prevalence of Elder Abuse and Neglect

Richard J. Bonnie and Robert B. Wallace, *Editors*

Committee on National Statistics

and

Committee on Law and Justice

Division of Behavioral and Social Sciences and Education

NATIONAL RESEARCH COUNCIL
OF THE NATIONAL ACADEMIES

THE NATIONAL ACADEMIES PRESS
Washington, D.C.
www.nap.edu

THE NATIONAL ACADEMIES PRESS • 500 Fifth Street, N.W. • Washington, DC 20001

NOTICE: The project that is the subject of this report was approved by the Governing Board of the National Research Council, whose members are drawn from the councils of the National Academy of Sciences, the National Academy of Engineering, and the Institute of Medicine. The members of the committee responsible for the report were chosen for their special competences and with regard for appropriate balance.

This study was supported by Contract/Grant No. N01-0D-4-2139 between the National Academy of Sciences and DHHS/National Institutes of Health. Any opinions, findings, conclusions, or recommendations expressed in this publication are those of the author(s) and do not necessarily reflect the views of the organizations or agencies that provided support for the project.

Library of Congress Cataloging-in-Publication Data

Bonnie, Richard J.
  Elder mistreatment : abuse, neglect, and exploitation in an aging
America / Richard J. Bonnie and Robert B. Wallace, Editors.
     p. cm.
Includes bibliographical references and index.
  ISBN 0-309-08434-2 (hardback)
  1. Aged—Abuse of—United States I. Wallace, Robert B. II. Title.
  HV6626.3+
  362.6—dc21
                                    2002012762

Additional copies of this report are available from The National Academies Press, 500 Fifth Street, N.W., Lockbox 285, Washington, DC 20055; (800) 624-6242 or (202) 334-3313 (in the Washington metropolitan area); Internet, http://www.nap.edu

Printed in the United States of America

Suggested citation: National Research Council. (2003). *Elder Mistreatment: Abuse, Neglect, and Exploitation in an Aging America.* Panel to Review Risk and Prevalence of Elder Abuse and Neglect. Richard J. Bonnie and Robert B. Wallace, Editors. Committee on National Statistics and Committee on Law and Justice, Division of Behavioral and Social Sciences and Education. Washington, DC: The National Academies Press.

THE NATIONAL ACADEMIES
Advisers to the Nation on Science, Engineering, and Medicine

The **National Academy of Sciences** is a private, nonprofit, self-perpetuating society of distinguished scholars engaged in scientific and engineering research, dedicated to the furtherance of science and technology and to their use for the general welfare. Upon the authority of the charter granted to it by the Congress in 1863, the Academy has a mandate that requires it to advise the federal government on scientific and technical matters. Dr. Bruce M. Alberts is president of the National Academy of Sciences.

The **National Academy of Engineering** was established in 1964, under the charter of the National Academy of Sciences, as a parallel organization of outstanding engineers. It is autonomous in its administration and in the selection of its members, sharing with the National Academy of Sciences the responsibility for advising the federal government. The National Academy of Engineering also sponsors engineering programs aimed at meeting national needs, encourages education and research, and recognizes the superior achievements of engineers. Dr. Wm. A. Wulf is president of the National Academy of Engineering.

The **Institute of Medicine** was established in 1970 by the National Academy of Sciences to secure the services of eminent members of appropriate professions in the examination of policy matters pertaining to the health of the public. The Institute acts under the responsibility given to the National Academy of Sciences by its congressional charter to be an adviser to the federal government and, upon its own initiative, to identify issues of medical care, research, and education. Dr. Harvey V. Fineberg is president of the Institute of Medicine.

The **National Research Council** was organized by the National Academy of Sciences in 1916 to associate the broad community of science and technology with the Academy's purposes of furthering knowledge and advising the federal government. Functioning in accordance with general policies determined by the Academy, the Council has become the principal operating agency of both the National Academy of Sciences and the National Academy of Engineering in providing services to the government, the public, and the scientific and engineering communities. The Council is administered jointly by both Academies and the Institute of Medicine. Dr. Bruce M. Alberts and Dr. Wm. A. Wulf are chair and vice chair, respectively, of the National Research Council.

www.national-academies.org

v

Acknowledgments

The Panel to Review Risk and Prevalence of Elder Abuse and Neglect wishes to thank the many individuals who contributed to the preparation to this report. The project was sponsored by the National Institute on Aging, National Institutes of Health, U.S. Department of Health and Human Services, with additional support from the Office of Behavioral and Social Science Research and the Office of Research on Women's Health of the National Institutes of Health and the Agency for Health Care Research and Quality. Sidney Stahl served as project officer and was very helpful in orienting the panel to the major issues on elder abuse and neglect that needed to be considered.

The panel also expresses its appreciation to Laurence Branch, Duke University; Larry Corder, Duke University; and Brian Kemp, University of California, Irvine, who prepared background papers in addition to those included in this volume. Thanks are also due to those who reviewed the papers commissioned by the panel and provided many helpful comments— Barbara Altman, National Center for Health Statistics; Jack Guralnik, National Institute on Aging; Jane Tilly, Urban Institute; Jordan Kosberg, University of Alabama; Kenneth Minaker, Massachusetts General Hospital; Carla VandeWeerd, University of South Florida; Richard Schulz, University of Pittsburgh; and George Annas, Boston University.

The panel also wishes to thank Marie-Therese Connolly, U.S. Department of Justice; Patricia McFeeley, University of New Mexico; Joanne Otto, Colorado Department of Human Services; and Patsy Klaus, U.S.

Department of Justice, for their presentations of background information to the panel.

The panel is also grateful to the staff of the National Research Council for its superb support throughout the course of the study. Study Director Earl Pollack, ably assisted by Marisa Gerstein, Danelle Dessaint, and Tanya Lee, helped the panel stay well-informed, on track, and on time. Constance Citro, senior project officer, provided many helpful suggestions. Lora Hamp, a third-year student at the University of Virginia Law School, provided valuable research assistance on elder mistreatment legislation and on legal and ethical issues in elder mistreatment research.

This report has been reviewed in draft form by individuals chosen for their diverse perspectives and technical expertise, in accordance with procedures approved by the Report Review Committee of the National Research Council. The purpose of this independent review is to provide candid and critical comments that will assist the institution in making the published report as sound as possible and to ensure that the report meets institutional standards for objectivity, evidence, and responsiveness to the study charge. The review comments and draft manuscript remain confidential to protect the integrity of the deliberative process.

We thank the following individuals for their participation in the review of this report: Ira Ralph Katz, Institute on Aging, University of Pennsylvania; Jennifer M. Kinney, Department of Sociology, Gerontology, and Anthropology, Miami University; Jill E. Korbin, Office of the Dean, College of Arts and Sciences, Case Western Reserve University; Kenneth Minaker, Massachusetts General Hospital, Boston; Becky Morgan, Stetson College of Law; and Stephen Zarit, Gerontology Center, Pennsylvania State University.

Although the reviewers listed above have provided many constructive comments and suggestions, they were not asked to endorse the conclusions or recommendations; nor did they see the final draft of the report before its release. The review of this report was overseen by Robert Butler, International Longevity Center-USA, Ltd., New York City. Appointed by the National Research Council, he was responsible for making certain that an independent examination of this report was carried out in accordance with institutional procedures and that all review comments were carefully considered. Responsibility for the final content of this report rests entirely with the authoring committee and the institution.

Contents

PART II: BACKGROUND PAPERS

Preface

Reports of this kind typically begin by calling attention to the magnitude and social cost of the problem being explored. The fact that equivalent statements cannot be made with any confidence about elder mistreatment is a telling indication of the need for the report, as well as for an intensified program of research. No survey of the U.S. population has ever been undertaken to provide a national estimate for the occurrence of any form of elder mistreatment; the magnitude of the problem—among community-dwelling elders, as well as those residing in long-term care facilities—is basically unknown. The best estimates, based on figures extrapolated from local studies, suggest that the national prevalence of elder mistreatment (including physical abuse, psychological abuse, and neglect) is between 1 and 2 million.

The occurrence and severity of elder mistreatment are likely to increase markedly over the coming decades, as the population ages, caregiving responsibilities and relationships change, and increasing numbers of older persons require long-term care.

Although the magnitude of elder mistreatment is unknown, its social and moral importance is self-evident. However, there is no solid understanding of the nature, causes, and consequences of elder mistreatment, the effectiveness and cost of current interventions, or measures that could successfully be taken to prevent it or to ameliorate its effects. The purpose of this report is to help the nation remedy this deficiency.

In *Understanding Child Abuse and Neglect* (1993) and *Violence in Families* (1998), the National Research Council was able to map out a comprehensive blueprint for research in the adjacent domains of child mistreatment and intimate partner violence. However, so little is now known about elder mistreatment that it would be premature to draw up a detailed research agenda for this nascent field. Instead, this report is best seen as laying the foundation for a much-needed scientific effort. The panel emphasizes the need to develop a better understanding of elder mistreatment in its different forms, to develop better measures for it, and to undertake a variety of population-based studies to ascertain prevalence and risk factors. Several priorities for research are identified in relation to the determinants of elder mistreatment, clinical screening and case identification, and preventive interventions.

We are not the first to lament the poor state of knowledge about elder mistreatment. In 1986, a consensus conference of leading researchers (including two of our panel members) was convened at the University of New Hampshire to point the way toward advancing knowledge. The conclusions and recommendations reached at that conference are strikingly similar to those appearing in this report.

One of the participants at the New Hampshire conference was Rosalie Wolf, by all accounts one of the founding leaders of the elder mistreatment field. The panel expressed its deep gratitude to Dr. Wolf for presenting her views at our initial meeting, despite her poor health, and was devastated when she passed away within weeks of her appearance at our meeting. We are publishing the remarks that she delivered at that meeting as an appendix to this report. Indeed, our report is in many ways a tribute to Dr. Wolf's heroic efforts over three decades to nurture the field of elder mistreatment research.

Abuse and neglect of older individuals in society breaches a widely embraced moral commitment to protect vulnerable people from harm and to ensure their well-being and security. To carry out this commitment, one cannot rely on good intentions alone. A substantial investment in scientific research along the lines outlined in this report is imperative to enable society to enhance its understanding of elder mistreatment and to mount an effective response to it in the 21st century.

Richard J. Bonnie, *Chair*
Panel to Review Risk and Prevalence
of Elder Abuse and Neglect

ELDER MISTREATMENT

Executive Summary

Elder mistreatment is a recognized social problem of uncertain, though probably increasing, magnitude. According to the best available estimates, between 1 and 2 million Americans age 65 or older have been injured, exploited, or otherwise mistreated by someone on whom they depended for care or protection. The frequency of occurrence of elder mistreatment will undoubtedly increase over the next several decades, as the population ages. Yet little is known about its characteristics, causes, or consequences or about effective means of prevention. This report is intended to point the way toward better understanding of the nature and scope of the problem, a necessary condition for the development of informed policies and programs.

As defined in this report, "elder mistreatment" refers to (a) intentional actions that cause harm or create a serious risk of harm (whether or not harm is intended) to a vulnerable elder by a caregiver or other person who stands in a trust relationship to the elder or (b) failure by a caregiver to satisfy the elder's basic needs or to protect the elder from harm. The term "mistreatment" is meant to exclude cases of so-called self-neglect—failure of an older person to satisfy his or her own basic needs and to protect himself or herself from harm—and also cases involving victimization of elders by strangers.

While elder mistreatment has attracted sustained efforts from practitioners and some interest from policy makers over the past two decades, it has not received concomitant attention from researchers or from the agencies that provide research funding. No major foundation has identified this field as one of its priorities, and the federal investment has been modest at

1

best. For example, fewer than 15 studies on elder mistreatment have been funded by the National Institute on Aging (NIA) since 1990, and support from other agencies has been even less substantial. As a result, elder mistreatment research has thus far been confined to a small community of investigators who have produced a modest body of knowledge concerning the phenomenology, magnitude, etiology, and consequences of elder mistreatment. Estimates of mistreated elders have been based on sample surveys in local areas and projected to the total U.S. population. Preventive and remedial interventions have been unsystematic, episodic, and poorly evaluated. In recognition of these deficiencies, the National Institute on Aging requested the National Research Council, through the Committee on National Statistics, to establish a panel of experts to assess the current state of knowledge in the area of elder mistreatment and to formulate a set of recommendations for a research agenda in that field.

When the body of published and unpublished research reports on elder mistreatment is examined as a whole, a number of weaknesses emerge:

- Unclear and inconsistent definitions
- Unclear and inadequate measures
- Incomplete professional accounts
- Lack of population-based data
- Lack of prospective data
- Lack of control groups
- Lack of systematic evaluation studies

Among the factors accounting for these deficiencies are:

- Little funding and few investigators
- Methodological uncertainties, especially about surveys
- Ethical uncertainties regarding research practices
- Inadequate links between researchers and service agencies
- Impoverished theory
- Intertwined and varying research definitions and statutory definitions
- Divergent research traditions in gerontology and family violence

In order the rectify these problems and to propel the field forward, the panel recommends the following agenda for research.

RECOMMENDED RESEARCH AGENDA

Basic research on the phenomenology of elder mistreatment is a critical early step in the further development of the field. Such research will lead to a much better understanding of the key elements of elder mistreatment, which in turn will facilitate the development of broadly accepted operational definitions and the development of research and clinical measures for these phenomena. Examples of such research include studies of: (1) the kinds of trust relationships that older persons enter into, the other parties involved in these relationships, the foundations of these relationships, and their association with different types of mistreatment; (2) the different types of harms that mistreated older persons may suffer, the interrelationship of the different harms (e.g., relationship of physical to emotional to financial), the severity of harms, their temporal characteristics, and their natural history; (3) the injurious conduct or omissions of other parties in trust relationships, how they manifest themselves, and their natural history; (4) the psychological effects of mistreatment, including types of psychological harm, their presentation, and their natural history; and (5) the circumstances under which harm is most likely to have been caused by the acts or omissions of another person.

Development of widely accepted operational definitions and validated and standardized measurement methods for the elements of elder mistreatment is urgently needed to move the field forward. The field must develop widely accepted operational definitions of the elements of elder mistreatment, its different forms, and associated risk factors and outcomes. The field must also develop a series of measures for these elements, with good (and known) reliability and validity. A menu of measures is necessary for each of the multiple contexts of research, including screening and case identification in clinical settings as well as studies of elder mistreatment in populations.

Population-based surveys of elder mistreatment occurrence are feasible and should be given a high priority by funding agencies. Preparatory funding should be provided to develop and test measures for identifying elder mistreatment. There is inadequate information on elder mistreatment occurrence among both community-dwelling and institutionalized elders. However, before embarking on such surveys, the aims and rationale for them should be clearly delineated, and the strengths and weaknesses of the survey methodology fully understood. Different methods and approaches may be required for various types of mistreatment, and multiple modes of case ascertainment should be considered and evaluated. Survey-acquired information could be enhanced by appropriately applied record linkage techniques. Complementary study of biomarkers that may enhance elder mistreatment case identification should be explored.

Funding agencies should give priority to the design and fielding of national prevalence and incidence studies of elder mistreatment. These studies should include both a large-scale, independent study of prevalence and modular add-ons to surveys of aging populations. Acquiring valid national elder mistreatment occurrence rates is critically needed for improved policy formulation. After appropriate methodological development, a national survey of elder mistreatment occurrence and risk factors, designed to inform important policy issues relevant to elder mistreatment prevention and treatment, should be conducted.

It is logistically feasible to add elder mistreatment case screening or detection modules to existing, comprehensive geographic health and social surveys, including longitudinal studies of aging populations, and attempts should be made to further this application. Those surveys that have access to frail, vulnerable elders and that contain study variables related to the risk or outcomes of elder mistreatment are the ones most likely to be fruitful. Such piggybacking of elder mistreatment items and instruments could also serve as a test bed for developing methodology intended for national surveys.

In addition to improved household and geographically referent sampling techniques, new methods of sampling and identifying elder mistreatment victims in the community should be developed in order to improve the validity and comprehensiveness of elder mistreatment occurrence estimates. It is likely that household sampling, while extremely useful, will be incomplete to some degree because of difficulty in gaining access to those households and respondents most at risk of elder mistreatment. A particular problem is accessing and characterizing the wide variety of assisted living and related residential facilities where many vulnerable elders are located. Developing additional ways to approach and access these populations may require other sampling techniques, such as through social networks and institutions, or the health care system.

The clinical course, antecedents, and outcomes of the various types of elder mistreatment occurrence are poorly understood, necessitating more longitudinal investigations, including follow-up studies of the clinical, social, and psychological outcomes of elder mistreatment cases detected. Many elder mistreatment situations are recurrent and may have various incarnations over long periods, making the definition of an elder mistreatment "event" difficult to define. Thus, further work on the nature, periodicity, variation, and triggers for elder mistreatment are needed and will require longitudinal investigations. Furthermore, the health and social outcomes of elder mistreatment are not well studied and require further investigation, an absolute requisite for prevention and intervention research.

The occurrence of elder mistreatment in the institutional setting, including hospitals, long-term care and assisted living situations, is all but uncharacterized and needs new study sampling and detection methods. Sampling and surveillance techniques may be different from those employed in community-based elder mistreatment detection, and considerable innovation may be required.

Studies are greatly needed that examine risk indicators and risk and protective factors for different types of elder mistreatment. It may make little conceptual sense to combine, for example, physical violence and neglect as subsets of the same phenomenon. Because of the relatively larger number of case-control studies focusing on physical violence, more reliable information regarding risk factors has emerged for that manifestation of elder mistreatment. Research is needed on risk factors for neglect, psychological mistreatment, sexual abuse, and financial abuse. Further, studies of the co-occurrence of different abuse types, and risk factors for such co-occurrence, are needed. This research should not neglect the study of protective factors for elder mistreatment. A particularly critical need exists for studies of risk factors for elder mistreatment in institutional settings.

Research on risk factors should be expanded to take into consideration the clinical course of elder mistreatment. Although longitudinal data are absent, it seems probable that elder abuse situations may follow a pattern similar to disease progression, which would include lead time prior to the manifestation of active signs and symptoms of mistreatment; periods of "remission"; and critical points in which mistreatment becomes more intensive or acute. Some have speculated that mistreatment typically increases in severity and intensity over time, but no empirical data demonstrate this pattern or individual differences in progression. Clinical accounts suggest that situations of mistreatment include cases that resolve on their own, cases in which mistreatment intensifies, and cases in which the situation remains abusive but stable. It is therefore both possible and important to identify risk factors for an increase or intensification in mistreatment. For these reasons, cohort studies are of great importance in determining risk factors for elder mistreatment.

Substantial research is needed to improve and develop new methods of screening for possible elder mistreatment in a range of clinical settings. These methods should be able to detect a broad range of categories of mistreatment and be highly accurate and efficiently deployed. Candidate techniques might include improved questionnaire designs; record linkage to other clinical, public health, social, and legal databases; automated alerts based on concurrent clinical records; and previously defined risk status based on prescreening methods. Special attention should be placed on the predictive value of various clinical injuries and other relevant clinical findings as indicators of mistreatment for therapeutic, social, and forensic reasons.

Research is needed on the process of designating cases as incidents of mistreatment in order to improve criteria, investigative methods, decision-making processes, and decision outcomes. The absence of a gold standard for case identification, and the momentous consequences of inaccurate decisions, highlight the need for studying and improving the process of case investigation and designation. Research assessing the capacity of older persons with cognitive impairments to provide accurate testimony is needed for improving the accuracy of case identification, not only in clinical settings, but also in legal settings, including prosecutorial decision making and formal adjudication.

Research on the effects of elder mistreatment interventions is urgently needed. Existing interventions to prevent or ameliorate elder mistreatment should be evaluated, and agencies funding new intervention programs should require and fund a scientifically adequate evaluation as a component of each grant. Specifically:

- Research is needed on reporting practices and on the effects of reporting, taking maximum advantage of the opportunity for comparisons of practices and outcomes in states with and without mandated reporting.
- Research is needed on the effectiveness of adult protective services interventions, ideally in study designs that compare outcomes in cases in which services were provided with those in which eligible recipients declined offered services or other cases in which mistreatment of an equivalent nature has been identified.
- Intervention or prevention research in existing health care environments that come into contact with mistreated elders, such as hospitals, emergency departments, and emergency response services, should be a priority, as it takes advantage of the existing expertise and resources of these services.
- The development of adult protective services/university research teams should be encouraged in order to evaluate existing data, recommend improvements in the collection of data, analyze incident reports, and design the studies of outcomes urged in this report.

Investigators and institutional review boards (IRBs) need clearer guidance (without rigid rules) concerning two issues that tend to recur in elder mistreatment research: conditions under which research can properly go forward with participants whose decisional capacity is impaired, and the proper responses to evidence of mistreatment elicited during the course of the study. In the absence of better guidance, IRBs are left setting their own criteria, leading to inconsistencies and confusion. Cooperative research between agencies or organizations is also difficult, if not impossible, since different IRBs often take different positions on these issues, including what information must be disclosed to obtain informed consent.

As a first step in this direction, the panel has sought to clarify some of the issues in these two areas and to provide some needed guidance. Eventually, the National Institute on Aging, in consultation with the Office of Human Research Protections and other federal partners, should take steps to promote further clarification, thereby helping investigators and IRBs to achieve the proper level of participant protection while enabling important research involving older and vulnerable adults to move forward.

An adequate long-term funding commitment to research on elder mistreatment must be made by relevant federal, state, and private agencies to support research careers and to develop the next generation of investigators in the field. Knowledge about elder mistreatment will advance only if its importance is recognized by policy makers and funding agencies, if stable research support is provided, and if useful theories and methods are successfully extrapolated from relevant disciplines and adjacent fields of research.

Recognizing that elder mistreatment crosses categorical boundaries in both health research and social science research, federal funding agencies (e.g., the National Institute on Aging, the Administration on Developmental Disabilities and Rehabilitation Research, and the National Institute of Justice) should work collaboratively to promote research on the abuse and financial exploitation of vulnerable adults, including older persons as well as younger adults with disabilities.

One promising approach for strengthening the scientific and political foundation of the caregiving aspects of elder mistreatment research would be to locate it in the domain of quality assurance in long-term care. It is already understood that prevention of mistreatment is a core element of quality assurance in nursing home regulation. Protecting elderly people in community settings, including their own homes, represents a parallel challenge for public policy and an overlapping agenda for researchers aiming to understand the phenomenology, etiology, and consequences of mistreatment and the interventions that can reduce it. By viewing elder mistreatment through the prism of quality assurance (safety and security) in long-term care, it is possible to draw together the frameworks and methods of researchers studying the needs of, and services provided to, vulnerable elderly people in various long-term care settings, as well as those used by researchers studying power and conflict in human relationships.

CONCLUSION

Systematic implementation of these recommendations will help establish a sound foundation for advancing knowledge on elder mistreatment. A genuine long-term commitment of resources to this important, though understudied, area will also help to recruit a new generation of scientists to field. By the same token, however, it is clear that, in the absence of the kinds of investment recommended in this report, knowledge and understanding of elder mistreatment will remain thin, even as the population ages and the occurrence of mistreatment increases. A substantial commitment to research is needed to inform and guide a caring society as it aims to cope with the challenges ahead.

1

Introduction

Elder mistreatment is a recognized social problem of uncertain, though probably increasing, magnitude. Based on the best available estimates, between 1 and 2 million Americans 65 or older have been injured, exploited, or otherwise mistreated by someone on whom they depended for care or protection (Pillemer and Finkelhor, 1988; Pavlik et al., 2001). The number of cases of elder mistreatment will undoubtedly increase over the next several decades, as the population ages. Yet little is known about its characteristics, causes, or consequences or about effective means of prevention or management. This report is meant to point the way toward better understanding of the nature and scope of the problem, a necessary condition for the development of informed policies and programs. After summarizing the social context within which the field has developed, this chapter assesses the present state of knowledge, identifies some of the problems that must be addressed if the field is to move forward, and locates the problem of elder mistreatment in a larger set of challenges confronting an aging society.

AN AGING AND VULNERABLE POPULATION

The aging of the population of the United States is a well-recognized demographic fact. The life expectancy of people born in the United States has been rising throughout the past century. The proportion of the population age 65 and older has increased dramatically since 1950. Between 1950 and 2000, the total population of the country increased by 87 percent, the population age 65 and older increased by 188 percent, and the population 85 and older increased by 635 percent (Eberhardt et al., 2001, Hetzel and Smith, 2001). Over this same period, the life expectancy of people at age 65 increased from 13.9 to 17.9 years (Natonal Center for Health Statistics, unpublished data, 2001). These trends will likely be accentuated by the aging of the post WWII baby boom generation. The U.S. Bureau of the Census predicts that by 2030, the population over age 65 will nearly triple to more than 70 million people, and older people will make up more than 20 percent of the population (up from 12.3 percent in 1990) (Population Projections Program, 2000).

It is heartening that large proportions of the nation's older people are living without substantial disability. Among people age 75 and older in 1999, 70 percent described their health as good or excellent (Eberhardt et al., 2001). Inevitably, however, the aging of the population is also associated with increases in age-related diseases and disabilities. Of the estimated 12.8 million Americans reporting need for assistance with activities of daily living (ADLs—eating, dressing, bathing, transferring between the bed and a chair, toileting, controlling bladder and bowel) or instrumental activities of daily living (IADLs—preparing meals, performing housework, taking drugs, going on errands, managing finances, using a telephone), 57 percent (7.3 million people) were over the age of 65 (Administration on Aging, 1997). Dementia is present in approximately 5 to 10 percent of persons age 65 and older and 30 to 39 percent of persons age 85 and older (Rice et al., 2001; Henderson, 1998). Among people age 85 and older in 1999, 33 percent reported themselves to be in fair or poor health, 84 percent had disabilities involving mobility (unpublished data Natonal Center for Health Statistics, 2002), and 16 percent had Alzheimer's disease (Brookmeyer et al., 1998).

Given the projected growth in the elderly population, long-term care for elderly people with disabilities has become an increasingly urgent policy concern (Institute of Medicine, 2001; Stone, 2000). The settings in which long-term care is provided depend on a variety of factors, including the older person's needs and preferences, the availability of informal support, and the source of reimbursement for care. An increasing number of elderly people reside outside traditional home settings in highly restrictive institutional environments (such as skilled or intermediate nursing facilities) or in less restrictive community-based residential settings, such as assisted living facilities, board and care homes, and adult foster homes. Among the 34 million persons over age 65 in 1995, 5 percent were nursing home residents, and 12 percent lived in the community setting with ADL or IADL limitations. The number of nursing home residents increased between 1973–1974 and 1999 from 961,500 to 1,469,500 among those age 65 and older, and from 413,6000 to 757,100 among those 85 and older (Eberhardt et al., 2001). In 1999, another 500,000 elderly people were living in assisted living facilities (Hawes et al., 1999). Among people age 85 and over, 21 percent were in nursing homes in 1995 and 49 percent were community residents with long-term care needs (Alecxih et al., 1997).

The nursing home population tends to be older and more severely disabled than elders residing elsewhere, with about half of the residents being 85 or older and about half having five ADL limitations, in 1996 (Stone, 2000); still, four out of five elderly persons with ADL or IADL impairments lived in the community setting (Alecxih et al., 1997). Approximately 17 percent of these community-dwelling older persons are considered severely disabled, with limitations in three or more ADLs. Of those ADL-impaired elderly people living in community settings, 37 percent report that they need help but do not receive it or receive less help than is needed (Stone, 2000).

Most long-term care for community-dwelling elders is provided in a traditional home setting, either in an older person's own home, with or without a spouse, or in the home of a close relative. The 1994 National Long Term Care Survey indicated that more than 7 million Americans, mainly family members, provided 120 million hours of care to elders with functional disabilities living in the community. However, the nature and character of the informal networks now providing long-term care services may change (Stone, 2000). The potential pool of adult children who can serve as caregivers is already decreasing, as a result of a variety of demographic trends, including divorce, smaller families, and increased workforce participation (Himes et al., 1996). These factors increase the pressures on families caring for their elderly relatives and also are likely to increase the demand for institutional care.

These trends highlight the growing challenge of ensuring the safety and protecting the other interests of elderly people in the diverse settings in which long-term care is provided. No matter where they reside, older people are vulnerable not only to the infirmities and suffering associated with disease and disability, but also to neglect, victimization, and exploitation by others, including their caregivers. In this respect, protecting older people from mistreatment is an important element of the broad challenge of ensuring quality services in long-term care.

While elder mistreatment has attracted sustained efforts from practitioners and some interest from policy makers over the past two decades, it has not received concomitant attention from researchers or from the agencies that provide research funding. No major foundation has identified this field as one of its priorities, and the federal investment has been modest at best. For example, fewer than 15 studies on elder mistreatment have been funded by the National Institute on Aging (NIA) since 1990, and support from other agencies has been even less substantial. As a result, elder mistreatment research has thus far been confined to a small community of investigators who have produced a modest body of knowledge concerning the phenomenology, magnitude, etiology, and consequences of elder mistreatment. Preventive and remedial interventions have been unsystematic, episodic, and poorly evaluated. In recognition of these deficiencies, the National Institute on Aging requested the National Research Council to commission this study as the first step in an effort to broaden and deepen knowledge about the mistreatment of elders. Support was also provided by the Office of Behavioral and Social Science Research on Women's Health of the National Institutes of Health and the Agency for Health Care Research and Quality. This report presents a research agenda for consideration by the National Institute on Aging and other potential sponsors of research on elder mistreatment—a term we explain more fully in Chapter 2.

HISTORICAL AND SOCIAL CONTEXT

Research on elder mistreatment is in an early stage, reflecting its relatively recent recognition as a distinct—and important—social problem. The prevailing understanding of the problem, and the social response to it, have gradually emerged over the past half-century, shaped by evolving social responses to child protection and family violence as well as by an intensifying concern about neglect and victimization of vulnerable elderly people.

Family discord and mistreatment of its vulnerable members were outside the public domain for much of this country's history. Responsibility for assisting families in need was assumed mainly by religious organizations and private charitable institutions. Although many states established asylums for people with mental illness during the 18th and 19th centuries, thereby providing some custodial protection for dependent or neglected adults, there was no legal basis for intervention into families until the late 19th century, when industrialization, immigration, and urbanization exacerbated family problems, including poverty and internal conflict, and also exposed them to public view—especially when its victims were children. The emergence of the juvenile court in the early part of the 20th century represented a significant assertion of collective responsibility for protecting and "saving" children who had become ungovernable by their parents; over the following decades, the jurisdiction of the juvenile courts gradually reached children who were neglected or abused by their parents (Platt, 1969).

The legal foundation for modern policies and programs for elder protection was put in place after World War II, particularly during a burst of national energy geared toward remediation of endemic social problems during the 1970s. Although the threads of child protection, adult protection, and family violence were intertwined in the history of that period, they are summarized separately below.

Origins of Child Protection

The current system for protection of elders and other vulnerable adults grew from the child protection system, which itself is only about 40 years old in its modern form. The seminal event in the formation of the modern child protection system was the publication of an article in the *Journal of the American Medical Association* by a team of physicians at the University of Colorado, who proclaimed the existence of a "battered child syndrome" (Kempe et al., 1962). Pediatrician Henry Kempe, the leader of the group and founder of the International Society for Prevention of Child Abuse and Neglect, spearheaded a movement to adopt mandated reporting laws. These laws, which were quickly adopted in all 50 states, rested on the premise that the abused child was an aberrant problem (amounting to several hundred egregious cases each year in the United States), and on the belief that the problem could be solved if health professionals brought those cases to the attention of social service authorities. Although initial federal action did not occur until significantly later, with the adoption of the Child Abuse Prevention and Treatment Act of 1974 (Nelson, 1984), that legislation also required states to adopt mandated reporting and investigation as the primary strategy for protecting children.

Origins of Adult Protection

Drawing on their *parens patriae* authority to protect helpless citizens, a few states developed new public welfare programs during the 1940s and 1950s to protect adults who could not manage their own resources or protect themselves from harm. New adult protective services units were established not only to provide social services, but also to provide legal services, such as guardianship. Aroused by these state innovations, federal interest in the problem first appeared in the 1960s. Legislation was directed at all adults who were seen as defenseless and susceptible to being hurt by others. In 1962 Congress passed the Public Welfare Amendments to the Social Security Act, authorizing payments to the states to establish protective services for "persons with physical and/or mental limitations, who were unable to manage their own affairs . . . or who were neglected or exploited" (U.S. Department of Health, Education, and Welfare, 1966).

One of the demonstration projects funded by this new program was operated by a team at the Benjamin Rose Institute in Cleveland under Margaret Blenkner and her associates (Blenkner et al., 1974; Anetzberger et al., 2000). She matched a group of elders receiving protective services with a group from the community who were receiving traditional services, finding that those who were receiving protective services had a higher mortality rate and higher nursing home placement rate than those who were receiving traditional services. This study raised important questions: Was the higher risk attributable to the intervention or to selection bias, and if the former, what aspect of the intervention increased the risk? Was it the nursing home placement? Notwithstanding this puzzling finding from the Blenkner study and other studies questioning the cost-effectiveness of protective services (Wolfe, this volume), advocates for the system continued to press for broader congressional action. Eventually, in 1974, Congress amended the Social Security Act to require states to establish protective service units for adults with mental and physical impairments, who are unable to manage on their own, and who were victims or were being exploited or neglected. Funding for the protective services was to come from social services block grants (SSBG) given by the federal government to the states. Until this time, most SSBG funds had been used exclusively for child protective services.

This new federal program directed the states to provide protective services to adults who, "as a result of physical or mental limitations, are unable to act in their own behalf; are seriously limited in the management of their affairs; are neglected or exploited; or are living in unsafe or hazardous conditions." A number of states then codified this federal mandate and, by 1978, 20 states had legislation establishing adult protection units as part of their social services agencies. This trend was accompanied by increasing use of SSBG dollars for adult protection: in 1980, 38 states reported that 83.3 million SSBG dollars were spent for adult protective services. As SSBG appropriations declined during the 1980s, however, funding for adult protective services declined; by 1985, it had declined by 42 percent.

Spotlight on Elder Protection

Scarce attention was paid to the problem of elder abuse before 1978 except for some intermittent articles published in British and American medical and social services journals. In the late 1970s, the national spotlight was directed for the first time at what was characterized as systematic mistreatment of elderly people. Congressman Claude Pepper held widely publicized hearings, calling attention to the "hidden problem" of elder abuse in the nation's families, including what one witness characterized as "granny battering" (Wolfe, this volume). Although the Pepper hearings did not lead immediately to federal action or funding, they stimulated additional state action. As the state response continued to evolve in the early 1980s, many states required reporting of abuse, bringing the problem within the purview of adult protective services. By 1985, 46 states had designated a responsible agency. Meanwhile, Congressman Pepper continued to agitate for a federal response to elder mistreatment. In a 1981 report (Pepper and Okar, 1981), he stated that elder abuse was increasing and recommended that Congress act immediately to help the states identify and assist elder abuse victims. Again, however, Pepper's plea was unheeded by the Congress. Finally, in 1989, Pepper succeeded in including creation of a national center on elder abuse as an amendment to the Older Americans Act. Although various versions of a national center followed, the current National Center on Elder Abuse was established in 1998.

In retrospect, it appears that elder mistreatment became identified as a national concern when it was conceptualized as an "aging" issue, rather than as an undifferentiated component of adult protection. This also helped to broaden the constituencies interested in research and program development to include gerontologists and the expanding network of service providers and advocates for the elderly. The Pepper hearings also cast the problem of elder abuse in a particular light—as a complication of caregiving. The emerging image was that of an impaired victim, usually an elderly parent being cared for by an adult caregiver who wasn't able to manage the caregiving because of stresses in life, on the job, and in the family. Even though it is only a partial explanation of elder mistreatment, this picture seemed to resonate with Congress and the media (Wolfe, this volume).

Emerging Conceptions of Family Violence

The evolving understanding of elder mistreatment as a social problem has more recently been shaped by another image—the trapped victim of family violence. Spouse abuse and other varieties of intimate partner violence have received increasing professional and political attention since the 1980s, leading to a wide variety of interventions and a substantial investment in research (National Research Council, 1996; National Research Council and Institute of Medicine, 1998). Prevention, protection, and punishment are necessary components of a comprehensive social response, requiring the participation and coordination of a broad array of public agencies. As the consciousness of health professionals has been raised, family violence has been embraced as a public health problem, thereby recruiting researchers and advocates in injury prevention and public health to the field (Institute of Medicine, 1999). Many of the preventive and protective tools developed in the context of intimate partner violence have now been directed to violence against elders. Bringing elder mistreatment into the domain of family violence widens the angle of the lens and thereby brings new ideas about etiology and prevention into view. However, it also exposes some tensions between social services agencies, with their traditional helping orientation, and many family violence specialists, with their greater emphasis on criminalization and punishment of perpetrators.

The Crisis in Child Protection

Evolving conceptions of elder mistreatment, and the appropriate social responses to it, will also be shaped, inevitably, by the deep concerns that have emerged over the past decade in the field of child protection. In 1990, the U.S. Advisory Board on Child Abuse and Neglect issued a highly publicized and rarely disputed declaration of a national emergency in the child protection system. By that time, the number of cases reported annually to state and county social service and law enforcement agencies in the United States approached 3 million—a number enormously discrepant from the 1962 estimate of Kempe et al. of approximately 300 cases annually. Moreover, the advisory board found that, by state social service agencies' own admission, many children officially found to have been maltreated received no services other than the investigation itself.

The U.S. Advisory Board on Child Abuse and Neglect (1990) attributed the emergency to the errant design of the child protection system itself: the system has become preoccupied by investigation (rather than prevention and treatment), and community responsibility for ensuring the safety of dependent children has effectively, if unintentionally, been diverted to a small social service agency. In response, the board (U.S. Advisory Board on Child Abuse and Neglect, 1993) proposed a new national strategy designed to rely on voluntary action to make child protection a part of everyday life (see Melton and Barry, 1994, Melton et al., 2001, for edited books articulating the social science foundation for this approach). As Wolfe notes in his paper in this volume, several states have attempted to deemphasize investigation in their state child protection statutes, and some major foundations have undertaken initiatives to demonstrate the feasibility of a neighborhood-based, largely voluntary, and largely preventive and supportive child protection system. Nonetheless, modal practice is largely unchanged, and the enormity of the problem remains (Melton, 2002).

The tensions in child protection policy (as well as the number of reported cases) have intensified as the scope of problems defined as child maltreatment has expanded. Although the modern system was created in response to the image of battered children, neglect has long been the modal reason for referral to child protection (Peddle and Wang, 2001), and most such cases involve complex social and economic problems, not willful neglect (Pelton, 1994). Similarly, the biggest increase in reporting occurred when sexual abuse was "discovered" early in the 1980s (Weisberg, 1984), and criminal prosecution became a common feature in the child protection system.

Recognition of the frequent linkage between intimate partner violence and child maltreatment (see Carter et al., 1999) has also challenged the child protection system, which generally (except to some degree in cases of sexual abuse and severe physical abuse) has not adopted the "perpetrator-victim" model commonly embraced by advocates for battered women (Melton and Andrews, 2000). There are some signs of an uneasy rapprochement between the two systems (see, e.g., Schechter and Edleson, 1999), as some child protection authorities have adopted safety planning, a feature of victim empowerment in programs for battered women, as a potentially useful element of intervention in cases of child maltreatment.

Even this development, however, has illustrated the field's vulnerability to unintended side effects. For example, a legislative determination in Minnesota that exposure of children to intimate partner violence is per se evidence of child neglect led to an immediate doubling of referrals to child protective services, a huge increase in expenditures, and increased stress and loss of confidentiality for women and their families living in shelters (Edleson, 2000). It was also speculated that this policy, soon retracted by the legislature, deterred some battered women from seeking protection for themselves and their children.

These tensions and policy adaptations in the field of child protection appear to be highly relevant to elder protection at this moment in the evolution of research and public policy in this nascent field. As discussed further in Chapter 6, adult protection services agencies grapple daily with the tensions between investigation and service, and prosecution and protection. Agency caseloads reflect the highly diverse problems within their jurisdictions, ranging from intentional partner violence to far more numerous cases of caregiver neglect (as well as problems not arising in child protection, such as financial exploitation). The recent history of child protection offers many lessons for specialists in elder mistreatment.

Looking Ahead

Prevailing conceptions of elder mistreatment draw on a diverse array of images (the forgotten and helpless nursing home resident, the battered granny, the stressed caregiver, the abusing spouse). Moreover, the system of adult protection that has emerged to respond to these varied problems (as well as other problems relating to adults with disabilities) is based on ideas and structures borrowed from policy and practice in child maltreatment and, more recently, intimate partner violence. Yet prevailing policies and practices in these adjacent domains are not fully applicable to elder mistreatment and have been controversial on their own terms. Repeatedly, National Research Council and Institute of Medicine panels have called attention to the need for sustained and aggressive research on the phenomenology, magnitude, etiology, and consequences of these problems and on the effects of interventions (National Research Council, 1993, 1996; National Research Council and Institute of Medicine, 1998). In so doing, they have noted that very little is known about the phenomenology, magnitude, etiology, and consequences of elder mistreatment, and that almost nothing is known about the effects of interventions. Although the body of evidence remains sparse, researchers have recently begun to raise doubts about the cost-effectiveness of current interventions (Dyer et al., 1999; Harrell et al., 2002; Pavlik et al., 2001; Hajjar and Duthie, 2001; Wolf and Li, 1999).

Overall, the national response to elder mistreatment still remains weak and incomplete. Adult protection is a poorly funded system, and Congressman Pepper's single-minded emphasis on the abuse, exploitation, and neglect of vulnerable elderly people has not been sustained by his successors in Congress or by a public preoccupied with youthfulness and ill at ease with aging. As a result, elder mistreatment remains hidden, poorly characterized, and largely unaddressed—more than two decades after the Pepper hearings first exposed it to public view. It is long past time to move the field forward in a careful and systematic way, drawing on the knowledge already generated in the domains of child maltreatment and intimate partner violence, while remedying the weaknesses that have so far plagued the field.

WEAKNESSES IN EXISTING RESEARCH

Although there is a sizable body of unpublished reports and commentary on elder mistreatment, fewer than 50 peer-reviewed articles based on empirical research have been published in the field. (A summary of these studies appears in Appendix A.) Although these studies provide a foundation for further work, it is not a strong one. National Research Council (1993) and Institute of Medicine reports (2001; National Research Council and Institute of Medicine, 1998) and other authoritative reviews (e.g., Pillemer, 2001; National Institute of Justice, 2000) have repeatedly lamented the weakness of the research base for designing programs and informing policy on the wide variety of overlapping problems, ranging from granny battering to neglect by nursing homes, that are grouped under the rubric of elder mistreatment. A systematic program of research is needed to better describe the many facets of the problem and to explore their causes and consequences.

Understanding the nature and scope of the problem is prerequisite to designing and implementing solutions. In the absence of the necessary research, interventions have been designed and implemented in the dark, so to speak. Almost every state has required reporting of suspected cases of elder mistreatment, but little is known about the effects of these requirements (National Research Council and Institute of Medicine, 1998). A few states and localities have mounted some creative interventions, but these few initiatives have been poorly evaluated. It has often been said that elder mistreatment, as a field of research, is at about the same embryonic stage of development as child mistreatment was about 30-40 years ago.

Some of the weaknesses of elder mistreatment research are summarized below.

Unclear and Inconsistent Definitions

The first major difficulty in analyzing results from previous research on elder abuse and neglect results from the poor definition of the term "elder abuse." To some extent, this problem is a reflection of conceptual confusion: What type of behavior or condition is denoted by the concept of "abuse"? To some extent, it is also traceable to the variations and ambiguities of the state statutes that direct or authorize interventions in cases of elder abuse or neglect. (The statutes are discussed in Chapter 2.) However, researchers have often exacerbated the problem by failing to define or operationalize their terms in a clear and objective way. For example, many researchers refer to the entire range of problems experienced by elders as "abuse," including lack of proper housing, untreated medical conditions, and lack of social services. Most of the studies are weakened by their undifferentiated treatment of various types of abuse and neglect. That is, all forms of mistreatment are lumped together, despite evidence that the forms of abuse and neglect differ substantially. In some studies, for example, it is difficult to determine whether financial exploitation is included in the research definition. Studies are especially weakened by their inclusion of the category "self-abuse" or "self-neglect." As discussed below, these terms refer to a category of conditions that has little in common with the conditions that bear on abuse and neglect of elder persons by other people.

Researchers have also diverged widely in their definitions of the pertinent component terms and have frequently used confusing and unclear definitions. For example, some researchers have used the term "abuse" tautologically; for example, one group of researchers defined elder abuse as "an abusive action inflicted by the abusers on adults 60 years of age or older." Another group called elder neglect and abuse "a generic term that refers to the neglect and/or physical, psychological, or financial abuse of the older person." Furthermore, definitions have differed so widely from study to study that the results of research are almost impossible to compare. While one set of investigators calls "withholding of personal care" physical abuse, a second researcher calls it active neglect; a third subsumes such actions under physical neglect; and yet a fourth considers such behaviors to be "psychological neglect." Similarly, some researchers define physical abuse in terms of actions: hitting, pushing, choking, etc. Others, however, use lists of injuries to define physical elder abuse, such as cuts, fractures, bruises, and burns.

The development of better definitions of mistreatment of the elderly should be an extremely high priority for researchers. In particular, it is critical to differentiate among various types of mistreatment. Researchers must be clear and explicit regarding what is included and excluded from the category of elder abuse in order to conduct any meaningful meta-analyses. The panel addresses this problem in the next chapter.

Unclear and Inadequate Measures

Related to the definitional issue is that of measurement. This is an equally vexing problem, since the definitions of the varying elements of elder abuse must be operationalized through the design and administration of a research instrument. Many studies have not developed separate research instruments at all; instead, they have simply analyzed the forms used by agencies. These forms are not designed for research and rarely provide data of the type and quality to be of use to researchers. Or studies use as a "measure" of abuse whether a professional has identified an elderly person as "abused"—thereby embracing without further clarification the discretionary judgments of clinicians and caseworkers applying the ambiguous statutory definitions. Few attempts have been made to create reliable and valid instruments for the studies. Even when research instruments have been used, researchers have used highly varying approaches.

An example to illustrate this point may be in order. Researcher A includes physical abuse in her definition of elder abuse. She is using the Conflict Tactics Scale, which measures physical acting out in response to conflict. She then proceeds to define physical abuse as a single incident in which the elder is hit, bit, punched, kicked, threatened with a weapon, or has a weapon used on him or her. Researcher B also includes physical abuse in his definition of elder abuse. However, he has developed his own scale, similar to the Conflict Tactics Scale but more broadly constructed, so that it measures any assaultive behavior of hitting, biting, kicking, punching, threatening with a weapon, or using a weapon regardless of the reason for the behavior. Furthermore, he decides that there must be at least two episodes of this behavior for it to be called physical abuse except for those items dealing with weapons, in which case one incident is sufficient. Thus both researchers have included physical abuse in their studies—indeed, it may be the sole focus of each researcher's study—but the measure of physical abuse differs across the two studies.

This problem arises for all of the types of elder mistreatment typically investigated, including neglect and financial exploitation. The lack of definitional consistency poses issues for interpretation and understanding across studies, including determining prevalence and risk factors. However, even if researchers embraced a common set of definitions for the elements of elder mistreatment and operationalized them the same way, that would still leave the problem of determining whether the instruments actually measure what they purport to measure (validity) and whether they can be reliably administered. At the present time, no measure of elder mistreatment has been validated, nor has any instrument been embraced by the field as a definitive measure of mistreatment, even within a narrow sphere.

All this suggests that researchers, policy makers, and other consumers of research on elder mistreatment must pay careful attention to the definitions and measures of any studies on which they rely. In most cases, the measures will not be comparable.

Incompleteness of Professional Accounts

Since the earliest stages of elder abuse research, surveys of professionals have been used to shed light on the prevalence of elder abuse and on risk factors. Investigators typically mail surveys to professionals and paraprofessionals, asking them about contacts with cases of elder abuse or neglect during a given time period. To provide a typical example, in a survey on elder abuse funded by the Administration on Aging, a sample of professionals, including administrators and direct service workers from 16 types of agencies, was surveyed in each of Pennsylvania's 67 counties. Overall, one-half of the responding agencies reported encountering elder abuse, ranging from over 90 percent of domestic violence agencies, to less than 30 percent for law enforcement, emergency services, medical clinics, and drug/alcohol agencies (Fiegener et al., 1989). Similarly, a survey of Alabama physicians and registered and licensed practical nurses found that 38 percent of the physicians and 53 percent of the nurses had seen cases of elder abuse in the previous year (Clark-Daniels et al., 1990).

At best, studies of professional experience provide impressionistic estimates and opinions about the prevalence, correlates, and consequences of elder mistreatment. Although such data may be useful for generating hypotheses for further research, they do not provide a sound basis for designing programs or formulating policies.

Elder mistreatment researchers have also relied on samples of cases that have come to the formal attention of a social agency or reporting authority. For example, records of patients at hospitals or social service agencies have been reviewed, and the percentage of elderly persons judged to have been abused is established. A more controlled version of this kind of study provides agency caseworkers or health professionals with a standardized assessment tool, which they are trained to fill out for clients. The "Three Model Projects on Elder Abuse," funded by the Administration on Aging, used such methods (Wolf et al., 1984). In both types of studies, however, researchers obtained data from professional accounts of mistreatment rather than from interviews with victims themselves.

It is widely recognized that reported cases are highly selective samples, and that there is a large reservoir of unreported and undetected cases of elder mistreatment about which very little is known. Although unreported cases may be similar to reported cases, they also may be quite different. Samples of reported cases may suggest common patterns and correlates of mistreatment, especially when paired with a control group, but the data must be interpreted with great care. Most important, the question of the extent of elder mistreatment cannot be answered by studies of reported cases. There are major problems with focusing on reported cases:

• The studies are primarily based on cases uncovered through surveys of community professionals—public health nurses, social workers, legal aid lawyers, etc. They are thus cases that have come to public attention in one way or another. However, we know from other studies of family violence using nonclinical populations that only a fraction of cases involving serious mistreatment comes to public attention and that these cases are not necessarily representative of the problem at large. (In relation to child abuse, for example, see the 1995 Gallup Poll, finding that far more of America's children are victims of physical and sexual abuse than officially reported—Gallup Poll, 1995.)

• Similarly, in most cases, the research data on elder mistreatment have not come directly from victims, but instead from professionals and outside observers. Such secondhand knowledge may distort the actual dynamics of mistreatment by failing to present the problems and their effects, as the actual participants perceive them.

• Case reports have little value in studying some forms of mistreatment that are rarely reported to adult protective services agencies, such as mistreatment in institutional settings.

Because elder mistreatment studies have relied so heavily on reports from professionals, crucial data about abuse situations have been missed. Community professionals in general do not collect data useful to researchers and policy makers. Thus, previous research using agency records has rarely been able to obtain detailed information about family history, attitudes, and consequences of mistreatment and other issues. Some researchers (e.g., Lachs et al., 1997a) have made effective use of these weak datasets by matching cases with higher-quality datasets.

In an effort to generate a national estimate of the occurrence of elder abuse and neglect based on case-identification by professional "sentinels," the National Center of Elder Abuse, in conjunction with Westat, Inc., conducted the National Elder Abuse Incidence Study (National Center on Elder Abuse, 1998). In this study, modeled after recent incidence studies of child abuse, the researchers identified a nationally representative sample of 20 counties in 15 states; for each county sampled, they collected data from the local APS agency as well as approximately 1100 professional "sentinels" having frequent contact with the elderly. In 1996, according to the projections based on this study, about 450,000 persons age 60 or older experienced abuse or neglect in family settings, about 16 percent of whom were in the APS report files. It is generally acknowledged that these findings detect only the most overt cases and thus significantly underestimate the incidence of elder mistreatment.

Studies of professionals and agency records are justified in those situations in which investigators specifically want to know how professionals view elder mistreatment. But researchers have too often used these professional surveys to estimate the incidence or prevalence of elder mistreatment, or to establish its causes. They are not appropriate for these purposes. Future research in this area should go beyond archival data and should rely to a much greater extent on elder persons' accounts of their experiences and on their perceptions regarding their own security.

Lack of Population-Based Data

Data on the extent of elder mistreatment in the general population are sparse. Representative sample surveys of community populations are urgently needed. Over the past two decades, knowledge about violence in families and the victimization of children and other vulnerable people has improved significantly. A major advance has been the fielding of major population-based victimization surveys that have helped to establish reliable prevalence estimates of select problems, such as intimate partner violence and child physical and sexual abuse. Similar progress has not occurred in the field of elder mistreatment.

In the earliest research about two decades ago, studies were generally conducted on small, nonrandom samples, with little generalizabilty to the population. Furthermore, research in the field was conducted independently by investigators from different disciplines, using different methods and without recognizing the problems faced by other investigators. For example, the medical community focused on clinical signs and symptoms that could not be explained by disease markers, and this was a daunting task. Very often, older adults who had multiple chronic diseases or conditions might have symptoms that could mask or mimic mistreatment. Using a patient-based approach to study elder mistreatment is also fraught with potential for sample bias, in that if an older adult does not have a doctor or does not come to the emergency department, mistreatment cannot be evaluated.

Although some population surveys have subsequently been fielded, many of them have excluded from the sample potential respondents who may be at high risk for abuse or neglect—e.g., older adults with profound dementia, severe hearing or speech impediments, or advanced problems with mobility who are unable to participate in survey research. Although some investigators have tried to use proxy respondents, this method poses even more challenging issues, because the proxy may be implicating him or herself in mistreatment.

Prevalence information (for one community in the United States) was best established by Pillemer and Finkelhor (1988), who used a stratified random sample of community dwelling older persons (65 or older) in the Boston metropolitan area. A two-stage interview process was used: screening to determine if the person was a victim of mistreatment (defined to include physical abuse and psychological abuse and neglect but excluding financial abuse), followed by in-depth interviews by telephone or in person. Since 1988, there has been no effort in the United States to obtain better prevalence data using large-scale random samples on either a locally or nationally representative sample. However, four such studies have been undertaken in Canada (Podnieks, 1992), the United Kingdom (Ogg and Bennett, 1992), Finland (Kivela et al., 1992), and The Netherlands (Comijs et al., 1998). Despite using different methods, these studies each reported that the prevalence of elder abuse falls in the 3-5 percent range. (It should be noted, however, that the scope and content of the definitions used in these studies vary, particularly with regard to financial abuse.) Despite attempts to estimate incidence and prevalence in other ways, random sample surveys of the elderly population alone allow for a more accurate assessment of the rate of elder mistreatment. In the United States, a national survey is urgently needed to estimate the prevalence of different types of elder mistreatment in the general population, and in specific regions and subgroups, as well as the co-occurrence of different forms of mistreatment (see Chapter 4).

Lack of Prospective Data

Prospective studies are powerful designs, in that they can overcome the recall bias inherent in retrospective studies based on self-reported mistreatment. Studies of this kind are urgently needed: to date, no prospective study of elder abuse has been conducted. However, in a pioneering study, Lachs and colleagues retrospectively linked Adult Protective Services data to a prospective study—the New Haven EPESE study (Established Population for Epidemiologic Studies in the Elderly) as the basis for this research, one of four cohorts funded by NIA (Lachs et al., 1996). In inception year 1982, the study sample consisted of 2,812 community-dwelling older adults over age 65. A manual record matching of EPESE and Connecticut ombudsman/elderly protective service records was done to determine if any cohort members had been seen by ombudsmen over an 11-year follow-up period from cohort inception (1982-1992 inclusive). After cohort members who were seen by protective services for the elderly were identified, weighted survival curves from cohort inception were constructed for three subgroups of subjects: (1) those found to have sustained verified elder mistreatment (abuse, neglect, or exploitation) by another party (i.e., nonself-neglect), (2) those seen by protective services for corroborated self-neglect, or (3) other members of the cohort who had no contact with elderly protective services.

Lack of Control Groups

Much of the data on risk factors and consequences of elder mistreatment are drawn from studies of clinical case samples. However, few of these studies have used controlled designs. For this reason, generalizations made from the existing studies are necessarily suspect. For example, some investigators have asserted that the abused elderly tend to be physically or mentally impaired or both. However, without a comparison group, it is impossible to know if they are more or less impaired than other persons. Several studies have attempted to go beyond previous efforts by interviewing the victims themselves and including a control group of nonabused elderly persons (Bristowe and Collins, 1989; Paveza et al., 1992; Pillemer and Finkelhor, 1988). These are still few and far between, however. Interestingly, although a number of controlled studies were conducted in the late 1980s and early 1990s, there are virtually no examples of more recent case-control studies of elder mistreatment.

Lack of Systematic Evaluation Studies

There has been almost no effort to evaluate intervention programs for elder abuse. Certainly, no study has as yet attempted a randomized control group design in this area. Any kind of experimental demonstration project is rare. Little is known about the relative effectiveness of various programs.

Summary

Due to such shortcomings, existing studies have not provided adequate data needed to answer three important public policy questions about elder abuse and neglect:

First, is the problem of sufficient magnitude to warrant large-scale public concern, including such measures as mandatory reporting laws and protective services? Better data on the true prevalence of elder mistreatment are needed in deciding what action government ought to take.

Second, what are the characteristics of locations, conditions, situations, and relationships in which the elderly are most vulnerable to mistreatment? To design and implement intervention programs, policy makers and service providers must learn more about the factors that increase or decrease the risk of mistreatment and the conditions that ensure safety.

Third, what interventions prevent elder mistreatment and ameliorate its effects? Extensive evaluation research using scientifically sound research designs is critically needed.

IMPEDIMENTS TO ELDER MISTREATMENT RESEARCH

Why is knowledge about elder mistreatment so underdeveloped? What accounts for the paucity of sound research in this important area? The panel has identified a number of explanatory factors.

1. Many investigators believe that victims and family members are not suitable respondents for interview studies of elder mistreatment, because they are not reliable respondents, because they are not willing to be interviewed, or because they are incapable of giving the necessary consent. In fact, many victims are more than willing to be interviewed and are reliable respondents able to give the necessary consent. Surveys including such respondents have uncovered serious cases of mistreatment, and a variety of studies have been conducted in which victims have been interviewed.

2. In general, methods that have been used successfully to investigate other forms of family violence have not been applied to research on elder mistreatment. Gerontologists who study elder mistreatment have tended to follow their interests in family caregiving and have seen the problem in this context. However, because much elder mistreatment does not occur in family caregiving situations, this has been a serious limitation. Furthermore, the technology for studying family violence has been developed and refined not by gerontologists, but by child abuse and intimate partner researchers. Elder mistreatment researchers have not been trained in methods of studying other forms of family violence, including sampling methodologies and measurement techniques.

One example of this problem is the lack of studies using the Conflict Tactics Scale (Straus, 1978; Straus and Gelles, 1990, 1992) to study elder mistreatment. Regardless of the occasional controversy over the scale, it is a hallmark instrument that has been used in scores of studies of child abuse and intimate partner abuse. It is to some extent the state of the art, but some elder mistreatment researchers do not seem to be aware of it.

3. It is very difficult to obtain access to perpetrators of mistreatment. In intimate partner studies, a number of researchers have used treatment programs for batterers as sources of research subjects. These do not exist for elder mistreatment.

4. The exclusion of some victims can seriously bias samples. The problem is most evident when residents of institutions are excluded altogether from population samples. However, even within the targeted study population (whether community dwelling or residing in institutions), exclusion criteria based on cognitive deficiencies can seriously skew the findings.

5. There is some anecdotal evidence that institutional review boards have interpreted the Common Rule (the governing regulations on research ethics) in an unduly restrictive fashion, impeding potentially valuable research on elder mistreatment (see Chapter 8).

6. Few investigators have been drawn to this field of inquiry. Reviews of the literature reflect the same small set of names time and again, with few new researchers selecting and remaining in this field. One of the reasons for this situation is that so little funding has been available for research on elder mistreatment. Although more outstanding investigators might have attracted more funding, dedicated funding also could attract more and better investigators. Although the total federal contribution to research on elder mistreatment is uncertain, expenditures by NIA, the lead agency for aging research, have totaled $10 million during the last 12 years (1990–2001). Annual expenditures have increased from less than $300,000 per year in 1990 to over $1.3 million in 2001; this is a modest sum even in comparison to the underfunded domain of child abuse research, on which federal agencies spend $3.8 million each year.

7. The existing body of research is largely descriptive and pragmatic, taking the concepts and definitions used in practice or in statutes as given, rather than deriving the concepts and measures from theoretical premises or hypotheses. The atheoretical nature of the research is reflected in the tendency to lump all forms of mistreatment within a single category.

8. Individuals who have attempted to conduct research on elder abuse report that they have sometimes been hindered by a lack of cooperation from agencies responsible for identifying and treating victims of mistreatment. Adult protective services programs and other elder abuse service programs have been characteristically reluctant to assist researchers in research activities, and especially research that involves interviews with victims and their families. Reasons for lack of agency cooperation include a desire to protect their clients' privacy and to prevent additional disruption in their lives, fear of evaluation research, and a shortage of staff time to devote to research.

9. Although every state has enacted a statute authorizing or directing intervention in cases involving vulnerable adults, including the elderly, these statutes vary widely in almost every respect (see Appendix B and tables in Chapter 2). They specify different ages or circumstance under which a victim is eligible for protective services, often differentiating between in-home and institutional abuse. They also vary in definitions of abuse, classification of abuse as civil or criminal, whether reporting is mandatory or voluntary, and the remedies or resources available when abuse is documented.

Each of the statutes defines conditions or circumstances that warrant intervention. The statutes typically define abuse or mistreatment as a series of broad categories, such as physical abuse, psychological or emotional abuse, sexual abuse or exploitation, and fiduciary abuse or exploitation, as well as neglect. However, not all states include all of these categories, and others are sometimes added. For example, some states do not include psychological abuse within the definition, while others add more specific forms of mistreatment such as "unreasonable confinement" or "abandonment." Moreover, statutes sometimes distinguish between degrees of mistreatment according to the perpetrator's culpability or state of mind; for example, the law may distinguish among willful infliction of physical abuse, negligently causing physical injury, and failure to prevent it.

In addition to variations in the types of mistreatment included in the statutory definition, the statutes also differ substantially in defining the common categories. For example, the definition of emotional abuse in several states includes "ridiculing or demeaning an infirm adult, making derogatory remarks to an infirm adult or cursing or threatening to inflict physical or emotional harm on an infirm adult," whereas other states require proof of "extreme emotional distress or harm" (see Appendix B).

These statutory variations in definitions and obligations create innumerable opportunities for confusion and lack of comparability, especially if reported cases are being studied. When data are reported to some central repository, unless the repository has imposed a specific definition for each of the forms of abuse, the same statutory element will trigger reports in different categories of cases in different states. Interpretation of combined statistics is treacherous, even if the only objective is to compare trends across states.

OUTLINE OF REPORT

Keeping in mind the impediments to research identified in this chapter, the panel decided to concentrate its attention on the tasks that are most urgently needed to propel the field forward. Chapter 2 addresses the problem of inconsistencies in definition and measurement that have thus far characterized research on elder mistreatment. Chapter 3 sketches a theoretical framework that may be useful in organizing research on the phenomenology and etiology of elder mistreatment in different settings and contexts. Chapter 4 addresses the challenge of measuring the occurrence of elder mistreatment in the population, highlighting important epidemiological considerations in elder mistreatment research. Chapter 5 summarizes what is now known about risk factors for elder mistreatment and identifies priorities for future research. Chapter 6 addresses research needed to improve screening and case identification in clinical settings. Chapter 7 reviews policies and programs aiming to prevent or respond to elder mistreatment and identifies priorities for future research. Chapter 8 addresses concerns about protecting human subjects in elder mistreatment research, and Chapter 9 identifies some necessary conditions for moving the field forward. The panel's conclusions and recommendations are presented in Table 1-1.

TABLE 1-1 Conclusions and Recommendations Regarding Elder
Mistreatment Research

Conclusion or Recommendation	Page Number
Concepts, Definitions, and Guidelines for Measurement: Chapter 2	
Basic research on the phenomenology of elder mistreatment is a critical early step in the further development of the field.	58
The development of widely accepted operational definitions and validated and standardized measurement methods for the elements of elder mistreatment is urgently needed to move the field forward.	58
A Theoretical Model of Elder Mistreatment: Chapter 3	
The panel recommends systematic, theory-driven longitudinal research, both qualitative and quantitative, exploring the changing dynamics of elder people's relationships and the risk of mistreatment, as they are affected by changing health status, social embeddedness, and caregiving and living arrangements, in both domestic and institutional contexts.	70
The Occurrence of Elder Mistreatment: Chapter 4	
Population-based surveys of elder mistreatment occurrence are feasible and should be given a high priority by funding agencies. Preparatory funding should be provided to develop and test measures for identifying elder mistreatment.	84
Funding agencies should give priority to the design and fielding of national prevalence and incidence studies of elder mistreatment. These studies should include both a large-scale, independent study of prevalence and modular add-ons to other surveys of aging populations.	85
In addition to improved household and geographically referent sampling techniques, new methods of sampling and identifying elder mistreatment victims in the community should be developed in order to improve the validity and comprehensiveness of elder mistreatment occurrence estimates.	86
Supplemental modules pertaining to elder mistreatment should be included in existing comprehensive geographic health and social surveys, including ongoing longitudinal studies of aging populations.	86
Once the measurement issues have been satisfactorily addressed, a comprehensive national prevalence study of elder mistreatment should be undertaken.	86

TABLE 1-1 Continued

Conclusion or Recommendation	Page Number
Research is needed on the phenomenology and clinical course of elder mistreatment. The occurrence of elder mistreatment in institutional settings, including hospitals, long-term care and assisted living situations, is all but uncharacterized and needs new study sampling and detection methods.	86, 87

Risk Factors for Elder Mistreatment: Chapter 5

Studies examining risk indicators and risk and protective factors for different types of elder mistreatment are urgently needed. A particularly critical need exists for such studies in institutional settings. Research on risk and protective factors should take into consideration the clinical course of elder mistreatment. Advances in measurement in risk and protective factor research are needed.	101, 102

Screening and Case Identification in Clinical Settings: Chapter 6

Substantial research is needed to improve and develop new methods of screening for possible elder mistreatment in a range of clinical settings.	120
Research is needed on the process of designating cases as incidents of mistreatment in order to improve criteria, investigative methods, decision-making processes, and decision outcomes.	120
Research assessing the capacity of older persons with cognitive impairments to provide accurate testimony is needed for improving the accuracy of case identification, not only in clinical settings, but also in legal settings, including prosecutorial decision making and formal adjudication.	117
Research is needed to help illuminate the characteristics of common injuries, such as their etiology, natural course, distribution, and severity so that the process of identifying cases of elder mistreatment can become more accurate and reliable.	120

Evaluating Interventions: Chapter 7

Research on the effects of elder mistreatment interventions is urgently needed. Existing interventions to prevent or ameliorate elder mistreatment should be evaluated, and agencies funding new intervention programs should require and fund a scientifically adequate evaluation as a component of each grant.	139

TABLE 1-1 Continued

Conclusion or Recommendation	Page Number
The panel strongly recommends systematic studies of reporting practices and the effects of reporting, taking maximum advantage of the opportunity for comparisons of practices and outcomes in states with and without mandated reporting.	124
Research is needed on the effectiveness of adult protective services interventions, ideally in study designs that compare outcomes in cases in which services were provided with those in which eligible recipients declined offered services or other cases in which mistreatment of an equivalent nature has been identified.	126
Prosecutorial response to elder mistreatment is an understudied area that should receive heightened attention by the National Institute of Justice and other funders of criminal justice research.	129
Research about the use of civil justice interventions and their effectiveness in preventing exploitation and other harm to elders should be jointly sponsored by the National Institute of Justice and the Administration on Aging.	131
The panel strongly encourages government agencies and private sponsors of elder mistreatment programs to give priority to interventions that emphasize specialized professional training and interdisciplinary collaboration. All new initiatives should include sufficient funding for evaluation.	133

Research Ethics: Chapter 8

Investigators and institutional review boards (IRBs) need clearer guidance (without rigid rules) concerning two issues that tend to recur in elder mistreatment research: conditions under which research can properly go forward with participants whose decisional capacity is impaired, and the proper responses to evidence of mistreatment elicited during the course of the study. The panel recommends that the National Institute of Aging, in collaboration with the Office of Human Research Protections and other sponsors of elder mistreatment research, undertake a consensus project to develop ethical guidelines and provide necessary clarification.	144
Whenever feasible, investigators should consult representative members of the populations being studied (elder persons and caregivers, nursing home residents and staff, etc.) to ascertain their perspectives and preferences regarding the proper responses to evidence of mistreatment (and the related ethical issues raised by the proposed research), and should take this information into account in developing the protocol.	144

TABLE 1-1 Continued

Conclusion or Recommendation	Page Number
Elder mistreatment reporting statutes should be amended to exempt researchers from their mandatory requirements.	145
NIH should issue certificates of confidentiality designed to insulate elder mistreatment researchers from any legal obligation to disclose possible cases of mistreatment that otherwise may arise under state law, including tort "duty to protect" obligations as well as reporting statutes. Issuance of these certificates should be predicated on the assumption that IRBs will carefully scrutinize the protocols to ensure that participants are protected from harm and that, under appropriate circumstances, IRBs will permit investigators to take voluntary steps to protect subjects in danger.	145

Moving Forward: Chapter 9

An adequate long-term funding commitment to research on elder mistreatment must be made by relevant federal, state, and private agencies to support research careers and to develop the next generation of investigators in the field.	151

2

Concepts, Definitions, and Guidelines for Measurement

As noted in Chapter 1, one of the complexities of research on elder mistreatment is that researchers have used varying definitions of mistreatment. To some extent, this problem has been traceable to statutory definitions that are highly variable and ambiguous. Because legal definitions of abuse and neglect vary widely from state to state, efforts to match research definitions in any given state with the statutory definitions tend to undermine efforts to achieve comparability in research designs. In addition, legal definitions ultimately depend on value judgments (initially by clinicians and then by judges and juries) about the seriousness of the perpetrator's conduct; these value judgments are contingent social facts that are themselves subject to empirical investigation.

One of the most urgent challenges confronting the field is the need to develop objective, uniform research definitions that are disentangled, to the greatest feasible extent, from state statutory variations, as well as from the contingent and subjective value judgments that inevitably characterize the application of vague statutory language. At the same time, however, the research definitions should also be logically connected to common statutory concepts so that they can inform policy and practice. Accordingly, the panel has reviewed state laws on elder abuse and neglect for the purpose of identifying common patterns and providing a concrete context for thinking about the core concepts and boundaries of the field of elder mistreatment. (Appendix B summarizes state statutes as of December 2001.)

Most state statutes include in some form (either under an umbrella definition of "abuse" or as separately defined elements) at least the following types of mistreatment: (1) physical acts causing pain or injury; (2) conduct inflicting emotional distress or psychological harm; (3) sexual assault; (4) financial exploitation; and (5) neglect. Some states also include other conduct and conditions, such as "isolation" or "unreasonable confinement." In most, but not all, states, abuse and neglect of elders fall under the general adult protection statute, whereas some states have enacted specific provisions for elder protection. In almost all states, protective interventions are authorized or required only if the adults (or elders) are mentally or physically impaired. In some contexts, the nature of the relationship between the elder person and the alleged perpetrator also matters. On one hand, "neglect" (by definition) usually is associated exclusively with persons who have a legal duty to provide care, but some states direct or authorize intervention in cases involving adults found to be neglecting their own basic needs ("self-neglect"). On the other hand, in most states, anyone, even a stranger, can be found to have committed "abuse." The common statutory patterns in definitions of abuse, neglect, and financial exploitation are depicted in Figures 2-1, 2-2, and 2-3.

TOWARD A SCIENTIFIC VOCABULARY

The scientific vocabulary and measures that are used to study elder abuse and neglect must diverge from the legal definitions in three important respects: First, the conduct (by a perpetrator) and harms (to the elder) being studied must be objectively ascertainable based on observation, record review, or direct questioning of relevant parties. Second, although abuse and neglect represent dichotomous (yes/no) judgments from a legal standpoint, most of the underlying behaviors fall along a continuum and must be analyzed empirically as dimensional variables in terms of frequency, intensity, and severity (or riskiness)—even though the data may often be subjected to dichotomous judgments. Third, the range of conduct being measured should be more inclusive than the behaviors or harmful consequences that would indisputably amount to abuse or neglect under the applicable law.

In other words, researchers should investigate all the conduct and harms that *could* amount to abuse or neglect if the perpetrator had the necessary intention or culpability and if other statutory conditions are met. Some subset of this all-encompassing category could be disaggregated in data analysis to represent "core" cases of abuse or neglect, based on suppositions about the presence of the necessary intention and other conditions. The main point, however, is that the ideal empirical strategy would define the category of interest broadly in terms of conduct and harmful consequences, leaving further narrowing to the analytical and interpretive stages.

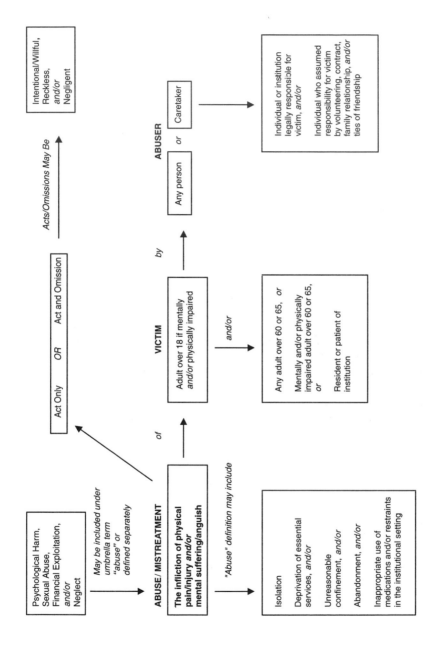

FIGURE 2-1 Summary of current statutory definitions of elder abuse.

37

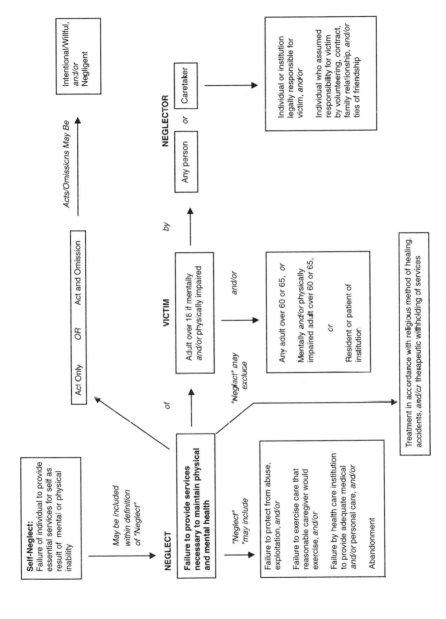

FIGURE 2-2 Summary of current statutory definitions of elder neglect.

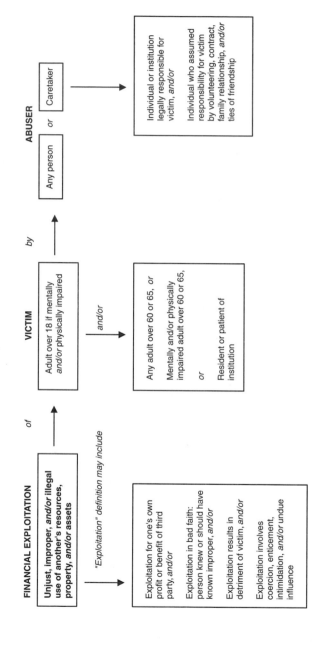

FIGURE 2-3 Summary of current statutory definitions of financial exploitation.

Elder Abuse and Neglect

In order to avoid unnecessary confusion, the panel has developed a research terminology to refer, descriptively, to the behaviors, relationships, interactions, and conditions of scientific interest, reserving the terms "abuse" and "neglect" to refer primarily to the legal category (recognizing that the statutory definitions vary). Box 2-1 presents the panel's glossary of terms. The term being used in this report to encompass the conduct and harmful consequences of scientific interest is "elder mistreatment." Although "mistreatment" is itself a value-laden term (and is used in some state statutes), the panel has selected it because it appears to have been least used as a statutory category.

The panel's definitions of elder mistreatment (and its constituent elements) have been guided entirely by scientific considerations. We have asked: What definitions will be most useful for facilitating advances in knowledge? It bears repeating that whether "mistreatment," as the panel is defining it, amounts to "abuse" or "neglect" in a legal sense depends on the statutory definitions in a particular jurisdiction, the actor's state of mind, and other factors.

BOX 2-1
Glossary of Research Terms

Abuse. Conduct by responsible caregivers or other individuals that constitutes "abuse" under applicable state or federal law.

Caregiver. A person who bears or has assumed responsibility for providing care or living assistance to an adult in need of such care or assistance.

Harm. Injuries or unmet basic needs attributable to acts or omissions by others.

Mistreatment. (a) Intentional actions that cause harm or create a serious risk of harm, whether or not intended, to a vulnerable elder by a caregiver or other person who stands in a trust relationship to the elder, or (b) failure by a caregiver to satisfy the elder's basic needs or to protect the elder from harm.

Neglect. An omission by responsible caregivers that constitutes "neglect" under applicable federal or state law.

Trust Relationship. A caregiving relationship or other familial, social or professional relationship where a person bears or has assumed responsibility for protecting the interests of the older person or where expectations of care or protection arise by law or social convention.

Vulnerability. Financial, physical or emotional dependence on others or impaired capacity for self-care or self-protection.

Elder Mistreatment

"Elder mistreatment" is defined in this report to refer to (a) intentional actions that cause harm or create a serious risk of harm (whether or not harm is intended) to a vulnerable elder by a caregiver or other person who stands in a trust relationship to the elder or (b) failure by a caregiver to satisfy the elder's basic needs or to protect the elder from harm. "Mistreatment" conveys two ideas: that some injury, deprivation, or dangerous condition has occurred to the elder person and that someone else bears responsibility for causing the condition or failing to prevent it.

Two features of this definition merit emphasis. First, the term "mistreatment" is meant to exclude cases of so-called self-neglect—failure of an older person to satisfy his or her own basic needs and to protect himself or herself from harm. Self-neglect may often be a proper occasion for intervention, at least of a temporary nature—for the purpose of determining whether the elder has the capacities for self-care and, if appropriate, of designating a caregiver, but the panel regards self-neglect as a separate domain of elder protection, not as a component of mistreatment.

Second, elder mistreatment, as defined by the panel, excludes victimization of elders by strangers. In the panel's view, ordinary predatory victimization of elders merits empirical attention as a species of criminal behavior, but it should not be regarded as a component of the distinct domain of elder mistreatment. We say this because the nature of the relationship between the elder and the perpetrator lies at the heart of common understanding of the concept of mistreatment (and in most statutory definitions of abuse and neglect) and therefore should guide the definitions used in empirical research.

Caregiving and Other Trust Relationships

Although we have excluded ordinary victimization by a stranger, thereby narrowing the boundaries of the field, what types of relationships are relevant? In the panel's view, the range of relevant relationships depends on whether the victim's condition was caused by an intentional act (typically causing an injury) or by a failure to satisfy a legal duty of care (leading to unmet needs). If the elder has been injured—we refer here to financial injury as well as physical and emotional injury—or otherwise put at risk by the actor's intentional conduct, the category of relevant relationships includes not only caregivers, but also other family members or even unrelated people (e.g., lawyers) who are aware of the elder's vulnerability and exploit it. The panel uses the phrase "trust relationships" to denote the relevant relationships. Financial exploitation is illustrative: the conduct of interest is exploitation by family members and others who may have assumed fiduciary obligations for elders with diminished capacity for financial decisions. As noted above, however, it does not include exploitation by other predatory parties; these victimizations would amount to legal harms (financial injuries) but not to mistreatment.

By contrast, if the presenting condition relates to the elder's unmet needs, a de facto caregiving relationship (or expectation of care) is required in order to preserve the boundary between neglect by responsible others (mistreatment) and self-neglect. Professionals who are clinicians, such as physicians, nurses, psychologists, or social workers, are de facto in trust relationships with elders for whom they care. In this context, the relevant relationships include only those people who have assumed the responsibility for caregiving or are expected to do so. Obviously this characterization ultimately depends on highly contextual social facts that are not easily ascertained in surveys or observations.

Vulnerability Associated with Aging

Vulnerability is another core concept in elder mistreatment. Its importance can be seen by asking whether intimate partner violence constitutes elder mistreatment simply because the victim is older than a designated age (e.g., 65). In the panel's view, the answer is "no" (although the issues may overlap when the victim is older and vulnerable). A predicate feature of elder mistreatment is that the victim has a diminished capacity for self-care or self-protection. Thus, a chronic pattern of intimate partner violence that has persisted into older age is not, by itself, "elder mistreatment." Conversely, if violence against an intimate partner is initiated or becomes more frequent or severe due to the older partner's age-associated vulnerability, then it is properly characterized as "elder mistreatment."

Although vulnerability is a core concept in the definition of elder mistreatment, the panel concluded that further specification would be premature at this time. Some aspects of vulnerability are indisputable, including financial dependence and impairments of mobility (being wheelchair-bound) or cognition (dementia). However, other factors that diminish capacity for self-care or self-protection have not been well characterized. For this reason, the panel regards the meaning of vulnerability as an empirical question—as a referent for the cluster of clinical or psychosocial risk factors associated with increased likelihood of mistreatment. For most research purposes, vulnerability should not be used as a selection criterion; instead, data bearing on vulnerability should be routinely collected and analyzed in most studies of elder mistreatment.

Finally, another boundary issue relates to the age cut off for being an elder. This is a complicated issue. Conceptually speaking, vulnerability, not age, is the determinative concept. There seems to be no important difference (conceptually or morally) between caretaker neglect of a 35-year-old with mental retardation and of a 65-year-old with dementia. So too with financial exploitation and other forms of abuse. Setting children to one side, the relevant population of vulnerable adults includes all persons with impairments or disabilities, such as mental retardation or impairments of capacity for mobility, associated with diminished capacity for self-protection. Not surprisingly, most adult protective services statutes include elder abuse and neglect within the broader category of vulnerable adults. Also, legislation designed to protect institutionalized persons (which includes psychiatric hospitals and mental retardation facilities as well as nursing homes) typically codify the right to be free of "abuse and neglect."

Having said this, however, the panel recognizes that the categorical channeling of research funding (as well as protective legislation) along the path of aging gives particular salience to vulnerability associated with aging (as opposed to other conditions). The National Institute on Aging has commissioned the panel's study, and a special focus on elders establishes the policy framework within which we are working. Accordingly, within the larger domain of adult protection, this report gives special attention to the aspects of research that focus on people who are vulnerable to mistreatment due to aging. However, this does not mean that "vulnerability associated with aging" should be defined categorically in terms of some particular age cutoff, such as 65. Even for legal purposes, the age of eligibility for benefits tied to older age varies—e.g., 65 for social security, 60 for programs funded under the Older Americans Act, 60 or 65 under adult protective services statutes. (Interestingly, the threshold age of protection under the Age Discrimination in Employment Act is 40.) For research purposes, a category defined as persons 65 or over would be both overinclusive and underinclusive—since many people over 65 are not vulnerable and some younger than 65 are vulnerable due to aging (e.g., dementias). In sum, the panel regards "older age" as one of the risk factors that should be explored empirically under the rubric of "vulnerability associated with aging." As the field of elder mistreatment develops, surveillance and research must attend specifically to age as well as other indicators of vulnerability. (The panel's conceptual vocabulary is depicted in Figures 2-4 and 2-5.)

GUIDELINES FOR MEASURMENT

In science, good measurement has several prerequisites. The first is a concept of what is being measured. In this case the object of measurement is the occurrence of elder mistreatment using the vocabulary and definitions presented above. The second prerequisite is an operational definition of the concept being explored so that it is objectively ascertainable in the field. Operational definitions in the domain of elder mistreatment are compli-

**Elder Mistreatment and Adjacent
Domains of Research and Policy**

*When do harmful acts or omissions lie within the
domain of elder mistreatment?*

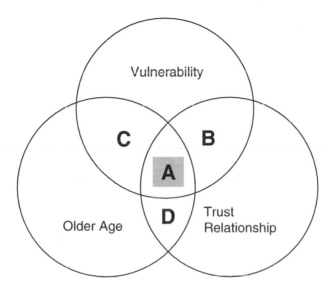

A = core area of elder mistreatment

Adjacent domains of research and policy interest:

B = mistreatment of adults with disabilities

C = "self-neglect" by elderly people; victimization by strangers

D = spouse or intimate partner discord or violence involving an
elderly partner

FIGURE 2-4   Elder mistreatment and adjacent domains of research and policy.

cated, in part because the relevant concepts are poorly developed, and in part because researchers' aims vary widely across studies. Operationalization answers questions such as: "How do we measure this or that aspect of mistreatment?" or "How will we know whether we should count this as a case of mistreatment?" Ideally, operationalization leads to the development of a set of criteria for answering this question and a process by which these criteria can be applied in the field—the measurement method.

<u>C</u>
Reported
Conduct   *Intentional acts*   *Failure to provide care*

or

Presenting   *Injury*   *Unmet [basic] needs*
Condition

<u>V</u>
Vulnerability *Impairment of capacity for self-protection or self-care*
Associated
with Aging

<u>R</u>
                  Person in trust   *Caregiver*
Relationship *relationship*

<u>LD</u>
Legal   *"Abuse"*   *"Neglect"*
Definition   (depends on definitions   (depends on definition
                  under applicable law)   under applicable law)

FIGURE 2-5   Basic elements of elder mistreatment.

Explanation

C + V + R represent a sequential analysis of the necessary elements of elder mistreaatment (conduct by people in caregiver roles or other trust relationships that injures a vulnerable elder, deprives the elder of basic needs, or exposes the elder to risks of injury or deprivation); each of these elements can be operationalized descriptively for research purposes.

C includes all injuries or threats to survival or health, by whomever caused, including self-inflicted injury or "self-neglect" and predatory conduct by strangers.

V excludes cases of "ordinary" victimization and self-injurious behavior not involving vulnerability associated with aging.

R excludes self-inflicted injury and self-neglect and predatory conduct by strangers.

LD represents the subset of cases defined by C+V+R that have been included in the definition of "abuse" or "neglect" under applicable state laws and practices. (A particular statute may also include cases that do not have all of these elements.)

Given the complexity of the definition of mistreatment, its operationalization is best approached in a stepwise fashion, with each step addressing a different aspect of the concept.

The next prerequisite involves the standardization of measures prior to their use in research. In many research settings, such as population surveys, it will be sufficient for the researchers to describe the conduct and other variables that have been measured in a way that reflects the relevant dimensions of mistreatment. As researchers continue the iterative process of conceptualizing and operationalizing the measures, a consensus will gradually emerge regarding the relevance and significance of the measures being used in the field for different aspects of mistreatment and its correlates and outcomes. In some clinical research contexts, however, it will be necessary for researchers to classify whether or not the data represent a "case" of mistreatment. Under optimal circumstances, there would be a method of measurement to definitively assess the presence or absence of elder mistreatment in such cases. Such a "gold standard" could be used to judge the value of other measures as well as to definitively determine the presence or absence of mistreatment for research purposes. Given the nature of the object of measurement, such a standard is not possible in the elder mistreatment field. There are two basic problems—contested facts and contested values. Irrespective of research methodology, uncertainties will arise regarding the conduct of the alleged perpetrator and the effects on the elder. Also, as already indicated, characterization of particular conduct as mistreatment requires value judgments, contestable at the margin if not at the core.

Using the example of other fields confronted with a similar problem, a "LEAD standard" (longitudinal, experts, all data) could be developed to serve in the place of a gold standard (Spitzer, 1983). A LEAD standard would use longitudinal observation, all relevant data, and the review by experts in the field to determine the presence or absence of mistreatment. A LEAD methodology typically involves two components. The first component is collection of data on the case that is to be classified (as mistreated or not mistreated). An expert in the area who investigates the case thoroughly collects the data. The investigation might include taking history from several sources, interviewing the person who may have been mistreated, interviewing the possible perpetrator(s), as well as reviewing medical and other pertinent records. The data collection focuses, as much as possible, on whatever longitudinal information is available on the case.

The second component of the methodology involves evaluation of the data by a panel of experts, who are asked to make a collective judgment about whether or not the case meets an a priori definition of mistreatment or a specific type of mistreatment. The definition is made available to the panel, often in the form of operational criteria. The panel, typically small—

5–7 members—for the sake of efficiency, includes interdisciplinary representation from professional backgrounds with expertise in the area of mistreatment. The expert who collected the data presents each case verbally and in the form of a structured case summary.

The panel then deliberates case-by-case to decide if a specific case meets the a priori definition. The decisions the panel makes in each case, such as judgments about which specific examples meet the definition and which do not, are recorded and eventually summarized in a workbook/minutes book reflecting the consensus process as applied to real cases. The latter can then be used to improve upon the definition, as precedent for future panels, or to train professionals in the recognition of elder mistreatment. This should be a process that (almost) everyone would agree is able to classify correctly individuals as mistreated or not mistreated without worrying about the resources or cost needed to make the determination. Put another way, if resources were not an issue, what would be done to decide if someone has been mistreated or not? Once a LEAD standard is in place, then several potential methods of determining mistreatment can be tested against this standard. And the LEAD method itself can be used in the context of research to definitively assess the presence or absence of elder mistreatment. Such an approach is already under way in the work of Fulmer and Wetle (1986).

The next step is the development of the measure. This involves deciding on the specific purpose of the measure and the measurement method, followed by an assessment of its reliability and validity. Measures may have different purposes, such as to ascertain occurrence of mistreatment in the population for research purposes or for surveillance, to assess the risk of mistreatment for early intervention, to screen for mistreatment in different settings (e.g., emergency department, long-term care), to determine whether mistreatment occurred in a given circumstance, to differentiate different types of mistreatment (e.g., physical or financial), to quantify the severity of mistreatment, and so forth. Clearly, different measures will need to be developed for use in these different research contexts.

Similarly, measures are likely to vary according to the method used to elicit the data. These include self-report, proxy or informant report, direct examination of the elder's physical and/or mental state, clinical observation, or a composite of these. The choice of assessment method will depend on the purpose of the measure, the risks of error associated with each method, the tolerance for error in measurement, and the research resources available.

The measure should be both reliable and valid. Reliability assesses how much agreement there is if different people are conducting the measurement (interobserver) or if a measure is applied at different points in time (test-retest). High interobserver reliability should be pursued. Test-retest reliability should also be pursued for all measures; short time intervals of test-retest are optimal, since the occurrence of mistreatment is transient in some cases.

Validity assesses how accurate a measure is of what we want it to measure, in this case some aspect of mistreatment. There are several types of validity: content, criterion, predictive, and construct validity. Content validity is an assessment of the measurement method's ability to measure mistreatment using logic and special expertise, typically by expert opinion. Criterion validity assesses the measure against a widely agreed-upon standard, in this case a LEAD standard. Predictive validity assesses the ability of the measure to make predictions about the future, such as predicting response to interventions or the course of mistreatment. Finally, any research evidence that tends to illuminate exactly what the instrument measures adds to its construct validity.

In sum, research measurement in the field of elder mistreatment is complicated for several reasons. First, several elements require measurement. Second, observations necessary to make a determination of mistreatment are usually not directly available to the researcher and must be inferred indirectly. Third, even with the necessary observations available, a determination of mistreatment is not immediately apparent but rather requires human judgment to assess whether these observations meet (a priori) definitions (operational criteria) of mistreatment derived from common sense, consensus, or law. Fourth, the definitions against which the observations are assessed appear to be variable in research conducted thus far. These issues greatly limit the ability of researchers to develop measurement tools that meet high standards of reliability and validity.

OPERATIONALIZING THE ESSENTIAL ELEMENTS

In the context of elder mistreatment, several variables are a target of measurement. These are listed in Box 2-2.

The items in this box merit initial comment prior to later detailed discussion. With regard to the first item, while the issue of who is an older person has no definitive answer for all purposes, the demographic category of interest needs to be defined explicitly for the purposes of research. The second item is the existence of a trust relationship between an elder and another person. As indicated above, the concept of elder mistreatment is predicated on the existence of such a relationship. Thus, a definition for what constitutes a trust relationship is needed. For both these items, operationalization is straightforward in the sense that an a priori definition, whatever its strengths and weaknesses, can be applied in the process of research so that a particular situation can be assessed against that definition (e.g., "Does this particular person meet the definition of being an older

---

BOX 2-2
Variables Requiring Operational Definition in
Research Involving Elder Mistreatment

1. Who is an older person?
2. What constitutes a trust relationship between an older and another person?
3. What is the relevant conduct of the "other" person in the trust relationship?
4. What harms has the older person experienced (or what dangers were created as a result of the conduct of the person in the trust relationship)?
5. Does this combination of conduct and harm constitute mistreatment, as that term has been defined in the study?
6. What are the risk and protective factors associated with the occurrence of mistreatment? Specifically, what aspects of the older person's condition make him or her more or less vulnerable to mistreatment?
7. What are the outcomes of mistreatment or of interventions aiming to prevent it?

---

person?" and "Does the relationship meet the definition of being a trust relationship?")

It is necessary to measure the relevant conduct (what was done or not done) of the other person, to assess whether or not the elder has been harmed, and, if so, to determine whether what the other person has done or not done has caused the harm. The definition of the relevant conduct and harm is a complex undertaking in that it is not always possible to anticipate in advance all conduct and consequences that might be of interest. Furthermore, in the process of assessment while in the field, it is highly unlikely that the conduct in question will be directly observable to those conducting the research and is therefore likely to be evaluated indirectly. This is often true for harms as well. Thus an operational definition of conduct and harm should contain a general description of the kinds of conduct and consequences that may be of interest as well as a description of the process used to determine the occurrence of relevant conduct and harms, constructed so that they can be assessed both directly and indirectly.

Determining whether a particular conduct caused a particular harm will not be necessary in most studies, especially those using survey methods. However, this task may be necessary in some studies, especially those relating to the factors that differentiate, clinically, between inadvertent injuries and intentional ones (see Chapter 6.). In some cases, when direct observation is available, it is possible to state unequivocally that a specific conduct caused the injury. For example, if a caregiver hits an elder on her upper right arm and there is a bruise where there the elder was struck, causality for the bruise is clear. However, if the elder also is anxious and scared, under what circumstances can one conclude that the striking of the arm caused these psychological consequences? Furthermore, if the elder has bruises elsewhere on her body, when might it be concluded that the same caregiver striking her at other times caused these other bruises? As should be apparent, the causal inference connecting conduct to consequences in many instances necessitates a judgment on the part of the researcher. Thus, for some studies, the researcher may have to specify an operational definition of causality and a process by which the determination of causality is made.

The next item in the box deals with the evaluation of information from the previous items in judging whether or not the combination of conduct and harm constitutes mistreatment. This requires operational definitions of the types of mistreatment against which the specific circumstances can be assessed. The panel encourages researchers to be as specific as possible in identifying which combinations of conduct and harm are being defined as mistreatment for purposes of the study. It may be helpful to define the category of mistreatment separately for (1) physical mistreatment, (2) sexual mistreatment, (3) emotional mistreatment (including isolation), (4) financial exploitation, and (5) failure to provide needed care, including abandonment.

As explained earlier, the panel recommends that researchers try to avoid stand-alone, unmodified use of the terms "abuse" and "neglect" because these terms require legal interpretations and community value judgments that inevitably vary across states and localities. In addition, it should be recognized that whether a case is found by the applicable authorities to constitute abuse or neglect also depends on the purpose of the intervention in a particular case and other aspects of the social context. In some situations, for example, the question being asked is whether an intervention or treatment might be implemented to help the elder. In other situations, however, a determination of abuse or neglect might lead to criminal prosecution of the perpetrator. These determinations are all rooted in value judgments made initially by the examining clinicians and subsequently by public officials and courts. These judgments are themselves subject to empirical study. In such investigations, what must be defined and measured are the variety of possible clinical, social, and legal responses that might be made to particular cases. If this type of research were added to the box, the question of interest would be "Was this combination of conduct and harm characterized as 'abuse' or 'neglect' by the relevant decision-makers?"

The sixth element in the box involves the operationalization and measurement of factors that increase or decrease the likelihood of elder mistreatment. Measurement of risk and protective factors is as important as measurement for mistreatment itself. Risk factors are factors that increase the probability of mistreatment, while protective factors are ones that decrease its probability. Their measurement is critical from the public health point of view for several reasons. Their identification is crucial to the detection of who is at risk for mistreatment so that preventive interventions can be applied. As well, their identification promotes understanding of the mechanisms leading to mistreatment. Because vulnerabilities associated with aging (and with disabilities) are of special concern in the fields of elder mistreatment and adult protective services, these risk factors require careful attention. (Research on risk and protective factors is discussed in Chapter 5.)

The final element in the box relates to the outcomes and consequences of mistreatment. Mistreatment has been associated with a series of consequences and adverse outcomes. For example, mistreatment can cause physical and mental morbidity that is at times sustained. It can lead to serious financial strain. As well, social isolation, loss of dignity, impaired quality of life can result. Research on the consequences of mistreatment is critical to understanding its individual and societal impact and to targeting and assessing the benefit of interventions. (A theoretical model linking mistreatment to its outcomes is discussed in Chapter 3.)

With this overview in mind, the discussion now turns specifically to the measurement of several of the elements involved in research on mistreatment as identified in Box 2-2.

Older Person

If an age cutoff is to be used, then the operationalization and measurement of who is an older person are straightforward and merit no further discussion. If, however, the definition is broadened to include other groups of vulnerable adults, operational definitions and specific measurement methods may be needed. For example, if the definition is broadened to include "adults with developmental disabilities," or "adults with mental illness," or "adults with physical disabilities," then a definition of each of these terms is necessary for research to go forward, as is a method of determining whether a specific individual meets the definition. It seems fair to assume that definitions and measurements for various types of disabilities exist in the relevant fields and can be imported with appropriate modification to research on elder mistreatment.

The panel favors specific definitions of disability if the population being studied is chosen on this basis, rather than use of a generic and vague category of all "vulnerable adults." Objective criteria of inclusion, such as cognitive impairment or frailty or disability impairing locomotion, should be used. However, if the study population is defined by age (e.g., everyone over 18 or 40 or 55, etc)., then the elements of vulnerability can be defined empirically according to the personal characteristics that emerge as risk factors for mistreatment.

Trust Relationship

A trust relationship is at the center of research in elder mistreatment. In the simplest terms, such a relationship exists when one party is charged with, or has assumed, the responsibility for caring for or protecting the interests of the older person, or when the relationship (in its social context) creates the expectation of care or protection. There are therefore at least two participants in such a relationship, the elder and the person—or persons—responsible for care or protection or expected to provide care or protection for the elder. Such a relationship may arise formally or informally and may be voluntarily undertaken or imposed by operation of law or social custom.

For example, the relationship may arise from a formal guardianship or a durable power of attorney in which the trusted person agreed to serve in that role in the event of the elder's incapacitation. Even in the absence of any formal designations, the relationship may arise out of kinship or friendship or professional roles. For example, a relative, caregiver, or other person may find himself or herself in the position of making health care or living decisions for the elder without any formal agreement or designation. Furthermore, someone may take on the responsibility to assist the older person in financial matters, such as an accountant, financial adviser, or friend with special knowledge in this area. Under certain circumstances, the existence of a trust relationship may be predicated on the fact that the other person is a health care professional who has taken on the care of the elder, as would happen in a nursing home, assisted living, or hospital with a nursing aide or licensed professional.

Different types of relationships may have different bearings on elder mistreatment, depending on the type of mistreatment. The threshold of involvement that constitutes a trust relationship may vary for physical mistreatment, emotional mistreatment, financial exploitation, or failure to provide needed care. For example, failure to provide needed care (neglect) depends on the existence of a de facto caregiving relationship and therefore would require a narrower range of relationships than the other categories of mistreatment. For example, any family member would be in a trust relationship for purposes of the basic expectation that they will not exploit or harm the vulnerable elder person. However, a family relationship clearly will not always amount to a relationship sufficient to give rise to a caregiver obligation; this is why the panel has distinguished between these two concepts and has defined trust relationships as a broad category that includes, but is not limited to, caregivers.

In some circumstances, of course, existence of a trust relationship is unambiguous and harm caused by the other person would always constitute mistreatment. These include legal guardians and professionals who enter into formal professional relationships with an older person. The case for a legal guardian should be obvious. Similarly, paid professionals, whether they be clinicians, attorneys, financial advisers, or accountants, enter into trust relationships by virtue of their professional activities. It should be apparent that relationships with paid professionals in all health care settings, such as hospitals, nursing homes, assisted living homes, adult day care programs, and the like, enter into trust relationships when they come into contact with older people. This includes not only licensed professionals such as doctors or nurses but also personal care workers (nursing aides), janitorial staff, escort staff, etc.

In other circumstances, whether a particular relationship amounts to a trust relationship for purposes of elder mistreatment research may be unclear. In the first instance, researchers should make every effort to determine the point of view of the older person regarding their trust relationships. In some situations, this may be determinative. However, in many situations, the elder person's point of view will not be ascertainable or will be superseded by social conventions or legal duties. For example, the older person may be suspicious of, and have no expectation of protection from, a home health care aide who has assumed a caregiving obligation. Conversely, the older person may develop a trusting relationship with a door-to-door vacuum cleaner salesman who, by law and social convention, bears no obligation to protect the older person's interests. Accordingly, applying the concept ultimately requires objective assessment and judgment.

In sum, empirical knowledge is lacking about the kinds of trust relationships that older persons enter into, the other parties involved in these relationships, the foundations of these relationships, and their association with different types of mistreatment. Therefore, an early priority of research in the field ought to be the conceptual and empirical development of different operational definitions of trust relationships.

Conduct of the Other Person in the Trust Relationship

The relevant conduct of the other party that may be of interest includes direct physical contact (hitting, pushing, shoving, etc.), verbal mistreatment (yelling, threatening verbally, criticism, etc.), placing restrictions on the older person (isolating to a room, unnecessary use of physical or chemical restraints), social embarrassment (berating the elder in public), depriving the older person of material possessions (restricting access to money, stealing from the elder, etc.), not providing necessary care (e.g., not providing medications, bathing infrequently, feeding a limited diet), and many more. The challenge for researchers is to define the conduct with maximum possible specificity to facilitate analysis and interpretation. Whether any such conduct amounts to mistreatment requires a value judgment based on context. For example, restricting access to money may be entirely appropriate conduct in caring for a person with dementia. (See further discussion of this point in the section on "mistreatment" below.) As noted earlier in this chapter, however, the most sensible strategy for research is to define the category overinclusively (with reference to the expected definition of mistreatment) for purposes of data collection and measurement and to refine it thereafter in analysis and interpretation.

Measurement of conduct is subject to a number of significant methodological limitations. Briefly, much of this conduct is not observed directly and relies for its detection on report by the elder, by the other party in the trust relationship—who may be the perpetrator of mistreatment— or by a third party, such as a colleague or supervisor of the other party in an institutional setting. Indeed, in the absence of direct observation, conduct is harder to assess than harm, since it may not leave evidence in the form of readily observable physical or emotional consequences, since it may be forgotten by the elder if she is cognitively impaired, since the older person may be reluctant to report the occurrence of such conduct, or since the other person may not report it out of conflict of interest.

The investigator is faced with the difficult task of detecting a "latent variable" requiring a research methodology that optimally employs several modalities of assessment and takes repeated observation. As with assessment of harm, there is a dearth of basic descriptive studies of conduct involved and of measurement methods.

Harm

As already noted, mistreatment (under any consensus definition) will include some types of conduct that have not actually caused harm—perhaps because harm was not intended or because the conduct creates an unacceptable risk of harm. However, many types of mistreatment do involve actual injury or harm, most notably physical assault and financial mistreatment (loss of property). To the extent that the definition includes harm, the measure of harm must be operationalized and measured.

The importance of measuring harm varies according to the type of research being conducted. For example, survey research and other studies in nonclinical settings (or not using clinical or legal records) are likely to focus mainly on the possible perpetrator's conduct; the presence of harm is likely to be ascertained on the basis of a few specific indicators (e.g., "Were you hurt?" "Did you have to go to the hospital?" "Did you lose any money?") However, in the context of research in clinical settings, such as identification of forensic markers for mistreatment, or development of improved screening tools, the assessment of harm may be a particularly important element of the study.

Pertinent types of harm to older persons include physical injury, emotional injury, and financial harm. Physical harm is the most straightforward, since its presence typically can be assessed reliably through examination, through laboratory tests (e.g., X-rays), or upon forensic assessment. Examples of physical harm include lacerations, burns, fractures, bruises, malnutrition, and others (Dyer et al., in this volume). Similarly, financial harm can typically be assessed reliably if access to the older person's financial records is available. Emotional harm is more difficult to assess. This may take on the form of mental distress and other psychological responses, post-traumatic symptomatology (social withdrawal, reexperiencing traumatic events, trouble sleeping or eating, etc.), or the onset (at times recurrence) of a psychiatric disorder, such as major depression, post-traumatic stress disorder, panic disorder, agoraphobia, among others. Measurement of harm must be able to determine the presence or absence of different consequences in the various domains above. Since many harms may not be anticipated prior to the initiation of the research, the measurement method must be general and flexible so as to detect a wide range of consequences that may be specific to the specific elder-trust relationship, and to the setting involved (home, hospital, long-term care etc.). The measurement method must also evaluate temporal aspects of the consequences (onset, frequency, duration) and quantify the severity of these consequences.

A key methodological issue in the measurement of consequences is that some of the harms involved are not always accessible to direct measurement. This is true for several reasons. First, in many cases, harms are transient and remit by the time an assessment occurs, as in the case of a bruise or a laceration. Second, many older persons who are mistreated are cognitively impaired and cannot recall past harms. Third, many older people are reluctant to report conduct of others who may have harmed them or that may constitute mistreatment out of embarrassment or for other reasons. Fourth, often the only other source of information about past harms may be the other person in the trust relationship, who has a conflict of interest regarding disclosure of the harm. Therefore, the best a researcher can do, as is customary when latent variables are being investigated, is to employ methods of assessment that are multimodal (e.g., self-report, observer report, data review, direct examination, laboratory studies, forensic assessment) and that are repeated with sufficient frequency to minimize the likelihood that relevant consequences are missed. The corollary to this is that measurement methods should include checks and balances so that false positives are minimized as well.

In general, methods to assess the presence or absence of physical injury, emotional disturbance, or financial injury are available and have been adapted to the elder mistreatment context. These methods generally are able to evaluate the presence or absence of injury (harm) and are also able to approach its temporal aspects and severity. The vast majority of measures have focused on the determination of whether elder mistreatment has occurred using a wide range of methods and definitions. Many studies have assessed the occurrence of mistreatment by review of protective agency records, study of sentinel reports (reports of professionals serving older adults), or criminal justice system statistics. These have used typically unstandardized or vague definitions of abuse and neglect, many based on the wording of state statutes, and have significant methodological weakness.

A few researchers have tackled the problem directly, but they have used definitions or measures that have varied from study to study. In some cases, methods have been developed to assess the occurrence of elder abuse using telephone or in-person interviews of family members or proxies or direct assessments of samples of older adults. However, there is a dearth of such measures, and most existing measures have had limited assessment of their measurement characteristics, reliability, or validity. Furthermore, the measures used have almost always been direct adaptations of measures intended for other purposes or for other settings (e.g., the Conflict Tactics Scale was intended to measure interpersonal violence for married couples and was modified by Pillemer and Finkelhor to assess abuse of older people by their caregivers). As well, existing measures are inadequately differentiated or specialized. They do not, for example, distinguish clearly the types of harm they are measuring (physical, emotional, etc.) or differentiate the measures according to whether they are intended to screen for harm, define its occurrence, or measure its severity.

The elder mistreatment field is lacking in descriptive methodological research on how to measure consequences that are related to mistreatment. As Dyer et al. (this volume) note, no studies have carefully described the different types of harms that mistreated older persons may suffer, the inter relationship of the different harms (e.g., relationship of physical to emotional to financial), the severity of harms, their characteristics, and their clinical course. In addition, few studies have compared different approaches to the measurement of harms. The greatest gap relates to psychological consequences of elder mistreatment. This sort of information is key to the ability to develop measures that are methodologically sound. Basic methodological research should also be an early priority in the field.

Mistreatment

Whether certain facts, collected using the methods discussed so far in this chapter, constitute mistreatment is a matter of definition and judgment. The researcher's main goal should be to make the process as transparent as possible. The facts, collected as above, must be assessed against an a priori

TABLE 2-1 Cross-Tabulation of Conducts and Harms

	Illustrative Conduct by Other Party					
Harm to Older Person	None or Unknown	Hit Once	Pushed Downstairs	Failed to Feed a Meal	Gave Wrong Medication Dose	Locked in Room
None						
Bruise						
Fracture						
Depression						
Dehydration						
Hospital admission						

NOTE: Intersecting sets may or may not constitute mistreatment depending on the definition used in the study.

definition. (The panel's preferred definition is set forth above.) Much of the time, the facts fit the definition with little doubt. In other cases, whether the facts should be characterized as mistreatment requires judgment. Thus the researcher must specify a process for making this determination.

This process works best if it has at least two characteristics. The first is a set of rules or guidelines specifying whether anticipated combinations of circumstances and conduct will constitute one form or another of mistreatment if detected in the field. A different cross-tabulation of conducts and harms is necessary for each type of mistreatment. This is illustrated in Table 2-1.

This approach illustrates several issues. While it is not possible to anticipate all combinations of conduct and harms that could be encountered, prior consideration of the types of issues that will come up in the course of the research will help standardize decisions in the conduct of the study. Also, the frequency of harms and conducts must be taken into account in the table. For example, a single instance of pushing an older person down the stairs may constitute mistreatment regardless of whether an injury occurs, whereas forgetting to feed her a meal now and then may not. Furthermore, the absence of both specific conduct and specific harms may, under certain circumstances, constitute mistreatment.

For example, as already mentioned, specific harms that could be due only to mistreatment (such as certain types of fractures) might be classified as mistreatment even if the relevant conduct were not detected. But conduct that has not resulted in any apparent harm may also at times be properly characterized as mistreatment. If a trusted person attempts to push an older person down the stairs but fails to succeed, thus causing no obvious harm, most would agree that this is physical mistreatment. What distinguishes this situation is the intent of the trusted person, so that if there is clear intent to harm, mistreatment may be present even if the harm did not occur.

While intent is important in limited circumstances, it should be kept in mind that intent to harm, which is very hard to determine (even in a courtroom, much less for research purposes), is not a necessary element of the definition of mistreatment, as defined in this report. Of course, when there is intent to harm that can be determined unequivocally, then in all likelihood mistreatment has occurred. While it would be interesting to study the relationship between intent of the trusted person and conduct or harms that constitute mistreatment (and that are characterized as neglect and abuse by social authorities) this is not a core aspect of the measurement of mistreatment.

An important caveat should be added at this point. One of the difficulties in elder mistreatment research so far has been the use of overly inclusive definitions of what constitutes mistreatment. Some writers have included the entire range of harms and conducts in Table 2-1 as mistreatment, including, in some cases, "social embarrassment" that may have been transient, or minor physical injuries that were clearly an accident. It is important for researchers to focus their attention on serious forms of mistreatment and not to define "normal" negative human interactions as pathological. The purpose of the cross tabulation is not to lay out all harms and consequences involved in interactions between an older person and another in a trust relationship; rather it is to limit the definition of elder mistreatment to a specific number of intersecting sets that have been defined by the researcher as plausible forms of mistreatment.

The second part of the assessment of mistreatment is the specification of a process used to apply the definition and guidelines to all cases under study. This process has as its starting point the facts in each case, the definitions of mistreatment being employed in the study, and the rules/guidelines derived from cross-tabulation of anticipated examples. This information is reviewed by designated individuals using a specified process. Typically, a trained expert looks at each case and decides the simple ones. A consensus panel then reviews the more complex cases, plus a sampling of the simpler ones classified by the individual reviewers. It bears emphasis that this classification is needed only if a dichotomous classification is required by the goals of a particular study. As already noted, the panel encourages study of a broad range of conducts and harms beyond those that could be classified as cases of mistreatment. The presence (or absence) of some of these might be predictive of the onset of mistreatment in the future. Also, even though they may not be mistreatment, some of these could affect the quality of life of the older person. Finally, these may be of interest to social scientists studying the relationship between conduct and consequence in older persons and their caregivers.

Risk and Protective Factors

A major purpose of research in elder mistreatment is to understand its causes so that it can be prevented, treated, or managed effectively. This line of inquiry typically begins with the study of factors that increase (risk) or decrease (protective) the probability that mistreatment will occur. As discussed earlier, it is the panel's view that one of the crucial risk factors involved is the vulnerability of the elder person. More research is needed on risk factors, including vulnerability, and protective factors for mistreatment. This issue is of such significance to the field that Chapter 5 has been devoted to it.

CONCLUSIONS

1. Further basic research on the phenomenology of elder mistreatment is a critical early step in the further development of the field. Such research will lead to a much better understanding of the key elements of elder mistreatment (see Box 2-1), which in turn will facilitate the development of broadly accepted operational definitions and the development of research and clinical measures for these phenomena. Examples of such research include studies of: (1) the kinds of trust relationships that older persons enter into, the other parties involved in these relationships, the foundations of these relationships, and their association with different types of mistreatment; (2) the different types of harms that mistreated older persons may suffer, the interrelationship of the different harms (e.g., relationship of physical to emotional to financial), the severity of harms, their temporal characteristics, and their clinical course; (3) the injurious conduct or omissions of other parties in trust relationships, how they manifest themselves, and their clinical course; (4) the psychological effects of mistreatment, including types of psychological harm, their presentation, and their clinical course; and (5) the circumstances under which harm is most likely to have been caused by the acts or omissions of another person.

2. The development of widely accepted operational definitions and validated and standardized measurement methods for the elements of elder mistreatment is urgently needed to move the field forward. The field must develop widely accepted operational definitions of the elements of elder mistreatment, its different forms, and associated risk factors and outcomes. The field must also develop a series of measures for these elements, with good (and known) reliability and validity. A menu of measures is necessary for each of the multiple contexts of research, including screening and case identification in clinical settings as well as studies of elder mistreatment in populations. To the extent that dichotomous classifications of mistreatment are needed, agreement must be reached on what LEAD-type methodology will be used in place of a gold standard for such studies.

Agreement on operational definitions for research may provide a useful foundation for developing standard definitions and classification criteria for surveillance and reporting. It is conceivable that a consensus conference could be convened to propel this process forward, although such an effort may be premature in the absence of greater experience in the field developing the approach outlined in this chapter. Another possibility would be to initiate a consensus process in a more limited domain—such as defining mistreatment in the context of developing definitions and measures of quality in long-term care, as recommended in a recent report on this subject by the Institute of Medicine (2001). (see Chapter 7 for further discussion).

3

A Theoretical Model of
Elder Mistreatment

The limited research on elder mistreatment lacks an overarching framework within which to understand the multiplicity of its ill-defined manifestations. Concerned citizens, clinicians of various sorts, including emergency room physicians, social workers, nurses, the police, and even the victims themselves report incidents of apparent mistreatment to the authorities (such as state adult protective services). They, in turn, investigate and classify them according to disparate legal definitions, collating them for reporting purposes but with only limited cross-state comparability. Academic researchers have tried their hand at identifying and cataloguing individuals subject to elder mistreatment in the population at large. But they too lack a fully developed theoretical framework that could serve to guide data collection efforts and permit a more effective assessment of (1) the differential prevalence of elder mistreatment by significant social attributes and (2) the causal sequences leading to enhanced risk of elder mistreatment.

As a result, the knowledge base about even the most elementary facts concerning elder mistreatment is incomplete, contradictory, misleading, and noncumulative. We are told, for example, that the majority of elder mistreatment cases are women. Yet we are not in a position to evaluate whether this is simply the result of the disproportionate number of elders who are women (due to differential mortality by gender) or whether women do indeed face a higher risk of elder mistreatment than men. Most studies reporting this finding simply lack a way of properly assessing the population base from which the clinical observations were generated.

RISK MODEL OF ELDER MISTREATMENT
IN DOMESTIC SETTINGS

Here we would like to propose, as a first approximation, a theoretical sketch for the study of elder mistreatment that in our view could help to codify the findings already in hand and to provide a framework within which to organize future research efforts.[1] It is offered in the spirit of starting a conversation about theoretically meaningful next steps rather than as a fully fleshed-out theoretical model. It draws its inspiration from George L. Engels's (1977) challenge to the reigning biomedical model of the time. He proposed a biopsychosocial model explicitly encompassing psychological and social factors in explaining biophysiological conditions, such as disease or aging processes. It has attracted increasing attention, most recently providing the framework within which a task force of the Institute of Medicine organized its discussion of sexually transmitted diseases (Institute of Medicine, 1997; see also Laumann et al., 1994:3-34, 541-548; Ensel and Lin, 2000). In Engels's view, the narrow biomedical model, with its highly individualistic, clinically centered presumptions, should be expanded to incorporate a multiperson interactional scheme with three sets of interrelated factors: the physiological, the psychological, and the social. What is missing from Engels's model is a fuller consideration of the environing cultural and social contexts in which these microprocesses are embedded.

The definition of elder mistreatment in Chapter 2 stipulates both a victim of mistreatment (the focal subject) and a responsible actor (a trusted other, typically the caregiver) that together lie at the center of analytic attention. The interaction between the characteristics of the potential victim of mistreatment (e.g., his or her changing health status, dependency, competencies) and those of the responsible actor (e.g., his or her care burden, stress, financial dependence) must be an essential feature of any analysis. In addition, contextual risk factors, such as those referring to location (type of institution, at home, etc.), social relationship (e.g., spousal, adult child caregiver, formal role caregiver like lawyer, nurse), and the broader sociocultural context (defined by race, ethnicity, religion, region, urban/rural location, and socioeconomic status), may set different generic levels of risk for the individuals embedded in them.

Figure 3-1 provides a bird's eye overview of the generic factors in the model of the risks for elder mistreatment, while Figure 3-2 presents a

---

[1] Several other theoretical sketches have been proposed in the research literature, including Ansello (1996); Phillips (1983); Schiamberg and Gans (1999); and Wolf and Pillemer (1989). The current framework attempts to be more comprehensive, including mistreatment both in domestic and institutional settings. In addition, it is applicable to multiple types of mistreatment. The sketches in the literature, however, are completely consistent in spirit and thrust with it.

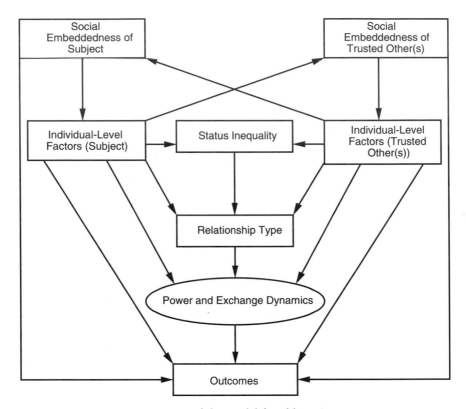

FIGURE 3-1   Summary overview of the model for elder mistreatment.

detailed specification of selected variables to be operationalized in applying the model to the empirical world.

It is fundamentally a model of a transactional process unfolding over time among the elder person, his or her trusted other, and other interested parties (stakeholders) concerned with his or her well-being in the context of changes in the physical, psychological, and social circumstances of the several parties as the result of the elder person's aging process and life course. This is called the microprocess, encompassing the factors that could be associated with the risk of mistreatment. In addition, this model should be understood as being embedded in an environing sociocultural context, such as the region of the country, the institutional or organizational locus (such as a nursing home, assisted living quarters, private household), and race or ethnic group of the elder person that are associated with

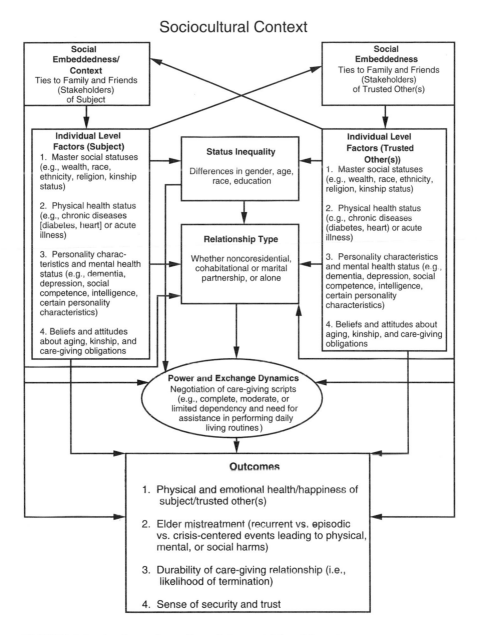

FIGURE 3-2 A schematic outline of the model for elder mistreatment.

different levels of risk for mistreatment. For example, it may be the case that different organizational settings (e.g., nursing homes, assisted living quarters) may have different characteristic levels of elder mistreatment risk. This feature of the model is the macrostructure in which the microprocesses described in Figure 3-2 occur. The risk of elder mistreatment can be conceptualized as the varying likelihood of an event or set of events causing harm to the elder person. This risk is a function of the various sets of variables depicted in the model at both the macro and micro levels.

The left side of the diagram includes the set of social, physical, and psychological attributes of the subject at risk of elder mistreatment, and the right side lists the pertinent attributes of the trusted other. The middle set of boxes represents the interaction of the two sets of individual-level variables that define the level of social or economic dependence (status inequality), type of social relationship in which the interaction between the elder person and the trusted other happens, with corresponding differences in the normative expectations held by different stakeholders and the power dynamics in negotiating the operative care-giving scripts (see Simon and Gagnon, 1987; Mahay et al., 2001). Note that we have also included "social embeddedness," which refers to the sets of people in the social networks of the elder person and the trusted other, respectively, constituting the social capital available in the dyadic transaction (see Sandefur and Laumann 1998). These two networks may overlap or not, with attendant consequences for their efficacy in exerting social control over the dyadic interaction of focal interest. Social networks can serve critical functions of monitoring the situation and informing relevant others when shortfalls or problems arise. Their presence may also serve as a form of social control on the behavior of the focal parties. Their absence greatly enhances the vulnerability of the elder person and the trusted other to the risk of elder mistreatment (see House et al., 1988; Lin et al., 1999). Finally, outcomes include the physical and emotional health and happiness of the elder person and the trusted other, the differential risks of elder mistreatment in its varied forms, and the durability (or risk of termination) of the caregiving relationship itself.

We should expect that all these outcomes have feedback effects on the variables above them—that is, the paths connecting outcomes to the boxes listing the independent variables are double-headed rather than unidirectional. For example, we might expect that the occurrence of an incident of elder mistreatment increases the odds of additional events of elder mistreatment, as it adversely affects physical, psychological, and social statuses for both the elder person and the trusted other. A mistreated elder is more likely to respond with depression, physical disability, or social withdrawal as a direct or indirect reaction to the mistreatment—each of which may enhance the likelihood of another incident. Similarly, the perpetrator may feel increased stress in his or her situation and become more likely to respond in an abusive manner to another challenge to his or her caregiving capabilities. In short, the overarching conception of the model is one of a time-dependent process with feedback loops that interact with the "independent" variables over time.

Such a conception highlights the critical need for longitudinal studies to gain a better understanding of the underlying dynamics. The clinically and forensically oriented literature often characterizes the issue as one of enhancing case identification methods so that "findings" of culpability can be established. But this leads to a focus on punishment and deterrence as the principal goals of intervention. A process-oriented account of elder mistreatment, in contrast, would lead to investigation of the reversibility of the process by providing a better understanding of the etiology of specific forms of elder mistreatment and therefore a better understanding of the preventive and remedial measures that could be undertaken.

Such a perspective would benefit from knowledge gained by qualitatively and phenomenally oriented research designed to flesh out the meanings of different forms of elder mistreatment. For example, how does spousal mistreatment differ from adult child mistreatment? What are the differences between one-shot or episodic mistreatment in response to a crisis situation that overwhelmed the caregiver and chronic or recurrent elder mistreatment in a long-term marriage characterized by recurrent physical conflict? We often speak of the heterogeneity of the phenomena of elder mistreatment, but there are literally no studies that attempt to explore the nature of that heterogeneity. At present, we are functioning at the level of commonsense classes, perhaps informed by legal distinctions rather than scientifically informed classification. Legal categories of elder mistreatment are highly heterogeneous in their phenomenal base and may thus arise from quite different etiologies, with correspondingly various implications for the kinds of interventions that might successfully be pursued. In regard to the potential opportunities and foci for prevention and intervention, the phenomena may be basically independent in cases of (a) battering by an intimate partner that persists as part of a long-term, even life-long pattern; (b) battering by an intimate partner that begins in late life (perhaps because of a transformation in the marital relationship as a result of changes in physical well-being or the social status and financial well-being of one or both spouses); (c) neglectful or abusive care by other kin who face a multiplicity of overwhelming care needs as well as other, perhaps unrelated problems; (d) neglectful or abusive care by employees of adult day programs, nursing homes, and hospitals; and (e) crimes of opportunity, in which dependent persons are exploited by caregivers who take advantage of access to financial resources.

RISK MODEL OF ELDER MISTREATMENT
IN INSTITUTIONAL SETTINGS

Figure 3-2 implicitly assumes that the trusted other (the right-hand side of the figure) was a family member or friend operating in the context of the informal provision of caregiving to the elder person in a private household. Let us now assume that the trusted other is an employee or volunteer working for an organization, such as a nursing home or hospice—that is, let us consider the model's applicability to institutional settings. Figure 3-3 specifies the set of variables (on the right-hand side of the model in Figure 3-1 down through individual-level factors) that are relevant to characterizing the organization as constituting the context within which trusted others (i.e., various staff members) are serving as the responsible care providers. We first note that there is a larger institutional context in which the organization is found—e.g., a particular region or state that has a stricter or more lax regulatory environment than other areas or a remote rural location (in comparison to an urban location) that hinders the access of the elder person's social network for visiting and monitoring what is going on. Next we can characterize the specific organizational facility with respect to its size, staff/resident ratios, per capita expenditures, etc.—all of which may be expected to be associated with different levels of risk of the caregivers in their employ engaging in elder mistreatment. For example, poorly managed and funded facilities with inadequate staff might be expected to pose a much greater likelihood of their staff engaging in elder mistreatment than the staff at well-run, well-funded facilities. Finally, we consider the individual-level attributes of the actual care providers themselves as affecting the relative risks of elder mistreatment. Can we, for example, expect more or less risk of elder mistreatment as a function of the training and experience of the care providers, or of racial, ethnic, or class differences between the elder person and the trusted other?

Figure 3-4 provides another take on the model that may help clarify what we have in mind. It can be regarded as a subsidiary process nested within the overarching model depicted in Figure 3-2. In this case, we consider an adverse physical change in the elder person's health status—e.g., the onset of vascular dementia. The risk of acquiring vascular dementia is shown to be a function of a set of prior factors, such as the subject's nutritional status, poverty, etc. With onset of the disease process, we expect a decline in physical function, including hypertension, depression, etc., that adversely affects the elder person's psychological outlook and social functionality (e.g., a decline in sexual interest and attractiveness to spouse). Diminished capacity to perform daily routines and increased demands on the spouse for help, combined with a loss of social facility and increased depressive behavior on the elder person's part, put increasing

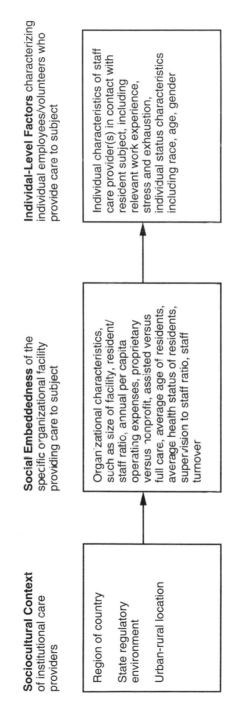

Elaboration of right-hand side of Figure 3-1 for institutional care providers

Sociocultural Context of institutional care providers

Region of country

State regulatory environment

Urban-rural location

Social Embeddedness of the specific organizational facility providing care to subject

Organizational characteristics, such as size of facility, resident/staff ratio, annual per capita operating expenses, proprietary versus nonprofit, assisted versus full care, average age of residents, average health status of residents, supervision to staff ratio, staff turnover

Individal-Level Factors characterizing individual employees/volunteers who provide care to subject

Individual characteristics of staff care provider(s) in contact with resident subject, including relevant work experience, stress and exhaustion, individual status characteristics including race, age, gender

FIGURE 3-3 Model of risk factors for different levels of risk for engaging in elder mistreatment by institutional care providers.

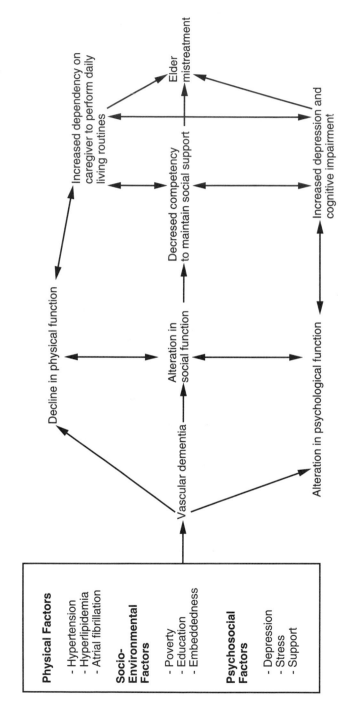

FIGURE 3-4 Impact of vascular dementia on risk of elder mistreatment in people age 55 and older.

stress on the caregiver, who feels captive to a deteriorating, "no-win" situation. He reacts with frustration and anger, finally physically hitting her in response to a "petty" demand for attention—an act that never occurred before in their many years of marriage. The figure attempts to identify the set of variables and their probable causal order; it also stresses the interactive character of the process over time. It should help guide the selection and measurement of the pertinent variables in evaluating this account of elder mistreatment risk.

RECOMMENDATION

The problem of identifying rare events like elder mistreatment is made more difficult because of its strong social stigmatization. It is quite analogous to the problem faced in studying AIDS infection in the population. AIDS is such a rare event (0.61 percent prevalence rate in the United States) that it is prohibitively expensive to get a sample size large enough to recruit sufficient cases for statistical analysis, even if one could assume that people would willingly disclose their infection status. Instead, analysis has focused on the prevalence of sexually transmitted diseases (STDs) inclusively defined, which have an estimated prevalence of 18 percent in the U.S. adult population age 18 to 59 (see Laumann and Youm, 2001:339), a much more workable situation from a statistical point of view. This could be done because the mechanisms implicated in STD transmission approximate fairly closely those implicated in AIDS transmission in the United States. A similar strategy could be undertaken for elder mistreatment, in which we could identify more broadly inclusive adverse events, for example, frequent and intense verbal arguments between the elder person and the caregiver, which are likely to include the events that meet a stricter definition of elder mistreatment.

The objective of this discussion has been to provide a comprehensive, flexible theoretical framework within which to organize research efforts employing qualitative as well as quantitative methodologies. Appropriately deployed in systematic empirical research, these methodologies can illuminate the fundamental processes generating the differential risks of elder mistreatment for both the elder population at large and for those who perform caregiving roles. Armed with a better understanding of the underlying processes, we will be in a much better position to devise more effective intervention strategies to reduce these risks.

In sum, we are unlikely to obtain much information relevant to prevention and post-mistreatment intervention in cases of elder mistreatment until the field moves toward a program of research that is grounded in an understanding of the everyday lives of older people in relation to their intimate partners and their other caregivers; the experience (phenomenology) of these relationships and their meaning to the people involved; the situational and motivational factors that tend to enhance or impair the cognitive performance of older people and their corollary capacity to protect their own interests; and the social factors driving—and potentially regulating—the settings in which older persons live, especially those who are cognitively impaired or financially dependent.

The theoretical sketch outlined in this chapter offers one approach for stimulating the thinking and research needed by the field at this stage in its development.

The panel recommends systematic, theory-driven longitudinal research, both qualitative and quantitative, exploring the changing dynamics of elder people's relationships and the risk of mistreatment, as they are affected by changing health status, social embeddedness, and caregiving and living arrangements, in both domestic and institutional contexts.

4

The Occurrence of Elder Mistreatment

This chapter reviews the scientific and logistical issues pertinent to the determination of mistreatment occurrence in the United States and elsewhere, identifies gaps in knowledge, and makes recommendations for possible research directions. Research to determine mistreatment occurrence rates or trends should, above all, be guided by the rationale for conducting the epidemiological inquiry. Is universal case finding critical within a population, or will probabilistic assessments to estimate incidence and prevalence suffice? Will the findings be used for specific local adult protective program design or as a guide to general policy formulation? Will there be a search for community indicators of elder mistreatment that are easily available or ascertainable if not totally accurate or precise? How will the findings inform clinical practice activities, particularly those related to frail older persons? Will private or governmental funds be allocated based on the findings, either for general prevention and control, criminal justice programs, or specific agency budgets? While the various available methods for determining occurrence estimates vary in precision and completeness, all may be of substantial value.

Basic to determining mistreatment occurrence rates is an understanding of sound epidemiological principles and vocabulary. While this is beyond the scope of this volume, an introduction to basic epidemiological study design is presented in Box 4-1 to enable the nonspecialist reader to better understand the discussion that follows.

BOX 4-1
An Overview of Epidemiological Study Designs

Epidemiology can be defined as the study of the distributions, determinants, and outcomes of health and disease in populations. These populations may be geographically defined, but they may also be clinical or institutional groups. Full population definition usually requires further demographic characterization, at a minimum. The determinants or causes of health and disease states are often referred to as *risk factors*. Outcomes of interest span a wide spectrum, including, for example, mortality, symptom severity, disease progression, other new mental and physical conditions (morbidity), the costs of illness, disability and dysfunction, and satisfaction with medical care. Epidemiology may be *observational*, wherein the world is observed as it is, or *experimental and interventional,* wherein experimental or quasi-experimental interventions are invoked. Within observational epidemiology, *descriptive epidemiology* generally refers to the quantitative occurrence of health and disease phenomena in characterized populations, often using rates over a specified period of time, and requiring a known population denominator. For example, a *prevalence rate* describes how frequently the event of interest, regardless of time of onset, occurs at any point within a specified time interval. An *incidence rate* is the rate of *new* events in the population occurring within that interval.

Epidemiology can also be *analytical* as well as descriptive. There are many analytical study designs to assess population phenomena; three are basic to assessing health and disease in populations. *Cross-sectional* assessments or surveys, at one defined point in time, can be used to determine prevalence rates, characterize those in whom the events of interest exist, and explore statistical associations among the study variables of interest.

The case-control, or *retrospective,* study takes many forms and is mainly intended to identify risk factors for diseases and conditions. In its simplest application, new cases of a disease are identified, a demographically similar control group is designated, and differences in prior "exposure" rates to the risk factors of interest are calculated. The *cohort* or *longitudinal study* in essence starts with a defined population in whom putative risk factor information has been well characterized, but in whom the disease or condition of interest has not yet occurred. The population is then followed for incident events of interest, which are then related to previously acquired risk factor information. Each type of study can be elaborated and each has strengths, weaknesses, and methodological nuances. Full descriptions of these epidemiological methods for both community and clinical settings can be found in standard textbooks of epidemiology and clinical epidemiology.

OCCURRENCE OF ELDER MISTREATMENT

While clinical descriptions of elder mistreatment are present in historical texts, even now there have been few population-referent, geographically based studies of elder mistreatment occurrence in the modern, peer-reviewed literature. The latter third of the twentieth century saw the description of the clinical syndrome and reports of various series of elder mistreatment victims, usually from geriatrically oriented facilities or programs managing chronic illnesses in older persons, and later from social service agencies. Gradually, recommended elder mistreatment definitions and criteria began to appear, and many of these recommendations have been published (see Chapter 2). Often, the basic demographic and clinical characteristics of elder mistreatment patients were defined in part by the nature of the study facilities as well by the patients/victims. Early clinical descriptions paved the way for later studies of elder mistreatment risk factors. Using case records from public health nurses, Phillips (1983) reported one of the first case-control studies of risk factors for elder abuse.

Estimates of the occurrence of abuse and neglect have varied from about 2–10 percent annual incidence, although the bases for these estimates are modest and uncertain (Branch, 2001). The issue of incidence versus prevalence and the recurrent nature of the problem among individual victims and other issues (discussed below) make these estimates very insecure. For example, Thomas (2000) reviewed both formally published and other data on elder mistreatment occurrence. The lack of population-based studies in this review is clear, and much of the information reviewed came from institutional and social service agency sources. Other than representative household samples, some research has explored samples of adult protective service workers, assessing their observations and experiences (Dolan and Blakeley, 1989) and other public and private institutional employees who may have contact with abused elders, such as police authorities, hospital personnel, and bank employees (National Center on Elder Abuse). While important, these approaches identify only those (potential or actual) elder mistreatment victims who have come to public attention and probably underestimate the true elder mistreatment occurrence rates.

One of the first and historically most important population-based studies of elder mistreatment was conducted by Pillemer and Finkelhor (1988). This was a prevalence study using a probability sample of noninstitutionalized persons age 65 and older residing in metropolitan Boston. Interviews were conducted over the telephone and in person using structured questionnaires and standardized criteria for three domains of elder mistreatment: physical abuse, psychological abuse, and neglect. About 72 percent of the eligible respondents were interviewed. Including all three elder mistreatment domains studied, they reported an overall rate of 3.2 percent.

A few other population-based studies have been published. Comijs et al. (1998) studied physical and psychological abuse in a cohort of Dutch elders in Amsterdam, using structured interviewing techniques. Overall, the one-year prevalence of elder mistreatment was 5.6 percent, with verbal aggression being the most common; the prevalence of physical aggression was 1.2 percent. In a telephone interview study of national samples from

Sweden and Denmark, Tornstam (1989) queried respondents about whether they had observed or knew about specific cases of persons who had been physically battered, threatened, economically abused, robbed, or severely neglected. The overall rate defined this way was 8 percent, but most cases were due to a single incidence of theft. The definitions were not always consistent with those used in other elder mistreatment studies, but most importantly, the individual respondent was not the unit of analysis.

Podnieks (1992) reported the findings from a representative telephone survey of Canadians age 65 and older. Domains included physical abuse, neglect, psychological abuse, and "material abuse." The overall prevalence rate was about 4 percent, but this was a cumulative experience since age 65, so the annual rates would be difficult to calculate; the most common form was material abuse (2.6 percent). Ogg (1993) attempted to repeat the Pillemer and Finkelhor survey in London but for methodological reasons was unable to obtain credible occurrence information.

Thus, based on the published, peer-reviewed literature and some efforts at obtaining unindexed, non-peer-reviewed studies, there appears to be little population-based information about elder mistreatment occurrence, including the clinical course and outcomes of proven events. It appears that more population-based approaches to elder mistreatment, including nationally representative samples, are needed. Even less information is known about elder mistreatment occurrence in institutional settings. Event detection is extremely challenging and to date only indirect approaches have been employed to make estimates.

The paper by Acierno (this volume) summarizes the primary ways in which elder mistreatment has been detected: (a) direct interview surveys of potential victims by telephone, personal interview, or self-administered questionnaire), (b) interviews of families or caregivers of possible victims or others with a trust relationship, (c) clinical or social service institutional record review, (d) placement of sentinel reporters within these agencies or organizations, and (e) acquisition of criminal justice information. Historically, these techniques have been applied most consistently and will be likely to continue to be important. Corder (2001) reviews many of the issues in population sampling and surveying relevant to household assessment of elder mistreatment occurrences. A summary of overall strengths and weaknesses of these approaches is shown in Table 4-1.

However, other, less explored methods for identifying elder mistreatment cases are available for research evaluation: (a) a two-stage process, beginning with screening potential victims for risk factors or risk indicators, using questionnaires, medical record review, and various biomarkers, with subsequent more intensive evaluation of high-risk persons, (b) screening fiscal records for types of behaviors associated with financial abuse, (c) active screening of older patients during general medical interactions, either inside or outside institutional settings, (d) provision of telephone hot lines, widely publicized and intended to attract victims who can then be further evaluated, (e) network sampling of social situations in which some forms of elder mistreatment are possible, (f) enhanced identification of high-risk persons or elder mistreatment cases using record linkage techniques, (g) the application of forensic techniques in medical settings, and (h) surreptitious surveillance of institutional staff in the work setting. None of these approaches is new, but they at least suggest that innovative approaches to case detection and surveillance are possible, and that is a needed research direction.

IMPORTANT EPIDEMIOLOGICAL CONSIDERATIONS

Important research issues relevant to defining, understanding, and advancing knowledge of elder mistreatment are discussed throughout this volume. These issues require detailed attention and are important requisites for planning population- and institution-based epidemiological research on elder mistreatment occurrence. The following sections synthesize and highlight some of these issues specifically with respect to determining elder mistreatment occurrence, adding further suggestions for conducting this research.

Defining the Situations and Circumstances Being Measured

Chapters 1 and 2 delineate the types and vocabulary of elder mistreatment. While no investigator must adhere to any particular elder mistreatment conceptualization, specification of the nature and types of mistreatment being assessed in a study is critical, both for understanding and interpreting the findings and for possible scientific replication. In particular, operational definitions are critical for quantitative studies under all circumstances, especially when multiple interviewers, geographic sites, institutions, or cultural groups are involved.

The structure of survey items eliciting elder mistreatment flows directly from the posited elder mistreatment definitions. Since it is axiomatic that in general survey responses will vary according the wording of survey items, it seems likely that this will be an issue here as well. Thus, careful item structuring will require consummate attention. In addition, item detail and explicitness may alter the type of responses. This was recently demonstrated in a related area—the survey of assessment of sexual victimization among college women (Fisher et al., 2000).

TABLE 4-1 Strengths and Weaknesses of Different Approaches to
Population-Based Elder Mistreatment Case Identification

Elder Mistreatment Case Identification Strategy	Strengths	Weaknesses
1. Interview of potential victims; all modes	-Victims can be identified with regularity through self-report. -Nature and severity of the mistreatment acts as well as many antecedents can be characterized. -Structured operational criteria for case definitions can be most rigorously applied.	-Some elder mistreatment victims will not admit mistreatment events for various reasons. -Cognitive impairment may preclude accurate reporting. -Interview setting in which perpetrators are present may deter reporting. -Access to some elder mistreatment victims may be limited by sampling incompleteness, household refusals, language barriers, or illness. -Not appropriate for study of fatal events.
2. Interview of families, other caregivers, and others in trust relationships	-Perpetrators are known to relate some elder mistreatment events. -Proxy respondents may report some elder mistreatment events more accurately, as well as some respondent characteristics (e.g., belligerent behavior). -Structured, operational criteria can be uniformly applied.	-Many perpetrators may not report elder mistreatment events. -Proxy respondents may have imperfect knowledge of events. -Some proxy respondents may have illness, frailty, or cognitive impairment. -Some characteristics of respondents can't be obtained by proxy interview (e.g., emotional status).
3. Clinical or social service institutional record review	-Level of objective documentation likely to be high. -Treatments and social interventions documented. -Historical data more likely to be obtainable.	-Only selected and more severe cases may be present. -Case definitions may not be consonant with those of investigators. -Clinical observations are often unstandardized in measures and notation. -Ancillary and risk factor information may not be collected in a systematic manner.

TABLE 4-1 Continued

Elder Mistreatment Case Identification Strategy	Strengths	Weaknesses
4. Placement of sentinel reporters within clinical and social agencies or organizations	-May identify cases that otherwise would not be detected or come to clinical attention. -Observers can be sensitive to case screening or detection criteria. -May be the most effective method in long-term care settings.	-Observers are often professionals who have other obligations. -Variation in personal powers of clinical observation. -Ethical issues in the insertion of observers in some settings.
5. Acquisition of criminal justice information	-Can identify some cases that otherwise may not be subject to clinical or social service detection. -Legal dimensions of elder mistreatment occurrence more fully documented.	-Cases likely to be a highly selective subsample of cases, more severe, and only of certain types. -Information may not be collected in a systematic manner.

Specifying the Unit of Measurement

As Acierno (this volume) and others suggest, the elder mistreatment "event" is not always easy to characterize. Target elder mistreatment events for detection may be single or multiple occurrences, happening over short or long periods of time, and involving one or more victims (particularly in the institutional setting) or one or more perpetrators, yielding potentially diverse clinical, social, or functional outcomes. Thus, a variety of events may make up the numerator of interest: a single act by a perpetrator, a single act on a victim, a series of elder mistreatment acts by a perpetrator regardless of the number of victims, a series of acts on one victim, and so on. Similarly, the denominator used in rate calculations may vary and requires clear specification. Is it all persons in an age group, all persons in a trust relationship, all persons exposed to a potential perpetrator, or persons with a particular risk profile? Will the analysis be presented as a "person-time" calculation, in which potential victims are at risk only during specified times, such as the night shift in a long-term care institution? The complex and fluid nature of social "exposures" requires great care in specifying both the numerator and denominators in occurrence rates.

Understanding the Clinical Course and
Outcomes of Elder Mistreatment

As noted above, clinical observation suggests that elder mistreatment may take place over a long period of time, and that only at certain times, such as when a severe injury or evidence of willful neglect increases, will the situation become clinically, socially, or legally apparent. As pointed out by Acierno (this volume) and suggested in other studies of later-life suicide attempts (Dube et al., 2001) and victimization from sexual or physical abuse (Cold et al., 2001), for some elder mistreatment victims the origins may reach back to youth or young adulthood, or they have been in place within a family relationship for many years, although the causal mechanisms are unclear. Ascertaining multiple events over long periods, particularly in retrospect, can understandably be extremely difficult. However, not only for defining the start of an "incident" elder mistreatment event, but more importantly for understanding the causes and trajectory of elder mistreatment, a broad, sometimes lifelong view of the problem seems essential. This amplifies the plea for more longitudinal studies of elder mistreatment. It is possible, for example, that retrospective medical record review, when available, may identify early elder mistreatment events that were unrecognized at the time. In medical parlance, it seems likely that many cases of elder mistreatment are remittent or recurrent but, with few exceptions (Lachs et al., 1997b), there is little quantitative work on this issue.

A similar issue relates to the short- and long-term impact of elder mistreatment on victims. A critical question that is almost unanswered is how elder mistreatment relates to the clinical, social, institutional, financial, psychological, and mortal outcomes of elder mistreatment victims and the overall impact of elder mistreatment on elder population health. For example, an important issue in gerontological public health is whether the mobility and functional status of elders in the United States has been improving, paralleling the increasing longevity seen in the latter part of the twentieth century (Manton et al., 1997; Freedman and Martin, 1999; Schoeni et al., 2001). This is important for forecasting and planning future health care and fiscal needs. Given the evidence that at least some population functional improvement has occurred, evidence to explain this phenomenon should be sought, in order to enhance preventive and therapeutic practice. It is at least a hypothesis that knowledge of elder mistreatment occurrence rates over time could be helpful in understanding secular trends in the prevalence and outcomes of elder population disability. In fact, elder mistreatment may be important and common enough to also consider when planning and evaluating long-term disease and disability prevention and treatment trials targeting vulnerable, dependent, and frail elders.

Clinical, functional, and population elder mistreatment outcomes could be studied in several research contexts. One set of relevant outcomes relates to the immediate consequences of mistreatment itself, including such factors as return to previous health status, wound or fracture healing rates, preservation or loss of psychological well-being, the status of general chronic disease control measures, and the immediate social and legal responses to mistreatment. Another set of outcomes relates to the effects of whatever interventions transpire, not only on the rates and intensity of further mistreatment, but also on new and preexisting medical conditions, victim satisfaction with the intervention, the types of medical service utilization engendered, the costs of the intervention process, and the long-term costs of social and medical care.

One particularly interesting question is whether, and under what circumstances, subjective measures of personal security or well-being could be developed as an ultimate outcome measure, both for the effects of mistreatment as well as for the effects of interventions. Obviously, many other factors affect an individual's personal sense of security, and studies using such a measure of outcome would have to deal with this problem methodologically, but this is a challenge worth undertaking. As a research question, it would be interesting to know whether this perception is related to the ability to restore optimal medical and mental health and well-being after elder mistreatment is detected and addressed.

Interface with the Public Health, Medical Care, and Social Services Systems

From a community perspective, it is clear that cases of elder mistreatment are underascertained by existing public health, social, medical, and legal activities and systems; this is understandable despite the need for improvement. Several papers in this volume acknowledge the important roles of these systems and programs in identifying cases as one technique for determining elder mistreatment occurrence. This is particularly true since a substantial proportion of elder mistreatment episodes appear to occur in frail elders, who are perhaps least likely to participate in household surveys. As reviewed by Acierno and Dyer et al. (this volume), there has been considerable work in trying to improve recognition of elder mistreatment in the formal program setting, especially within clinical health and social services. It seems clear that more research is needed on the interface of elder mistreatment with these services, and it is important to understand the nature and value of increased and more refined medical and social surveillance and screening practices on geographically based elder mistreatment rates. Health care settings could be particularly important, since each year approximately 85 percent of persons age 65 and older use formal ambulatory care services and 16–20 percent are hospitalized. With the inclusion of long-term care service use and the various forms of residential and assisted living that contain chore or clinical services, as delineated by Hawes (this volume), few elder mistreatment victims would be outside the reach of some type of screening, and most could be identified if accurate, inexpensive, and comprehensive methods were available.

As case detection and epidemiological research on elder mistreatment proceed, the importance of some basic public health notions becomes clear. It is important to distinguish between *screening*, where-by someone is put into an "elevated probability" group for further evaluation, and *case finding*, where-by an actual designation of elder mistreatment is made. Both in research and practice, the two approaches encompass different levels of rigor and investigation (see Chapter 6 for further discussion). Any substantial increase in either activity could lead to increased elder mistreatment detection rates and could lead to spuriously increased population occurrence rates; community-based elder mistreatment prevention and treatment programs should be alert for this. Screening research could usefully be applied to many settings, including all types of medical care sites, social service and adult protective service settings, and the legal and judicial systems. As this research progresses, it would also seem to be of value to monitor the extent of overall community elder mistreatment screening and case finding, to better understand whether observed changes in elder mistreatment secular trends may be due to variation in surveillance intensity. There may also be long-term variation in the propensity of elders to verbalize and report mistreatment.

Attention should also be given to the potential role of using existing or newly developed injury surveillance systems to measure and monitor trends in certain types of elder mistreatment. For example, violent deaths of elders will be included in a new National Violent Death Reporting System that will provide much richer information than is currently available from existing data sources on homicides and suicides (see Institute of Medicine, 1999). While current surveillance of nonfatal injuries is limited, even the existing data collected in emergency departments and through hospitals are not very sensitive for elder mistreatment. The panel encourages the National Center for Injury Prevention and Control of the Centers for Disease Control and Prevention (CDC) to study ways of enhancing the utility of existing injury surveillance systems for identifying elder mistreatment and of incorporating it into newly developed systems. Other types of public health surveillance could also be useful in measuring the occurrence of elder mistreatment. In many jurisdictions the public health system provides various levels of preventive and medical care, often emphasizing vulnerable populations, as well as inspecting and licensing long-term care institutions. Research on surveillance efficacy in these settings may also be of value.

Relation of Risk Factors to Occurrence

Chapter 5 delineates much of what is known about risk factors for elder mistreatment, and these are not reviewed here. Chapter 5 and the paper by Acierno make the important point that risk factors may be related to the environment or to the characteristics of the perpetrator, not only to those of the victim. Acierno also notes that some elder mistreatment research projects use "known" risk factors for case definition, such as dimensions of dependence and vulnerability, possibly limiting the ability to study these factors or to identify related risk factors. Investigators should be alert to this issue when conducting community surveys. For example, if an elder mistreatment case definition demands the presence of frailty or vulnerability, then risk factors for elder mistreatment that may be associated with more robust older victims cannot easily be explored.

A related issue is the problem of applying clinical risk factors to case definitions of elder mistreatment. Older persons, particularly frail elders, have many clinical problems and dysfunctions, and from both conceptual and statistical perspectives it may be challenging to use these risk factors for case ascertainment. For example, among general, community-dwelling populations over age 65, over half may have at least one chronic illness and at least one physical limitation or dependence. In addition, general symptoms such as pain, fatigue, and sleep problems abound, as well as organ-specific complaints, related, for example, to the skin and or the gastrointestinal tract. Thus, the specificity of these factors for case designation may be lower than hoped. This is discussed more fully in Chapter 6 on case ascertainment in the clinical setting.

It may also be useful to distinguish between a *risk factor*, for which a causal association to elder mistreatment is being sought, such as the social isolation of a victim, from a *risk indicator*, a certain characteristic that is associated with elder mistreatment but is not thought to be causal. An example of the latter is an environmental (contextual) factor, such as living in a community in which the police make frequent domestic violence calls. It is also possible that some putative risk factors, such as cognitive or other functional impairment, may in some instances result from elder mistreatment as well as being potential causes, as these impairments may be due to head trauma, misuse of medications, or some forms of bodily neglect. This is another reason why understanding the clinical course of elder mistreatment is critical to its detection. It may also be worth restating here that some risk factors may only be relevant to certain forms of elder mistreatment, and not to all of its forms and manifestations.

There still is a large amount of work to be done in defining risk factors for elder mistreatment. More community-based and institution-based studies are needed, and they should be done in geographically, economically, and culturally diverse populations. Also, much more work needs to be done on how elder mistreatment victims are detected and managed in various health care systems and in communities with varying levels of long-term care and adult protective service availability. Several papers in this volume note the use of qualitative techniques to further define the various elder mistreatment "syndromes" and characteristics; further application of these methods would seem to be of value. Finally, very little is known about elder mistreatment occurrence and related risk factor status among minority populations in the United States, including cultural variation in how mistreatment is defined and perceived. In general, a more diversified approach to research on risk factor and occurrence assessment would achieve several ends: (a) more critically defining populations with higher and lower occurrence rates, (b) determining the generalizability of putative elder mistreatment risk factor findings across such diverse populations, (c) more precisely providing sample size estimates for intervention studies within these populations, and (d) exploiting cross-cultural variation in elder mistreatment occurrence to better understand its causes.

Piggybacking Assessment Modules on Existing Population Surveys

One way to promote research on elder mistreatment occurrence is to add detection items and instruments to existing field surveys, particularly those that cover large geographic areas or are national in scope. This is discussed extensively by Corder (2001).

On one hand, this could provide several potential advantages: it may allow substantial resource savings when compared with conducting surveys de novo; national estimation of elder mistreatment rates could be substantially enhanced; existing surveys may contain important respondent and family health, social, and economic variables that can be explored as both risk and outcome variables; and some surveys may have longitudinal data collection, allowing a time dimension not otherwise available in cross-sectional surveys.

On the other hand, there may also be important limitations to this approach: sensitive assessment of elder mistreatment may not lend itself to certain modes of data collection, such as mail or telephone surveys; elder mistreatment themes may not be compatible with the other survey content; there may be different requirements and challenges in the use of proxy respondents; there may personal respondent resistance to items related to elder mistreatment; certain demographic or cultural groups may not be adequately represented in the parent surveys of interest; and content and sampling techniques may be unsuitable for many elder mistreatment scientific questions of interest. There may also be limitations on identifying or following up respondents, should substantial evidence of elder mistreatment events emerge. Still, the use of supplementary elder mistreatment modules within existing or planned large-scale or national surveys would seem to be a potentially fruitful approach that should be further evaluated.

The issue of household sampling is paramount in defining elder mistreatment occurrence rates. The general experience of household surveys targeting elders is that the older and more vulnerable potential respondents are the ones most difficult to access, leading to the potential for underassessment of elder mistreatment occurrence. Thus, in many instances, supplementary sampling approaches may be needed, such as through informal social networks, the health care system, or other social institutions.

Record Linkage

The limitations of interview data as the sole source of elder mistreatment occurrence are apparent. Some of those at greatest risk, as noted above, may not be able or willing to serve as survey respondents, and while Acierno (this volume) notes that family members and others may admit to elder mistreatment, the completeness and accuracy of such declarations are uncertain. Inaccurate recall among survey respondents in general and older respondents in particular is well described, and recall accuracy is further called into question by the increasing levels of cognitive impairment with advancing age. In fact, Acierno (this volume) begins his discussion of case detection methods by dichotomizing elder mistreatment victims into those with and without "significant" cognitive impairment. This may be a useful construct, but cognitive function is multidimensional and variably progressive, so from the perspective of studying elder mistreatment occurrence, it may not be easy to categorize case populations into those with and without cognitive decline in advance of applying the case ascertainment protocol itself. Clearly, the issue of determining instances of elder mistreatment among those cognitively impaired is an important research question.

One potentially important method for enhancing knowledge of the occurrence and clinical course of elder mistreatment is record linkage. Determining the health, social, and economic status of older persons may profitably be enhanced by compiling information from many sources, including information from prior surveys, vital records, health care and health administrative records, social service and criminal justice records, and records from other publicly available, potentially health-relevant sectors of society. The use of primary institutional records should increase the accuracy of the information available for analysis and could complement information gained from interviews. However, there are several potential challenges to record linkage, including additional costs, the availability of electronic record systems, increasing privacy concerns (National Research Council, 2000a), and the logistics of assembling data from multiple sources.

Details on the value of data linkage in research and policy formulation can be found in a report from the National Research Council (1988) and other sources (Kelman and Smith, 2000). A corollary issue is the need to determine the accuracy and completeness of the records being linked.

Potential Role for Biomarkers

An unexplored area in determining elder mistreatment occurrence is the application of biomarkers. A biomarker in this case is any physical, physiological, or biochemical measure that could assist in identifying victims of elder mistreatment and could most easily be acquired in field surveys via blood or urine specimens. Even if biomarker associations with elder mistreatment are proven, these are much more likely to indicate increased risk and would not lead to definitive elder mistreatment designation. Some biomarker applications may relate to undernutrition, such as blood cholesterol, albumen, or micronutrient levels. Others may relate to chronic psychological or physical stress, but as blood or urinary catecholamine or cortisol levels or markers of chronic immune dysfunction. Chronic blunt trauma may increase blood or urinary myoglobin or other muscle protein degradation products. Additional forensic techniques, both antemortem and postmortem, may be useful detecting elder mistreatment cases. It is not outside the realm of possibility that genetic markers may be candidates for elder mistreatment research, to the extent that they perhaps reflect particular behaviors, diseases, or responses to stress and trauma. As one example, somatic mutation rates in the genome have been proposed as an indicator of cumulative environmental exposures (Albertini, 1998). The application of biomarkers to elder mistreatment assessment could be an area for possible future research. A recent volume addresses many aspects of applying biomarker acquisition to population surveys (National Research Council, 2000b).

CONCLUSIONS AND RECOMMENDATIONS

1. Population-based surveys of elder mistreatment occurrence are feasible and should be given a high priority by funding agencies. Preparatory funding should be provided to develop and test measures for identifying elder mistreatment.

There is inadequate information on elder mistreatment occurrence among both community-dwelling and institutionalized elders. However, before embarking on such surveys, the aims and rationale for them should be clearly delineated, and the strengths and weaknesses of the survey methodology fully understood. Different methods and approaches may be required for various types of mistreatment, and multiple modes of case ascertainment should be considered and evaluated. Survey-acquired information could be enhanced by appropriately applied record linkage techniques. Complementary study of biomarkers that may enhance elder mistreatment case identification should be explored.

Efforts to improve research on incidence and prevalence must move ahead deliberately while new instruments and measures are being developed. As noted in Chapter 2, measurement of elder mistreatment has been hampered by a lack of well-validated and reliable instruments. Several instruments have been used in elder mistreatment research, but little more than face validity supports the assumption that they provide valid or reliable measures of elder mistreatment, and further instrument development is needed. As an example, one of the most frequently used instruments in elder mistreatment research, the Conflict Tactics Scale, has generally been accepted on the basis of its proven usefulness in other studies on violence in the family. However, its overall reliability for identifying physical mistreatment in older adults has not been adequately established. Other instruments that have been used in research were developed principally as clinical screening tools. While they have shown their adequacy in clinical situations, it is unclear whether they are fully valid measures for defining abuse and neglect in population or other research contexts, and whether they can be reliably administered in different research settings.

In the absence of fully validated instruments that are usable across settings and types of research, it will be difficult to make effective comparisons across studies, either in relation to incidence and prevalence or in relation to risk factors. With a set of common instruments that are valid and reliable, as well as criteria matched across instruments, it becomes possible for useful cross-study comparisons to be made. Furthermore, with such instruments in place, more rapid progress should be possible in identifying and confirming risk factors. Such instruments must be capable of differentiating among the varying forms of elder mistreatment as well as serving as a composite measure. Both for occurrence studies and risk factor studies, specificity for the various types of elder mistreatment is critical.

2. Funding agencies should give priority to the design and fielding of national prevalence and incidence studies of elder mistreatment. These studies should include both a large-scale, independent study of prevalence and modular add-ons to other national surveys of aging populations.

Acquiring valid national elder mistreatment occurrence rates is critically needed for improved policy formulation. After appropriate methodological development, a national survey of elder mistreatment occurrence and risk factors, designed to inform important policy issues relevant to elder mistreatment prevention and treatment, should be conducted. The panel recommends a two-pronged approach for obtaining the needed information:

- Supplemental modules pertaining to elder mistreatment should be included in existing comprehensive geographic health and social surveys, including ongoing longitudinal studies of aging populations. These studies will require the use of short instruments, or a series of questions, designed to identify likely victims of elder mistreatment. For reasons of economy, an alternative is to use these supplemental modules to target only selected forms of mistreatment, such as physical mistreatment, neglect, and financial exploitation. The unique contribution of such studies is to provide a large national sample from which reliable prevalence estimates can be drawn. Of equal importance, however, is the ability to use the longitudinal data to identify risk factors, further define health and social outcomes, and serve relevant policy needs. Elder mistreatment modules appended to existing national surveys can also serve as a test bed for new scientific approaches to data collection. Such piggy-backing of elder mistreatment items and instruments is logistically feasible in most contexts, and attempt should be made to further this application.

- Once the measurement issues have been satisfactorily addressed, a comprehensive national prevalence study of elder mistreatment should be undertaken. The purpose of this study would be to generate useable national estimates of prevalence and the critical demographics for each of the principal forms of elder mistreatment (physical mistreatment, sexual mistreatment, emotional mistreatment, financial exploitation, and neglect).

Both the supplemental module studies and the national prevalence study must ultimately address family and nonfamily settings, including nursing homes and the full range of assisted living arrangements and other community-based locations in which vulnerable older persons reside. Without such information, policy makers and program developers have no empirical basis for assessing the needs of elder mistreatment victims or for deciding how much to invest in research and prevention programs.

3. In addition to improved household and geographically referent sampling techniques, new methods of sampling and identifying elder mistreatment victims in the community should be developed in order to improve the validity and comprehensiveness of elder mistreatment occurrence estimates. It is likely that household sampling, while extremely useful, will be incomplete to some degree because of difficulty in gaining access to those households and respondents most at risk of elder mistreatment. A particular problem is accessing and characterizing the wide variety of assisted living and related residential facilities where many vulnerable elders are located. Developing additional ways to approach and access these populations may require other sampling techniques, such as through social networks, institutions, or the health care system.

4. Research is needed on the phenomenology and clinical course of elder mistreatment. The clinical course, antecedents, and outcomes of the

various types of elder mistreatment occurrence are poorly understood, necessitating more longitudinal investigations, including follow-up studies of the clinical, social, and psychological outcomes of elder mistreatment cases detected. The existing research appears to lack depth and texture. This is not surprising in light of the field's early stage of development and the emphasis thus far placed on occurrence of cases (in population-based surveys and in the clinical setting). If the field is to move forward, attention must be devoted to theory-driven efforts to identify the intersecting behaviors, relationships, and conditions that characterize mistreatment and to trace its clinical course.

Longitudinal studies are needed to explore the relationship among different forms of mistreatment, to place descriptive information about risk factors in context, to trace outcomes, to draw causal inferences, and to identify potential targets for intervention. For example, what are the individual and familial outcomes of elder mistreatment? What proportion of mistreatment cases result in emergency department visits? To what extent do persons who experience elder mistreatment develop post-traumatic stress disorder or other psychiatric conditions? Many elder mistreatment situations are recurrent and may have various incarnations over long periods, making the definition of an elder mistreatment "event" difficult to define. Thus, further work on the nature, periodicity, variation, and triggers for elder mistreatment is needed and will require longitudinal investigations. Such longitudinal studies could be enhanced by linkage of medical and social records, when feasible, to augment the range of available information.

5. **The occurrence of elder mistreatment in institutional settings, including long-term care and assisted living situations, is all but uncharacterized and needs new study sampling and detection methods.** Sampling and surveillance techniques may be different from community-based elder mistreatment detection, and considerable innovation may be required.

5

Risk Factors for Elder Mistreatment

$\mathbf{W}$hy do family members (or others in a trust relationship) mistreat elderly persons? What factors place older persons at risk? These are critically important questions, but finding answers poses a number of difficult challenges for researchers. Some of the difficulties are methodological: obtaining information on a hidden—and for most people, shameful—phenomenon is a daunting task at best. The search for risk factors has also been clouded by a 20-year history of elder mistreatment as a social problem: early assertions, founded on faulty data (or no data at all), have been frequently repeated and widely believed, despite the lack of evidence.

Thus, although fairly extensive research on risk factors for child abuse and intimate partner abuse has been conducted, the risk factor literature on elder mistreatment is both limited and inconsistent. It is important to remedy this situation, for several reasons. First, an understanding of associated factors and antecedents of elder mistreatment is necessary for the development of screening methods. Victims of elder mistreatment infrequently seek help for the problem on their own; therefore, by the time the case has progressed to the point at which it is detected by a service agency, it is often very complex and difficult to treat. Effective screening could result in a reduction of the negative effects of elder mistreatment and reduce the need for extensive treatment.

Second, specification of risk factors for elder mistreatment is needed to provide a rational basis for prevention programs. If the risk factors for elder mistreatment can be uncovered, we may be able to reduce or eliminate those factors and thus prevent the development of new cases of elder mistreatment or deter the progression of existing cases. Third, understanding risk factors is critical to the development of public policy initiatives. It is necessary to identify populations at higher risk, and the causes of that heightened risk, before the costs and benefits of reducing exposure can be determined (Gordis, 1996).

A note on terminology will be useful at the outset. For the purposes of this chapter, following Timmreck (1998), risk factors are defined as experiences, behaviors, aspects of lifestyle or environment, or personal characteristics that increase the chances that elder mistreatment will occur. Increased risk factor exposure increases the probability of the occurrence of elder mistreatment. As noted in Chapter 2, a distinction can be made between risk factors (factors that increase the probability that a problem will occur) and protective factors (factors that decrease the probability of occurrence). To simplify the discussion, in the rest of the chapter we refer to risk factors only, in part because most published work involves variables associated with an increased probability of mistreatment. The discussion of risk factors, however, may also hold for protective factors. In fact, research on protective factors may be as important as study of factors that increase risk, since it may suggest factors that can be put in place as a means of preventing elder mistreatment.

PROBLEMS IN THE RESEARCH BASE

Prior to summarizing the available findings, it is important to review briefly the problems in using existing research to establish risk factors for elder mistreatment. Problems exist in two areas: (1) the nature of the phenomenon of elder mistreatment itself creates challenges for risk factor research and (2) specific methodological limitations of existing studies limit the ability to integrate findings.

Nature of Elder Mistreatment

With some diseases or conditions, attribution of cause can be fairly simple and straightforward; a salmonella outbreak serves as an example. Other conditions have very complex causation, and indeed the condition itself may be difficult to define and identify. Elder mistreatment clearly fits the latter pattern.

The complexity of elder mistreatment can be highlighted by reference to the concept of a "geriatric syndrome"—that is, common clinical problems that typically do not have a single underlying pathophysiological process, but instead have several contributing factors that shape presentation

(Lachs and Pillemer, 1995). Examples of geriatric syndromes include falls, urinary incontinence, and functional decline.

Geriatric syndromes share several characteristics: environmental factors play an important role; interventions must be multifaceted and directed at both specific pathophysiological problems as well as at contributing factors in the environment; and such syndromes are often underdiagnosed and undermanaged by health and social service providers. Elder mistreatment shares these characteristics of a geriatric syndrome. Most important for the purposes of this chapter, contributing etiologies can be related to the relative (or person in a trust relationship), to the elder, or to the environment. Thus, the search for risk factors is both complex and challenging and necessarily must look for sources of risk in the host (the elderly person), the agent (the perpetrator), and the environment. As well, it must study the interplay of factors in these three domains in affecting the risk of elder mistreatment.

Weaknesses of Existing Studies

The first major limitation of previous risk factor research results from unclear definition of the object of study. Findings from most studies are confused in that they do not differentiate the various types of abuse and neglect articulated earlier in this report. It is likely that the etiology of these elder mistreatment types differs. Second, different criteria have been used to determine the population at risk of elder mistreatment. Some researchers have included persons under age 60 in their studies, while most others have chosen 60 or 65 as the entry point. Some researchers have restricted their studies to caregivers of elderly persons or to persons sharing a residence, while others have included all categories of elderly people.

Third, studies of risk factors have employed widely differing sampling methods, including random sample surveys, interviews with patients in medical practices or caregivers in support programs, and reviews of agency records. Fourth, few studies that have purported to address risk factors have in fact included control groups in their designs. In the absence of controls, the validity of associations between elder mistreatment and putative risk factors cannot be assessed. Furthermore, even those studies that have included control groups have often failed to ascertain that the controls were actually free of elder mistreatment. Fifth, a number of studies have not employed reliable and valid measurement of the indicators of risk.

Sixth, with one exception (Lachs et al., 1994, 1997a), prospective studies of elder mistreatment do not exist. As Lachs and colleagues (1994) point out, retrospective research designs contain several potential biases: recall bias—the respondent reinterpreting key facts or feelings from a later vantage point; information bias—the respondent (especially if cognitively impaired) may not be able to recall or provide valid information about exposure to maltreatment; and the failure of studies to take into account the timing and duration of events and their progression over time.

For these reasons, a clear framework of known risk factors for elder mistreatment cannot be derived from previous research on elder abuse. Despite a large number of review articles over the past two decades, it must be acknowledged that any statements about relative risk among the elderly should be viewed with caution.

However, the small number of studies using acceptable research designs do reveal some associations that are of interest. In this chapter, findings from these studies are summarized. For the purposes of the discussion, an attempt has been made to focus on studies that meet two criteria. First, priority was given to studies that involve a comparison group of some kind. In such studies, elderly victims (or perpetrators) have been compared to nonabuse cases uncovered in a survey or to a comparison group of some kind. Because the literature is so sparse, however, in a few cases, studies are referred to that have an "implied" comparison group. Second, the study must have collected information directly from victims and perpetrators and not from agency records (for problems with using agency records in elder mistreatment research, see Chapter 2).

FRAMEWORK FOR ELDER MISTREATMENT RISK FACTORS

The theoretical model for understanding the risk factors for elder mistreatment presented in Chapter 3 includes both the microprocess of generation of elder mistreatment risk, involving the individual and the trusted other(s), as well as the environing sociocultural context in which victims and perpetrators are embedded (such as living environment and social and economic characteristics). This model indicates the wide array of variables that could be included in risk factor research.

To date, a small number of this wide range of potential risk factors has been addressed in research. These factors, for each of which there is at least one study, fall into the following categories of the framework depicted in Figure 3-2:

Social Embeddedness/Context (subject): social isolation.
Social Embeddedness/Context (trusted other): social isolation.
Individual Level Factors (subject): gender, race, dementia, physical health status, personality characteristics.
Individual Level Factors (trusted other): mental illness, hostility, alcohol abuse, experience of violence or aggression in childhood.
Relationship Type: Shared living arrangement, relationship to victim (spouse or child).

Power and Exchange Dynamics.   Abuser dependency, victim dependency/caregiver stress.

For the purposes of this chapter, we review these risk factors based on the supporting evidence. It is possible to categorize risk factors for elder abuse into three general groups:

1. Risk factors validated by substantial evidence, for which there is unanimous or near-unanimous support from a number of studies.
2. Possible risk factors, for which the evidence is mixed or limited.
3. Contested risk factors, for which potential for increased risk has been hypothesized, but for which there is a lack of evidence.

As the earlier discussion makes clear, however, these categories are only loosely constructed. All findings should be taken with caution, due to methodological shortcomings in the studies. Furthermore, the evidence is generally too limited to make clear distinctions among abuse types. When such information is available and relevant, it is mentioned below.

RISK FACTORS VALIDATED BY SUBSTANTIAL EVIDENCE

Living Arrangement

Both clinical accounts and limited empirical research suggest that a shared living situation is a major risk factor for elder mistreatment, with older persons living alone at lowest risk (Pillemer and Finkelhor, 1988). Paveza et al. (1992) found that risk of mistreatment of Alzheimer's disease patients by caregivers was greatest when the patient resided with immediate family members (other than the spouse). Lachs et al. (1997a) found living alone to be an important protective factor against mistreatment. Pillemer and Suitor (1992) also found a shared living arrangement to be a risk factor for violence by Alzheimer's disease caregivers.

The mechanisms for the effect of living arrangement are straightforward. A shared residence increases the opportunities for contact, and thus conflict and mistreatment. Furthermore, tensions that may be relieved by simply leaving the immediate situation can escalate into mistreatment (see Wolf and Pillemer, 1989). Exploration of the differential role of living arrangement according to type of elder mistreatment needs to be conducted. For example, neglect (as the panel has defined it) by its very nature suggests a shared living situation, but financial exploitation may occur even when abuser and victim live apart.

Social Isolation

Social isolation has been found to be characteristic of families in which other forms of domestic violence occur. This is in part because behaviors that are considered to be illegitimate tend to be hidden. Detection of abusive actions can result in informal sanctions from friends, kin, and neighbors and formal sanctions from police and the courts. Thus, elder mistreatment is hypothesized to be less likely in families embedded in strong social networks.

Research provides support for this view. In the Lachs et al (1994) prospective, community-based study of risk factors for elder abuse, having a "poor social network" significantly increased risk of mistreatment. Compton et al. (1997) found low levels of social support to be associated with verbal and physical abuse by caregivers, as did Wolf and Pillemer (1989). Grafstrom et al. (1993) found both caregivers and care recipients to be more socially isolated in families in which abuse occurred. The case comparison by Phillips (1983) also found abused elder persons to be more socially isolated.

Dementia

There are two types of evidence that implicate Alzheimer's disease or related dementia as a risk factor for the mistreatment of elderly persons. First, several studies have estimated prevalence rates of elder mistreatment in samples of dementia caregivers; these rates can then be compared with rates in general population surveys. Coyne et al. (1993) found that 11.9 percent of the dementia caregivers in their sample reported having committed physical abuse. Paveza et al. (1992) found a rate of severe physical violence toward care recipients of 5.4 percent, which is close to Pillemer and Suitor's (1992) finding of 5 percent in a similar sample. Homer and Gilleard (1990) found physical abuse occurring in 14 percent of caregivers to Alzheimer's disease patients in a respite care program. Given the prevalence findings of rates of physical abuse in the 1-3 percent range in the general population, dementia patients would appear to be at greater risk of such mistreatment.

Second, a few studies have contrasted abusive and nonabusive caregivers, examining dementia in the victim as one among a number of risk factors. The results are contradictory. Lachs et al. (1994) did not find cognitive impairment to be a risk factor, and Reis and Nahmiash (1998) did not find dementia to discriminate between probable abuse and nonabuse cases. However, Lachs et al. (1997a) found that dementia predicted identification as an abuse victim.

One explanation for this contradictory set of findings comes from

Pillemer and Suitor's (1992) finding that Alzheimer's caregiver violence is strongly related to experience of violence from the *care recipient*, and Compton et al.'s (1997) finding that behavior problems are related to both verbal and physical abuse. It may be that dementia itself is not the risk factor, but rather disruptive behaviors that result from dementia. Such an explanation would be consistent with research that has shown disruptive behaviors by Alzheimer's disease patients to be an especially strong cause of caregiver stress. Future research of the relationship between dementia and elder mistreatment should differentiate the cognitive, functional, and behavioral effects of dementia and examine the independent association between each and the risk for elder mistreatment.

Intraindividual Characteristics of Abusers

Intraindividual theories of mistreatment locate the causes of abuse in some pathological characteristic of the abuser, usually mental illness, personality characteristics, or alcohol or drug abuse. This approach has a lengthy history in the study of child and intimate partner abuse, including a long-standing debate over the role of intraindividual factors as risk factors for the forms of mistreatment. In the field of elder mistreatment, there is compelling evidence that certain characteristics of perpetrators constitute major risk factors for elder mistreatment, with surprising unanimity on this issue among studies using different methods.

Mental Illness

Wolf and Pillemer (1989) found that 38 percent of abusers in three related samples had a history of mental illness and 39 percent had alcohol problems. Reis and Nahmiash (1998) attempted to validate a screening tool using a sample of 341 agency cases in which caregivers could be interviewed. The cases were classified as "likely" or "not likely" to involve abuse of the care recipient. They found that the caregivers' mental health and behavior problems were strong predictors of likely abuse. Pillemer and Finkelhor (1989) found in a case-comparison study that abusers were substantially more likely to have experienced psychiatric hospitalization than nonabusers.

These studies did not differentiate particular forms of mental illness. Several studies have specifically pointed to depression as characteristic of perpetrators of elder mistreatment. Paveza et al. (1992), in their study of Alzheimer's caregivers, found that caregiver depression predicted physical abuse. Coyne et al. (1993) compared physically abusive and nonabusive caregivers who called into a telephone helpline for family members of Alzheimer's disease patients; abusive caregivers were more depressed.

Homer and Gilleard (1990) found that among caregivers referred to a respite service, abusive ones scored higher on a depression scale. In a recent study, Williamson and Shaffer (2001) conducted structured interviews with 142 spousal caregivers regarding "potentially harmful behaviors"; these 10 items included verbal aggression, threats, and physical violence. Multivariate analyses found that more depressed caregivers were also more likely to treat their dependent spouses in potentially abusive ways. This finding is also supported by Fulmer and Gurland (1996). Of course, it is possible that depressed individuals may be more likely to report their own behavior as abusive. All of these studies were retrospective; prospective research will be needed to establish the causal direction.

In the only study to distinguish between abuse types, Reay and Browne (2001) found that physical abusers scored significantly higher on a depression scale than did perpetrators of neglect; thus, there may be a difference by type of mistreatment, which needs to be assessed in future research.

Hostility

A study of a sample of Alzheimer's disease caregivers found that abusive caregivers (a category that combined "emotional and/or physical abuse") scored higher on a hostility scale (Quayhagen et al., 1997).

Alcohol Abuse

Several studies of elder mistreatment suggest that alcohol abuse on the part of perpetrators was relatively common. For example, Greenberg and colleagues (1990) reviewed 204 substantiated cases of elder abuse; 44 percent were identified as having alcohol or drug abuse problems. Case-control studies have supported this assertion, finding that elder mistreaters were disproportionately more likely to be identified as having an alcohol use problem (Bristowe and Collins; 1989; Homer and Gilleard, 1990; Wolf and Pillemer, 1989).

In a study funded by the National Institute on Aging that directly addressed this issue, Anetzberger et al. (1994) compared a group of 23 adult children identified by agencies as perpetrators of domestic violence against an elderly parent with a group of 39 nonviolent caregiving children. Both alcohol use and abuse were more common among the perpetrators; for example, daily alcohol consumption was more than twice as likely among perpetrators.

It is possible that the role of alcohol abuse may differ by abuse type. Reay and Browne (2001) found that alcohol abuse by the caregiver (consumption of over 21 units of alcohol per week) occurred in seven out of nine of the physical abuse cases, but only one of the neglect cases.

Abuser Dependency

Related to the previous risk factor, findings from early research on elder mistreatment suggests that perpetrators tended to be dependent on the individual they were mistreating. In 1982, Wolf and colleagues surveyed community agencies in Massachusetts regarding elder abuse cases they had encountered (Wolf et al., 1982). The authors identified a "web of mutual dependency" between abuser and abused. In two-thirds of the cases in that study, the perpetrator was reported to be financially dependent on the victim. Another early study by Hwalek et al. (1984) also reported that financial dependence on a relative was a risk factor in abuse. Other studies, without control groups, have found substantial percentages of financially dependent abusers (Anetzberger, 1987; Greenberg et al., 1990).

A number of studies have confirmed this finding. Pillemer (1986; Wolf and Pillemer, 1989) found that abusers were substantially more dependent on the victim for housing and financial assistance than were members of a comparison group. In Pillemer and Finkelhor's (1989) analysis of cases from a random-sample survey, nearly identical results emerged.

POSSIBLE RISK FACTORS

Gender

Adult protective services reports and other studies of agency samples universally find that the majority of victims are female (Wolf, 1997b). However, it is not clear whether this is due to higher risk for victimization or to women's greater numbers in the population of seniors. Pillemer and Finkelhor's (1988) survey suggested that the latter may be the case; in their study, they found that the victimization rate for men was higher at 5.1 percent, compared with 2.5 percent for women. They attributed this in part to the fact that elderly women are much more likely to live alone, which reduces their risk. Furthermore, their sample included intimate partner abuse among the well elderly, in which the victim would not necessarily have been classified as vulnerable according to our definition.

Pillemer and Finkelhor (1988) also noted the important caveat that women tended to sustain more serious abuse and to suffer greater physical and emotional harm from mistreatment. This may in turn explain their greater representation as victims in adult protective services caseloads.

Relationship of Victim to Perpetrator

Despite suggestions that adult children are the most likely perpetrators of elder abuse, the only survey-based study of this topic found that spouses were more likely to be abusers (Pillemer and Finkelhor, 1988). However, there are insufficient data on this risk factor to make a determination.

Personality Characteristics of Victims

Comijs et al. (1998) found that certain personality traits of elderly persons increased their risk of being an abuse victim. In a community survey conducted in the Netherlands, they examined whether hostility and coping style were related to being a victim of chronic verbal aggression, physical aggression, and financial mistreatment. Victims of chronic verbal aggression scored lower on a locus of control scale than did the nonabused members of the sample and higher on one indicator of hostility. Victims of all three abuse types showed higher levels of aggression as measured by the hostility scales and were generally more likely to use passive and avoidant ways of coping, rather than active problem-solving strategies. Because of the cross-sectional nature of this study, it is impossible to determine whether these characteristics are indeed risk factors, or whether they are consequences of the abuse. However, the findings are sufficiently suggestive to merit further exploration of personality factors in longitudinal studies.

Race

Lachs and colleagues (1994, 1997a) found that being black was a risk factor for reported elder mistreatment. However, they noted that this may be an artifact of the definition of elder mistreatment, which was "being reported to an [adult protective services] agency." No other study has found significant differences in elder abuse risk based on race.

CONTESTED RISK FACTORS

Physical Impairment of the Older Person

The role of victim health and functional status as a risk factor for elder abuse is a complex one. For the purposes of this report, some degree of physical vulnerability is considered to be a necessary component of the definition of elder mistreatment. That is, mistreatment necessarily implies a weaker individual who is mistreated by a stronger one. Greater impairment diminishes the individual's ability to defend himself or herself or to escape the situation. It therefore is reasonable to consider physical health problems as a predisposing factor for elder mistreatment, which increases the likelihood of abuse in the presence of other risk factors.

However, research has generally failed to find support for the view that frailty of elderly persons is in itself a risk factor for elder mistreatment.

That is, case-control studies have not found a direct relationship between elder mistreatment and functional impairment or poor health. Reis and Nahmiash (1998) did not find impairment in activities of daily living to be associated with elder abuse. Neither Cooney and Mortimer (1995), Paveza et al. (1992), Bristowe and Collins (1989), nor Phillips (1983) in case-comparison studies found functional impairment to be a risk factor for abuse by caregivers. Lachs et al. (1997a) found that impairment in activities of daily living was associated with being an abuse victim, but the researchers acknowledged that the dependent variable—protective services intervention for elder abuse—may have led to these results, and that findings may differ for elder mistreatment that is not detected by an agency.

There is as yet no evidence as to whether this pattern of nonfindings holds for all types of mistreatment. In the only study to address this issue Wolf and Pillemer (1989) found that victims of elder neglect were more likely to be impaired than victims of either physical or psychological abuse.

Victim Dependence and Caregiver Stress

If there can be said to be a "traditional" view in the field of elder mistreatment, then it can be summed up in the following way. Elderly people become frail, difficult to care for, and sometimes demanding. These characteristics cause stress for their caregivers; as a result of this stress, the caregivers become abusive or neglectful toward the elder. In this view, elder mistreatment is seen as an outgrowth of the aging process, which leads to the need for care by others. Much early writing emphasized the dependence of the elderly person and resulting caregiver stress as the predominant (and sometimes sole) cause of elder abuse (Davidson, 1979; Hickey and Douglass, 1981; Steinmetz, 1988).

However, there is a lack of evidence that an older person's need for assistance or that caregiver stress in fact lead to greater risk for elder mistreatment. First, it is clear from the gerontological and geriatric literature that a substantial number of elderly persons are dependent on relatives for some degree of care. However, findings about the prevalence of elder mistreatment indicate that only a small minority of the elderly is mistreated. Since abuse occurs in only a small proportion of families, no direct correlation can be assumed between the dependence of an elderly person and abuse, as sometimes has been done.

Second, case-comparison studies have generally failed to find either higher rates of elder dependence or greater caregiver stress in elder abuse situations. Bristowe and Collins (1989), Homer and Gilleard (1990), Phillips (1983), Pillemer (1985), Wolf and Pillemer (1989), Pillemer and Finkelhor (1989), Pillemer and Suitor (1992), and Reis and Nahmiash (1997) did not find greater dependence or caregiver stress among victims and their family members, when compared with nonvictims. One exception, a study by Coyne et al. (1993), found that callers to a help line who had committed abuse had been providing care for a longer time and for more hours a day than nonabusers and had higher burden scores.

Intergenerational Transmission

Social learning theory gives rise to the hypothesis that when individuals experience violent behavior from parents or other role models in childhood, they tend to revert to these learned behaviors when provoked as adults. Indeed, it has by now become a commonplace that victims of child abuse may grow up to themselves become child abusers, a pattern often described as the "cycle of violence." The cumulative research evidence supports this hypothesis, with experiencing violence from parents or witnessing violence between parents in childhood strongly related to perpetrating child or intimate partner abuse (See Newberger, 1998; Stark and Flitcraft, 1998).

Despite this evidence from other fields, the only two studies that have addressed this issue (Anetzberger et al., 1994; Wolf and Pillemer, 1989) found no evidence of intergenerational transmission of physical violence against elderly relatives. This issue, however, is worthy of further study, given the importance of childhood experience of aggression as a risk factor for other forms of interpersonal violence. The importance of early childhood experiences of perpetrators as risk factors for types of elder mistreatment other than physical violence should be explored. In addition, given that in the elder mistreatment field the victim and perpetrator have been in a long-standing personal relationship, as spouses or as parent and child, it may be more important to assess the type of relationship between the abuser and the victim as a risk factor for elder mistreatment.

ELDER MISTREATMENT IN INSTITUTIONAL SETTINGS

Despite the likelihood that elder mistreatment in nursing homes is equally or more prevalent than abuse in domestic settings, only one study has been conducted that specifically addressed risk factors. Pillemer and Bachman-Prehn (1991) analyzed data from a survey of staff regarding self-reported psychological and physical abuse. Predictors of psychological abuse were staff burnout, experiencing physical aggression from residents, negative attitudes toward residents, and age of the staff member, with younger staff more likely to engage in psychological abuse. Risk factors for physical abuse were again staff burnout and resident aggression, as well as the reported amount of conflict with residents. This study is limited by the self-report method used to assess the occurrence of elder mistreatment. Self-report may be subject to bias, especially since the staff would often have to report themselves or their colleagues as abusers, which may well have affected ascertainment of occurrence of elder mistreatment.

A number of other potential risk factors can be derived from the more general literature on quality of care in nursing homes. Pillemer (1988) proposed four sets of variables that may be related to maltreatment: exogenous factors (including the availability of nursing home beds and the unemployment rate in an area); characteristics of the nursing home environment (such as size, reimbursement rates, ownership status, staff-resident ratio, and turnover rate); staff characteristics (including age, gender, education level, and burnout), and resident characteristics (health and functional status, social isolation, and gender). A full-scale test of this model remains to be conducted.

In her background paper for this panel, Hawes suggests risk factors derived from surveys of stakeholders in long-term care. She proposes three risk factors from these studies: stressful working conditions, particularly resulting from staff shortages; staff burnout; and the joint effects of resident aggression and poor training of staff in management of challenging behaviors. Pillemer (2001) combined insights derived from long-term care practice with the limited data on nursing home mistreatment to suggest four key factors: poor hiring and staff screening practices; chronic staffing problems; lack of administrative and supervisory oversight; and inadequate training. Taken together, these approaches suggest a number of avenues for studies of risk factors, at both the structural and the individual levels.

CONCLUSIONS AND RECOMMENDATIONS

Although risk factors at times are causes of mistreatment, this is not always the case. Some risk factors (preferably called "risk indicators") may be "markers" for unmeasured/unobserved causes (confounders); or risk factors may modify the relationship between causal factors and elder mistreatment (effect modifiers). For example, depression in a caregiver may be a causal risk factor in that a depressed caregiver may be more likely to neglect the care of an elder by virtue of the fatigue, social withdrawal, and uninterest associated with depression. Living with others has been associated with an increased probability of mistreatment. However, this may not be a direct causal relationship, because living with others is a contextual factor in which mistreatment is more likely to occur; it would be possible to reduce the risk of mistreatment by modifying other factors associated with living with others and not changing the living circumstances of the older person (which is often difficult and disruptive). To provide another example, frailty—a form of vulnerability—may be an effect modifier, such as at very high levels of frailty the probability of mistreatment may be much higher than at lower levels of frailty. Further study of issues such as these is absolutely critical to a research agenda on elder mistreatment.

A research agenda for risk factor research on elder mistreatment is to some degree straightforward, because it parallels our general recommendations for research on this topic. Studies using larger and more representative samples, as well as scientifically accepted epidemiological techniques, must be conducted before risk factors can be more accurately specified. The importance of case-control designs and cohort studies cannot be overemphasized. We do not reiterate all of these recommendations here.

The following are specific additional recommendations to advance knowledge of risk factors for elder mistreatment.

1. Studies are urgently needed that examine risk and protective factors for different types of elder mistreatment. Studies are needed to advance understanding of what places older and vulnerable adults at risk for mistreatment and what places persons at risk for becoming abusive. These studies can be carried out using well-established methods for determining risk factors, including epidemiological case-control studies. These studies must, however, use common measures that allow for comparison across studies. Moreover, they must focus not only on the composite concept of elder mistreatment, but also on its various forms.

Intensification of epidemiological research to establish risk factors will be facilitated by greater collaboration between researchers and the adult protective services and elder services systems. Researchers in the field have generally been hampered in their efforts to establish risk factors because they have often needed to find both mistreatment cases and "controls" in general population samples. Most retrospective epidemiological research has used readily available case populations for studies, while attempting to sample well-defined control groups. Many of the advances in understanding risk factors associated with child abuse and intimate partner violence occurred as the result of participation and engagement between the research communities and the service provider agencies. In the panel's view, advances in risk-factor research in elder mistreatment will require cooperation between adult protective services agencies and the research community, such as exhibited in the work of Dyer and her colleagues in Texas. By using persons clearly identified by some external source as victims of mistreatment, the focus can shift from concern about sample size to the identification of an appropriate group of controls.

Such studies have the potential for providing vital information for both policy makers and program developers to help define target behaviors for intervention. In addition, this information can be used to develop profiles of persons at risk for being mistreated, as well as to develop forensic markers. However, studies to identify protective factors from elder mistreatment should not be neglected.

2. **A particularly critical need exists for studies of risk indicators and risk and protective factors for elder mistreatment in institutional settings.** The available evidence reviewed by Hawes (this volume), combined with extensive professional and public concern about serious quality problems in long-term care (Institute of Medicine, 1996), suggests that a vast reservoir of undetected and unreported elder mistreatment in nursing homes may exist. Because nursing home residents as a class are both extremely physically vulnerable and generally unable either to protect themselves or report elder mistreatment they experience, the physical and emotional costs of elder mistreatment in such environments are likely to be very high. Prevention programs exist (see Pillemer and Hudson, 1993), but they have not been informed by rigorous risk factor research. Understanding the causes of mistreatment of this extremely fragile population is of the highest priority.

3. **Research on risk and protective factors should be expanded to take into consideration the clinical course of elder mistreatment.** Although longitudinal data are absent, it seems probable that elder abuse situations may follow a pattern similar to disease progression, which would include lead time prior to the manifestation of active signs and symptoms of elder mistreatment; periods of "remission" from elder mistreatment; and critical points in which elder mistreatment becomes more intensive or acute. Some have speculated that elder mistreatment typically increases in severity and intensity over time (Breckman and Adelman, 1988), but no empirical data exist that demonstrate this pattern or individual differences in progression. Clinical accounts suggest that elder mistreatment situations include cases that resolve on their own; cases in which mistreatment intensifies; and cases in which the situation remains abusive but stable. It is therefore both possible and important to identify risk factors for an increase or intensification in elder mistreatment.

For these reasons, cohort studies are of great importance in determining risk factors for elder mistreatment. Although prospective cohort studies would be ideal, the lengthy period needed for cases of elder mistreatment to develop is a deterrent. In the near term, retrospective cohort, or nested case-control studies using established study populations may be preferable, in which a preexisting data set is used and elder mistreatment measured at a later point (the technique used by Lachs et al., 1994, 1997a). There are a number of existing datasets involving elderly persons that could be used for such a purpose (for example, existing panel studies of caregivers could be assessed for incidence of elder mistreatment in a follow-up study).

4. **Advances in measurement in risk and protective factor research are needed.** The measurement of risk factors many times can be accomplished

adequately by importing measures for suspected risk factors from other settings. For example, good measures exist in the literature for cognitive impairment, dementia, handicap, and frailty. As well, some characteristics of individuals that may place them at increased risk of mistreatment, such as personality, stress, and the burden of caregiving, have been developed in the child mistreatment field and could be adapted to this research setting. For the most part, observational and hypothesis-driven research in the elder mistreatment field will have to develop measures that are specific to the field, such as measures of risk characteristics in trust relationships and aspects of settings that may be of interest. This is in addition to adapting measures of risk factors that have been developed in the child mistreatment field and in other research.

6

Screening and Case Identification in Clinical Settings

Elder mistreatment research must be conducted in a variety of settings in order to maximize understanding and make it possible to take proper measures for prevention and management. These settings include geographically defined communities and households, social service agencies, the law enforcement and judicial systems, and the health care system. Pertinent health service settings include all levels of primary, secondary, and tertiary care, including long-term care institutions. While it is important to understand the determinants and occurrence rates of elder mistreatment through population-based studies, it is also critical to identify victims in diverse settings where they frequently appear and where many of the consequences of mistreatment are likely to be manifest.

This chapter focuses on case ascertainment of elder mistreatment in the clinical setting. The American Medical Association's (AMA) *Diagnostic and Treatment Guidelines on Elder Abuse and Neglect* (1992) urge "every clinical setting" to utilize a protocol for the detection and assessment of elder mistreatment, following a "routine pattern" in each case (see Figure 6-1). Implementation of such a structured protocol, however well intentioned, could be costly and counterproductive in the absence of careful planning. Since most older patients are not mistreated, and mistreatment is probably uncommon in most general health service settings, any case ascertainment method or program must be accurate and efficient, because it will consume resources and have important consequences, especially if cases are misclassified. Also, many health care delivery settings are so complex that careful case ascertainment is difficult to achieve in practice.

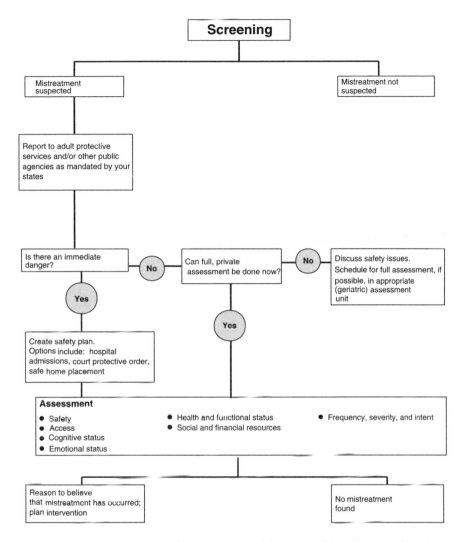

FIGURE 6-1 Diagnostic and treatment guidelines on elder abuse and neglect, Part I.
SOURCE: American Medical Association (1992:13).

Thus, research is needed to improve detection methods for elder mistreatment, particularly those that could lead to improved case management. The benefits of careful case finding go beyond protecting the victim. Accurate case identification can lead to rational resource allocation, creation and funding of specialized services, and improved professional and public education. Improving accuracy in case designation also has important implications for the social service and criminal justice systems, particularly in the areas of prevention and perpetrator prosecution. As noted in Chapter 1 and in the paper by Wolfe (this volume), however, a preoccupation with case identification can also have high costs; recent experience in child abuse indicates that a single-minded emphasis on case investigation (when accompanied by the threat of prosecution or other disruptive interventions) can undermine the goal of protection.

A FRAMEWORK FOR ELDER MISTREATMENT SCREENING AND CASE IDENTIFICATION

Several approaches are used to identify persons with important conditions or situations in the clinical setting, and general principles have been well developed (Rich and Sox, 2000; Neilsen and Lang, 1999). Figure 6-2 represents a framework for screening approaches, emphasizing that case screening and investigation are parts of a multistage process, although the nature and timing of each stage is varied. Validation of each step is an important aim of research. A LEAD standard would be the appropriate means of validating any proposed screening method prior to its widespread application. Typically, the process of clinical screening and case identification starts with designating appropriate settings and situations for carrying

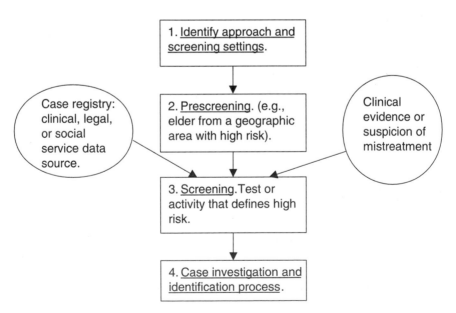

FIGURE 6-2   A framework for clinical screening and case identification.

out this important function. These may include emergency rooms, primary care settings, social service agencies, and public health clinics; research on the feasibility of other potential settings is indicated.

A Sequential Process

As shown in Figure 6-2, prescreening may occur, formally or informally, through use of warning signs thought to signal an elevated risk, such as being from a high-risk geographic area or having a certain cluster of clinical symptoms or conditions or repeated admissions. To the extent that clinicians rely on such a prescreening process, epidemiological research could improve the accuracy and efficiency of the process by helping to identify the warning signs. Another possible approach is the development and use of case registries. Appearance in a data repository of persons who have been suspected, evaluated, assessed and/or treated for elder mistreatment through the health, social, or justice systems could be used as a basis for initiating a more focused screening process.

The next level is the screening process itself (Figure 6-2). This may take many forms but most often has been based on short screening questionnaires (see detailed discussion below). Various approaches may be of value, however, and the potential utility of different approaches to screening aside from interviewing is an area in need of additional investigation. A critical feature of the screening process is the cutoff point for deciding whether the case is screened in or out; this task often involves considerable discretion, highlighting the continuing tension between statistical and clinical methods of screening. When the screening activity indicates a positive result, a case identification investigation is initiated in order to definitively confirm or refute the positive suspicion. While investigation of cases screened as positives is a general characteristic of screening programs, it is worth reiterating that this can be a time-consuming and difficult process; screening programs should be initiated cautiously (with a higher threshold of concern, for example) if resources for case investigation are scarce. For those cases that are identified after investigation, management programs and teams need to be available to address the demands of the particular situation.

Statistical Approaches to Evaluation

Standard statistical methods can be used to determine the accuracy of screening tests, including any that could be explored for elder mistreatment. Techniques include the use of such measures as sensitivity, specificity, predictive values of positive and negative tests, and receiver operator curves, all available in standard references. For example, the proportion of patients with proven mistreatment who are designated as positive on the screening test represents the *sensitivity* of that test. For that same test, the *predictive value of a positive test* is the proportion of persons who screen positive and have the condition being screened. This is not the same as sensitivity, and both are important properties to understand. The proportion of patients screened negative for mistreatment who have not been mistreated represents the *specificity* of the method; highly specific tests correctly identify those people who do not have the condition. While a detailed discussion of these measures is beyond the scope of this chapter, it should be noted that variation in screening test application, target conditions, and condition occurrence may alter the measurement properties of a given screening test.

These methods are more readily applied to conditions that can definitely be designated as being present or absent. For example, a clinical outcome such as a cancer, high blood pressure, or high blood cholesterol can be reliably determined in most circumstances, and the properties of screening tests are well understood. As long as researchers utilize the same cutoff points, outcomes can be compared across studies and conclusions based on data drawn from many studies may be reached in a reliable manner. However, the manifestations of elder mistreatment may be varied, depending on the type of victim and perpetrator and the social context. This variation in disease outcome across study settings may decrease the generalizability of screening test findings. Even with attempts at uniform case definitions, such as that used by Dolan and Blakely (1989:33) to describe elder neglect ("a pattern of conduct which deprives another person of the minimum amount of care which is necessary to maintain physical and mental health"), the definition may be interpreted in myriad ways. Each researcher's interpretation of phrases such as "pattern of conduct" and "minimum amount of care" will be different and hard to operationalize. It is thus extremely important that researchers explicitly and carefully state their operational definition of elder mistreatment when developing screening tools and assessing their accuracy.

SCREENING

Approaches to Screening

As noted above, although little research has been done in most of these areas, several approaches to screening and prescreening are possible: short questionnaires, geographic characteristics, the presence of certain types or patterns of injuries, clinical or research biomarkers, lack of adherence to or success with various medical regimens, unusual behavioral manifestations, or a history of prior victimization, either recent or remote (Bowen, 2000). Automated medical record systems may be developed that could flag certain patients who are at increased risk of mistreatment based on validated indicators and formulas. These are all in need of further exploration. Research is also needed on the best ways to verify and manage situations in which patients spontaneously report possible episodes of mistreatment. Many health centers have domestic abuse detection and management systems in place, providing an important opportunity for clinical research on elder mistreatment.

As noted, most efforts to screen elder mistreatment in the clinical setting have involved short, directly administered questionnaires. For example, the AMA guidelines (American Medical Association, 1992) encourage physicians to "incorporate routine questions related to elder abuse and neglect into daily practice." Table 6-1 contains a listing of published screening methods for elder mistreatment, along with information on their measurement properties. While several screening tools are now available to identify possible cases of elder mistreatment, it is not known if these tools are widely utilized; anecdotal evidence indicates they are not. Most emergency rooms, one logical place to institute screening procedures, do not routinely screen for elder mistreatment (Jones et al., 1997). The existing tools have rarely been validated in diverse clinical settings, and they have not been adequately validated overall. Some have been evaluated in the emergency room setting, others in the home setting, but none in the office, nursing home, or community settings (such as senior centers or adult day care programs). Several of the current tools depend on accurate responses from the possible victim, who may be unable to give reliable answers due to dementia, fear, or other cognitive or emotional factors. Others depend on responses from the caregiver or trusted other, who may not be willing to provide accurate, truthful responses or may be incapable of doing so. The caregivers of many frail and dependent elders may themselves be equally frail and impaired (Schultz and Beach, 1999).

Even among published screening tools, improvements in design and measurement properties may be indicated. There is also need for extending screening instruments into a wider range of settings, such as the physician's office, adult day care programs, and, despite the challenges, long-term care facilities. These instruments must be practical for those settings. While some of the existing instruments have been available for many years, few have received confirmatory validation by other investigators. Because some cases of mistreatment are obvious and overt, testing the current screening tools to see if they correctly identify these cases may be a reasonable starting point. Once we know that the clear-cut cases are identifiable, it should be easier to proceed to the gray areas where many cases of possible mistreatment lie.

In order for a screening tool to be practical in a clinical setting, it should not only be accurate, but also easy to use and efficient. Some of

TABLE 6-1 Maltreatment Screening Instruments

Instrument and Citation	Purpose	Type of Elder Maltreatment
BASE The Brief Abuse Screen for the Elderly Reis et al. (1993)	5 items Trained practitioner evaluation of caregiver and elder. To help the practitioner assess the likelihood of abuse.	Physical, psychological, neglect, financial
IOA Indicators of Abuse Screen Reis and Nahmiash (1998)	29 items Trained practitioner assessment of caregiver and elder. To enable practitioners to identify abuse cases among health and social services agency clients.	Physical, psychological, neglect
H-S/EAST Hwalek-Sengstock Elder Abuse Screening Test-Revised Hwalek and Sengstock (1986)	15 items Elder as respondent. To help agencies identify situations likely to be or become abusive or neglectful.	Physical, psychological, financial

Evaluation	Validation Method	Validation Setting	Reliability Estimates
Reis et al. (1993) Paper presented at the Canadian Association on Gerontology	Face Validity 86-90% agreement by 3 different trained practitioners.	Home assessment of health and social services agency cases.	Not analyzed
Reis and Nahmiash (1998)	Construct Validity The performance of the IOA was evaluated against the BASE measure. Scores of 16 and above have a sensitivity of 85% and a specificity of 99%.	Home assessment of 341 health and social services agency cases (55 and older).	Chronbach's alpha = 0.91
Hwalek and Sengstock (1986)	Predictive Validity services cases. Using known abuse cases and control cases, 9 items were 94 % accurate in classifying cases into abuse and nonabuse cases.	97 social-health 100 elders living in public housing	Not analyzed
Moody et al. (2000)	Predictive Validity Using known abuse/ nonabuse cases, discriminate function analysis showed that 6 items were as effective as the 9-item model in classifying cases (71.4%) as abused.		

continued on next page

TABLE 6-1 Continued

Instrument and Citation	Purpose	Type of Elder Maltreatment
EAI Elder Assessment Instrument (revised)	35 items Caregiver as respondent.	Abuse, neglect, exploitation, abandonment
Fulmer et al. (2000)	To identify individuals at high risk of mistreatment who should be referred for further assessment.	
CASE Caregiver Abuse Screen	8 items specifically worded to be nonblaming.	Physical, psychological, neglect
Reis and Namiash (1995)	Filled out by caregiver. To identify caregivers who are more likely to be abusers.	

those published, such as the Hwalek-Sengstock Elder Abuse Screening Test and the Elder Assessment Instrument, require referral to a more specialized assessment process. Often, no well-established or specialized assessment process is available in many clinical settings; putative cases are reported to the community adult protective systems, which may vary in assessment rigor and standardization, adding to the challenge of screening instrument evaluation. This referral and evaluation process could be another direction for research on the screening process for elder mistreatment.

Another important challenge is the design and validation of new instruments and approaches to detect the various types of elder mistreatment in addition to overt physical abuse in the home, particularly abuse in the institutional setting, intentional neglect, and financial abuse. While these types of mistreatment may overlap, it is likely that different markers will be

Evaluation	Validation Method	Validation Setting	Reliability Estimates
Fulmer and O'Malley (1987)	Content validity: 0.83	Acute care.	Chronbach's alpha = 0.84
Reis and Namiash (1995)	Predictive Validity Using known abusers and a control groups, overall scores of abusers were significantly higher on the CASE (mean 3.2) than nonabusers (mean 1.9). Construct Validity CASE scores were positively correlated (0.41) with IOA scores.	44 known abusive caregivers and 45 nonabusive caregivers receiving care from a social services center.	Chronbach's alpha = 0.71

present in the domains of subject, trusted other, and social embeddedness (see Chapter 3).

Challenges in Screening

A variety of factors make screening challenging and difficult. Mistreatment may occur as a single act or as a chronic, subtle series of events. In fact it is often difficult to know when an event or series of events have crossed the line from inappropriate conduct to actual mistreatment. At what point does inadequate care become intentional neglect? Expectations across different settings may also influence the identification and definition of cases. For example, different standards of care may be applied to the professional staff of a nursing home in contrast to a family caregiver or volunteer in-home helpers. In addition, common physiological changes in the elderly complicate the assessment of elder mistreatment. Bruises and fractures and even death may be indicators of abusive assaults, but they are also common occurrences in frail and dependent elders due to spontaneous falls and tissue fragility. How do we know when a bruise is an indicator of abuse rather than an expected result of a person's medical condition and functional status?

As is evident throughout this report, the context in which an injury occurs is often as important as the injury itself in screening for elder mistreatment. Instruments for screening and case identification would be likely to benefit from considering contextual risk factors as well as characteristics of the elder subject and characteristics of the trusted other. As an example, the places where elders reside and spend time may affect the risk for mistreatment. For those living in a skilled nursing facility or who are housebound, residential or institutional risk factors take on greater importance. Others may spend time in a variety of settings, such as senior centers or adult day care centers. The varied distribution of social environments may alter risk profiles and the performance of screening instruments. The sociocultural milieu in which elder mistreatment occurs is another potentially important contextual issue that has received little research attention. Understanding how variations in race, ethnicity, religious beliefs, and socioeconomic status affect the risk and occurrence of elder mistreatment is critical to improving screening and case identification methods.

Further complicating screening and case identification of elder mistreatment is the problem of cognitive impairment. Depending on the degree of impairment, different methods may be employed to elicit needed information. Some with mild impairment may be able to give a reasonably accurate history of neglect or abuse, but those with moderate or severe dementia may not be able to do so (see further discussion of this issue below). There is good evidence that mistreatment is a substantial problem among Alzheimer's disease patients (Paveza et al., 1992). Screening and diagnosis must then be done via interviews of caregivers or others who are knowledgeable about the elder's situation and via clinical evaluation of the patient. Screening the trusted other in these circumstances is an important research direction as environmental and social factors in elder mistreatment are ascertained.

CASE IDENTIFICATION

As emphasized throughout in this volume, the range of behaviors subsumed under elder mistreatment is large, diverse, and multidimensional. While some cases are obvious and easy to designate, many are not, and the definitions of elder mistreatment should be the subject of research, as noted in Chapter 2. That chapter also discusses use of the LEAD standard methodology to validate case identification methods. In addition, the clinical process of case investigation in the community practice setting has substantial implications for the social service (adult protective services) and justice systems. The Adult Protective Services experience is of particular interest. In a survey (National Association of Adult Protective Services Administrators) for 1999–2000 in which all 50 states responded, of the complaints received by adult protective services, only two-thirds were investigated. Of those investigated, half were substantiated for abuse or neglect. While the complaints and investigative processes are tracked by every state, the methods of case validation preceding the finding varies widely from state to state.

The starting point for adult protective services response to a complaint of alleged elder mistreatment is the state statute and administrative rules. A total of 26 states respond to complaints for people age 60 years and older, and 18 states respond to complaints for people age 65 and older. Two states include any adult who is vulnerable or has disabilities. As discussed earlier, state statutes also differ significantly in their definitions. For example, some statutes do not cover neglect.

If the complaint received by adult protective services meets the local statutory definitions, a caseworker is assigned to assess or investigate the situation, determine if the abuse is substantiated, and develop a plan to protect the person from further harm. The assessment-investigation process is often identified by adult protective services workers as one of the most difficult aspects of their work. There is a paucity of training for them prior to receiving a caseload, with only a handful of states requiring significant training. In addition, states differ in their emphasis on case identification versus provision of social services. Some states are more weighted toward investigation, that is, the process of making a finding about the allegation and abuse registries, while others spend more time on the provision of services and less on investigating.

Once a case of elder mistreatment has been assigned for investigation, most state statutes require a face-to-face visit with the alleged victim within a prescribed time period, more quickly depending on the seriousness of the report, but typically within 48 hours. Once at the home or residence, in the majority of instances, the adult protective services worker must first receive consent of the client for the assessment-investigation. If the client refuses, the worker cannot proceed. When conducting an assessment-investigation, the worker's task is not only to find out what happened and determine if it was abuse or neglect, but it may also include an evaluation of the person's functional capacity, and his/her ability to live independently (physical tasks) and to make judgments (mental tasks). This knowledge helps to determine what support should be offered so that the person can live as independently as possible, and it is also useful in determining their ability to protect themselves from further harm. The assessment should also include evaluation of the risk of future abuse.

While adult protective services units have developed several instruments and guidelines to carry out their state mandate—for example, screening, investigation and evaluation of mental competence—and have shared best practices among the states, they are well aware of the need for validation and research and of the subjective nature of the decision making often required in conducting assessments-investigations. The processes of case identification and case management are in need of research for all of its components. Some of the major challenges for both the clinical and community settings are discussed below.

Standardized Criteria for Case Identification

A major barrier to the identification of cases of elder mistreatment is that the researcher or clinician is rarely in a position to directly observe the relevant event(s). Most of the time, the identification of a case is made indirectly, relying on the report of the victim—or the perpetrator—or on the presence or absence of observable signs and symptoms believed to be indicative of mistreatment, such as emotional distress or bruises. However, indirect approaches may be uncertain. The accuracy of self-report by victims or perpetrators is not quantitatively established in most clinical settings. The value of self-report may be further undermined when the victim is ill or cognitively impaired.

The capacity of older persons to provide accurate accounts of their observations or experiences is an important area for research. In many situations, case identification is predicated largely on the injured person's account of the circumstances. Whether adult protective services or a prosecutor acts on the possible mistreatment is dependent in such an instance on the credibility of the victim.

If an allegation is brought, whether a court even hears the injured person's account may be dependent on a finding of his or her competence to testify. If the older person has cognitive impairments, then the admissibility of his or her testimony may be contingent on judicial findings that the witness had the ability to form a "just impression of the facts" (i.e., to perceive the situation) at the time that the injury occurred, that the witness has the ability to recall the situation and communicate that memory, that the witness understands the difference between truth and falsity, and that the witness knows the nature of an oath and understands the obligation to tell the truth in court (see Myers, 1993).

Ultimately, the application of these standards arguably depends on an assessment of the jury's ability to make sense of the witness's testimony. Given that time will be consumed in any event by a determination of a witness's competence, the victim's testimony should be heard if it is not likely to mislead or confuse the jury. In such a case, however, the jury still has to consider the witness's credibility, and expert opinions may be introduced about the possible effects of the witness's cognitive impairments (Melton et al., 1997, § 7.07).

There is now a large body of research on children's credibility and competence as witnesses. Many studies have addressed child witnesses' suggestibility and accuracy of recall (see Saywitz et al., 2002). Extension of this research to elders with dementia poses significant challenges, because the impact of the impairments to statements about victimization will be affected by medications, comorbidities, the experience of trauma, and the severity of the dementia itself. However, some of the methods used in research on child witnesses could be applied in studies of testimony by mildly or moderately confused elders.

Research assessing the capacity of older persons with cognitive impairments to provide accurate testimony is needed for improving the accuracy of case identification, not only in clinical settings, but also in legal settings, including prosecutorial decision making and formal adjudication.

Another impediment to accurate case identification is that many elders have conditions that are associated with physical frailty and other medical problems as well as psychological or emotional problems. For example, as many as 18 percent of seniors report depressive symptoms (although many of these are mild symptoms)—much higher than can be accounted for by mistreatment alone. Also, normal age-related changes make an elder more susceptible to serious consequences of seemingly minor illnesses. An older person with atrial fibrillation taking an anticoagulant may have easy skin bruising, and thus the presence of bruising will be less helpful than otherwise as a sign of possible mistreatment. This "fact" is clinically accepted and makes intuitive sense, yet no studies quantify bruising rates under normal circumstances, compared with cases of mistreatment. Fragile capillaries and thinner skin, both age-related changes, also make elderly individuals more susceptible to bruising. Quantification and standardization of mistreatment-related clinical observations are necessary to explore their utility in designating cases of mistreatment. Because so little is known about the signs and symptoms of mistreatment, it is easy to assume that an injury is due to a certain constellation of natural changes and illnesses rather than to mistreatment. There are no studies that help illuminate when to consider an injury as a marker of mistreatment. Retrospective studies may be a valuable tool in understanding markers, particularly in cases of ongoing abuse. If elders with severe injuries secondary to mistreatment are identified, one may be able to look at their histories and see if there were markers that would have made it possible to identify mistreatment at an earlier stage.

A critical step to advance the field is the development of a consensus around the determination of whether or not a case of mistreatment has occurred. Since elder mistreatment is almost always assessed by indirect means, a gold standard of case identification may not yet be possible. Investigators will need to create new approaches to case standardization and develop alternative benchmarks for case identification. One useful approach discussed in Chapter 2, applies the LEAD (longitudinal, expert, all data) standard. This method must be well described, widely accepted, and replicable in a variety of settings in which mistreatment might be encountered.

Applying Causal Logic to Case Finding

In addition to the determination of relevant conduct and harm, the occurrence of mistreatment requires a determination of cause, especially in studies aiming to improve clinical methods of case identification and screening. In some cases the co-occurrence of harm and relevant conduct is such that an unequivocal determination that the perpetrator's conduct caused the harm can be made. For example, a caregiver might be observed striking an elder. In many situations, however, the critical issue is whether the observed harm suffered by the victim was attributable to the trusted other's conduct. (As noted in Chapter 2, in some circumstances there is conduct of interest but no evidence of harm. The issue of causality is not relevant in such cases, unless there is concern that harm has not been detected, in which case the problem involves the detection of consequences.)

Determination of cause is most relevant in two types of situations. In one type, consequence and conduct could both be detected but neither alone would constitute mistreatment, unless the conduct was shown to have caused the consequence. This scenario is most relevant to neglect. For example, an older person might have fallen and fractured her hip at the same time that the caregiver was known to leave her alone at home for several hours during the day. If the elder had a problem walking and always needed help to get around, it might be concluded that the lack of supervision was critical to the older person's fall and thus constituted mistreatment. In contrast, if the elder had no problems walking and fell because she rushed to go downstairs to answer the phone, the caregiver's conduct would not constitute mistreatment.

Applying causal reasoning that meets research standards to this sort of circumstance is clearly complex. While logical inference is critical to determine whether certain prerequisites are met (e.g., "Did the conduct occur *before* the consequence?" or "Was the conduct such that the specific consequence would be expected to have resulted from it?"), ultimately, the determination of causality may often be judgmental, requiring a process by which the determination can be made. This decision process itself may be the object of important research and at a minimum should have high face validity and reliability and be sufficiently delineated so that it can be replicated.

The other situation in which causal reasoning could be called on is one in which a harm has been detected without a clear conduct that could have caused it. While this too could be considered a failure in the measurement of conduct, some research indicates that there are certain harms that older persons may suffer that can only have been by mistreatment (or have a such high probability of having been caused by mistreatment that they are presumed to be due to mistreatment until proven otherwise). An example of such a presumed case would be the presence of a clinical phenomenon that could only have occurred by the conduct of another person.

Identifying Physical Markers of Elder Mistreatment

Some physical findings in children, such as shaken baby syndrome, are considered to be hallmarks of abuse. Characteristic injuries in this syndrome include retinal hemorrhages, subdural hematomas, and rib or long bone fractures. Are there similar hallmarks that may comprise a syndrome of physical abuse or neglect in the elderly? Possible examples discussed by Dyer et al. (this volume) include lacerations of specific body parts, certain types of burns, dehydration in certain contexts, and possibly specific types of bone fractures. Further clinical, behavioral, and forensic research in this area is needed to determine what harms under what circumstances would constitute almost unequivocal evidence of having been caused by the conduct (acts or omissions) of another person.

There are to our knowledge no published studies of physical markers of elder mistreatment that help distinguish preventable, unavoidable signs from those that are intentional, inflicted, or avoidable. One study of skin tears in nursing home residents described the characteristics of the tears, but almost half (48 percent) of the tears had an unknown cause, and the possibility of mistreatment was not addressed (Malone et al., 1991). The only study on bruising that included elderly subjects did not address the influence of medications, functional status, illnesses, or living situation, nor did it address etiology (Langlois and Gresham, 1991).

Possible markers of neglect and abuse include bruises, pressure sores, fractures, burns, and abrasions. A key to interpretation of these markers is not merely their presence but their characteristics—such as anatomic location, extent, morphology, severity, and multiplicity—which may help differentiate between an intentional injury and an avoidable one. For example, a single bruise on the back of the forearm is probably common in cases of accidental bruising, but multiple bruises in various stages of healing on the neck, anterior upper arm, and abdomen raise a suspicion of physical abuse. Also, it is not known if hip fractures due to spontaneous falls have a different radiographic appearance than those due to an inflicted injury. Research is needed to help illuminate the characteristics of common injuries, such as their etiology, natural course, distribution, and severity so that the process of identifying cases of elder mistreatment can become more accurate and reliable. While certain physical signs (such as burns and ligature marks) are likely to be more reliable indicators of elder mistreatment than others (such as fractures and pressure sores), neither the challenge nor the importance of advancing knowledge in this area should be underestimated. Mistakenly characterizing a spontaneous bruise or other injury as intentionally inflicted may lead to substantial clinical, social, and legal jeopardy for all concerned.

CONCLUSIONS

The need for accurate and efficient screening and case identification methods for elder mistreatment is immense. We must minimize false negatives to protect the elder subject and minimize the false positives to avoid false accusations of the trusted other. Just as mistreatment can have devastating consequences for an elder, a false accusation can have devastating consequences for the trusted other. It is likely that screening and case identification will hinge on understanding the constellation and interaction of signs, symptoms, findings, and the context in which they occur.

Substantial research is needed to improve and develop new methods of screening for possible elder mistreatment in a range of clinical settings. These methods should be able to detect a broad range of categories of mistreatment and be highly accurate and efficiently deployed. Candidate techniques include improved questionnaire designs; record linkage to other clinical, public health, social and legal databases; automated alerts based on concurrent clinical records; and previously defined risk status based on prescreening methods. Special attention should be placed on the predictive value of various clinical injuries and other relevant clinical findings as indicators of mistreatment for therapeutic, social, and forensic reasons. Also, the panel sees value in economic analyses of cost-effectiveness for elder mistreatment screening in various clinical settings.

Research is needed on the process of designating cases as incidents of mistreatment in order to improve criteria, investigative methods, decision-making processes, and decision outcomes. The absence of a gold standard for case identification, and the momentous consequences of inaccurate decisions, highlight the need for studying and improving the process of case investigation and designation. The impact of resource constraints on the designation process and its consequences for affected persons should also be studied.

7

Evaluating Interventions

In this chapter we discuss policies and programs designed to protect older persons from mistreatment and to ensure their safety. Overall, the panel's conclusions can be easily summarized: no efforts have yet been made to develop, implement, and evaluate interventions based on scientifically grounded hypotheses about the causes of elder mistreatment, and no systematic research has been conducted to measure and evaluate the effects of existing interventions.

Mandatory reporting and interventions by adult protective services, the core elements of the current system for preventing and ameliorating elder mistreatment, have never been subjected to a rigorous evaluation. Nor have most other interventions targeted at preventing elder mistreatment or addressing the needs of victims and abusers. While intervention programs are presented at national and regional meetings, these programs have not been subjected to systematic evaluation. Without rigorous evaluation, reports of these programs are usually not accepted for publication. Moreover, lack of systematic evaluation can result in the duplication of programs in which the benefits of the program, if there are any, are attributable to the characteristics of the agency that carried it out, rather than the effects of the intervention itself. A secondary result of such duplication is the investment of resources, both public and private, for programs that have never been shown to work and that may be ineffective. This inevitably reduces the funding for new innovations.

The chapter briefly surveys existing interventions to highlight several important research opportunities. Mandatory reporting requirements are discussed first, since they lie at the center of current policy. The chapter then addresses community-based interventions—focusing on adult protective services, the health and criminal justice systems, and emerging examples of collaborative programs—before turning to mistreatment in institutional settings.

REPORTING ELDER MISTREATMENT

Reporting of suspected elder mistreatment is the most commonly used and most controversial intervention. The adult protection statutes of all states and the District of Columbia include provisions governing the reporting of suspected elder mistreatment. All but six of those jurisdictions mandate reporting of suspected mistreatment by specified categories of persons. The other six states—Colorado, New Jersey, New York, North Dakota, South Dakota, and Wisconsin—permit reporting but do not require it. In general, reports are to be made to the pertinent adult protective services agency; in some jurisdictions, however, reporters may be required to transmit their suspicions to a law enforcement agency or some other type of organization in lieu of or in addition to adult protective services.

According to a statutory analysis conducted by the American Bar Association Commission on Legal Problems of the Elderly (through December 2001), in eight of the mandatory reporting states (Delaware, Indiana, Kentucky, New Mexico, North Carolina, Rhode Island, Texas, and Wyoming), "any person" who suspects mistreatment is required to report it. In the other jurisdictions, the reporting obligation is directed to various occupational and professional groups. However, nine of those states take a hybrid approach, requiring "any person" and members of specific occupations to report, depending on the circumstances. In all, 14 states list between 1 and 10 categories, 9 states list between 11 and 20, and 14 states list 21 or more. The occupations and professions commonly mandated to report include:

- Health care professionals
- Mental health professionals
- Caregivers (whether paid or unpaid)
- Home care providers
- Employees of nonresidential programs for the elderly
- Employees of sheltered workshops and similar nonresidential programs
- Employees of residential facilities for the elderly
- Social workers
- Long-term care ombudsman program staff and volunteers
- Employees of adult protective services programs

- Employees of area agencies on aging and other aging service providers
- Employees of human services, social services, or health departments
- Law enforcement and public safety employees
- Attorneys
- Guardians and conservators
- Teachers and educators
- Financial profession employees

The concept of mandatory reporting of suspected mistreatment was borrowed from the child abuse laws without research demonstrating its applicability to older persons. The ongoing debate concerning mandated reporting raises many empirical questions about the effects of these laws on the behavior of mandated reporters and about the consequences of reporting on the lives of people affected by them. Yet virtually no research has been conducted on these important issues. For example, to what extent are mandated reporters aware of their legal obligations? To what extent do they comply with them? What factors affect reporting behavior? What are the motivations, concerns, and expectations of those who report and those who decline to do so? Does reporting behavior vary significantly among the professions and occupations required to report under state law? Hawes (this volume) discusses some studies indicating significant underreporting of elder mistreatment by physicians and other health care professionals, long-term care ombudsmen, and residents of long-term care facilities and their family members. The panel is not aware of studies of other professions or occupations. There is much anecdotal evidence of underreporting, but systematic study of reporting behavior is needed—not only to assess compliance but also to provide the necessary foundation for critical evaluation of the effects of mandated reporting.

Many questions have been raised about the effects of mandated reporting. What actually happens as a consequence of a report, compared with informal interventions that might otherwise have occurred? What are the consequences (both positive and negative) of being reported on the lives of the victim, the perpetrator, and the family? To what extent does the threat of being reported (and the ensuing intervention) affect the behavior of potential (or previously reported) perpetrators and victims? These important issues can be addressed in well-designed studies comparing responses to suspected mistreatment in jurisdictions with and without mandatory reporting. The fact that six states do not require reporting affords an unusual opportunity for cross-jurisdictional comparisons. Before-and-after designs may also be possible as some of the six states with voluntary reporting schemes consider adopting mandatory reporting and other jurisdictions reevaluate their existing reporting requirements.

The panel strongly recommends systematic studies of reporting practices and the effects of reporting, taking maximum advantage of the opportunity for comparisons of practices and outcomes in states with and without mandated reporting.

ADULT PROTECTIVE SERVICES

Adult protective services agencies are the backbone of community-based efforts to respond to elder mistreatment. Statutes require every state to respond to reports of abuse of vulnerable adults. The laws generally establish a system for reporting and investigation of alleged abuse or neglect and for providing protective services to help the victim and ameliorate the abuse. Most laws pertain to adults who have a disability, vulnerability, or impairment that reduces their capacity to protect themselves. All states include the elderly population that may be eligible by virtue of age or age in combination with disability (see Chapter 2 and Appendix B).

The important, and sometimes exclusive, role of adult protective services in responding to reports of abuse and neglect warrants closer examination. After receiving a report, adult protective services serve three main functions. The first organizational function is to receive, assess, and triage abuse and neglect reports. The initial response includes screening the report to evaluate its fit with the applicable abuse and neglect definition. Once a referral is accepted, most states require a response within 24 hours. Many offices have crisis intervention services available through a hotline or on-call system so that an initial determination can be made about the need for emergency services and referrals to other services or providers.

A face-to-face visit with the alleged victim is required in most states. This often includes an assessment of risk (of further abuse) along with an assessment of cognitive ability and the ability of a person to function independently. Although three states (Arizona, Delaware, and Louisiana) use risk assessment tools for which there is some evidence of reliability and validity, the instruments being used in about one-third of the states have not been tested for reliability or validity. The risk assessment instruments in use evaluate client and environmental factors, availability and adequacy of support services, current and historical abuse factors and perpetrator factors. As discussed in Chapter 6, the utility of screening instruments is an important area for research. With regard to adult protective services screening in particular, the panel recommends studies tracking samples of individuals excluded or included for further action.

After providing any needed emergency services, the second function of adult protective services is to investigate abuse or neglect reports. Agencies differ in their approach to finding out whether abuse or neglect occurred. Some are heavily investigative, and others focus on providing social services. Some rely exclusively on law enforcement to conduct investigations. The balance between investigation and social services may also be influenced by other factors, such as federal statutes (e.g., requiring investigation and placement on a registry for nursing assistants and the ombudsman program, which responds to complaints of abuse in nursing homes) or Medicaid rules on abuse (which must be followed in order to receive reimbursement for services). Several states, including Ohio and Wisconsin, have recently evaluated their entire systems of response to elder mistreatment. Wisconsin's review concluded that the role of the adult protective services system should be focused exclusively on providing social services and that investigations should be conducted solely by law enforcement agencies (Wisconsin Department of Health and Family Services, 2001).

In the context of investigations, a method being increasingly used, modeled on the child protective system, is the state abuse registry. As mentioned above, a federal law requires a registry to be kept for certified nursing assistants who have been substantiated for abuse. Long-term care providers are required to check this registry before hiring an employee. These registries are most often maintained by the state nursing board, but a number of states have developed similar registries for any caregiver substantiated for abuse. Maintaining a registry can be an expensive activity, especially if substantial procedural protections are accorded to people whose names are listed. Florida and Minnesota have well-developed systems but, as is true with other interventions, the effects of maintaining a registry have not been studied. The unanswered questions include whether people are safer and, ultimately, whether these interventions are cost-effective.

The third, and often most time-consuming, function of adult protective services is to develop a protective services plan aiming to terminate mistreatment and ensure safety. Assessments of the individual's need for help with activities of daily living and of his or her support network are conducted as part of the overall plan. Additional services can include attendant care, food, housing, rent or mortgage payments, transportation, money management, changing of locks, cleaning, respite care, and ongoing counseling and case management. Adult protective services programs have also tried to adapt the domestic violence model of offender treatment described by Wolfe (this volume) to perpetrators of elder mistreatment. San Francisco and Los Angeles have experimented with small groups targeting perpetrators and using cognitive behavioral techniques to affect the violent behavior.

Although reporting is mandatory in most states, a critical principle embodied in most state statutes is client autonomy. Simply put, services cannot be provided to clients without their consent. The policy of least restrictive intervention is generally embraced, along with the goal of maximizing client independence. These principles are laid out in the National Association of Adult Protective Services Administrators statement on ethics (2002). Although the vast majority of services are based on consent of the client, about 10 percent of interventions are provided without client consent. Involuntary intervention is legally authorized in most states if the refusing client is exposed to a substantial risk of harm or if the client lacks the capacity to make an informed decision to accept or reject protective services. Available interventions typically include guardianship and conservatorship. In addition, emergency protective placements, which are usually limited to 24–72 hours and provided only with judicial approval, may be available. Courts may also issue restraining orders to caregivers and members of the elder's family.

For difficult cases, adult protective services agencies often convene or participate in multidisciplinary review teams. These teams represent the best effort to offer a coordinated community response to elder mistreatment.

Many would agree that adult protective services is an underfunded and overworked system, often operating in a crisis management mode (as did children's protective services in its earlier years). However scarce the resources, choices are inevitably being made about their allocation. It does not appear that any of the adult protective services activities, including triage, investigation, and service planning and delivery, have ever been evaluated. When surveyed by Rosalie Wolf in 1999, state administrators wanted research to define outcomes and measure them, to identify the best practices for intervention, and to help design effective training for their workers (Wolf, 1999). Research is critically needed on the effectiveness of the interventions that are now being deployed. How well, and at what cost, do interventions improve the safety, security, and independence of older persons who have come to adult protective services attention for mistreatment?

Research is needed on the effectiveness of adult protective services interventions, ideally in study designs that compare outcomes in cases in which services were provided with those in which eligible recipients declined offered services or other cases in which mistreatment of an equivalent nature has been identified.

It should be noted that a large proportion—in some states, more than half—of the reports coming into adult protective services concern elderly persons who are neglecting their own care. A typical scenario includes an elderly person with dementia who is losing the ability to cook or take care of a serious medical condition and who has no natural support to call on for assistance. The panel has decided to exclude cases of self-neglect from this report in order to concentrate its attention on the need to develop knowledge about elder mistreatment. However, the inclusion of self-neglect within the jurisdiction of adult protective services can easily confound research on elder mistreatment. Thus it is essential for researchers studying adult protective services interventions (or studying other interventions derived from adult protective services activity or using subjects identified in adult protective services databases) to exclude cases of self-neglect or segregate them from cases involving harm or neglect by others.

HEALTH SYSTEM INTERVENTIONS

Wolfe (this volume) describes the progress made in child abuse detection when health care professionals began to routinely screen for child abuse indicators and to report worrisome cases. Family physicians and the emergency room physicians are ideally situated to see mistreated elders and to refer suspected abuse and neglect for appropriate action. The task of designing and implementing an elder mistreatment screening program for health care professionals presents special challenges. It will require educating health care professionals about the normal changes of aging and how these changes may influence the appearance of forensic markers of elder mistreatment, such as bruises, fractures, and pressure sores (see Dyer et al., this volume.) They must be able to distinguish between cases in which an injury is accidental or unpreventable and those in which it is inflicted or otherwise preventable.

Research on the effects of training health care professionals in responding to family violence indicates that the best practices are based on adult learning theory—that is those in which the curriculum is attached to screening instruments and the ability to practice the skills. The same is likely to be true for neglect cases. Several initiatives are under way to provide specialized training to health care professionals. For example, the geriatric program at Baylor University is developing a curriculum on elder mistreatment for medical school use and is involving medical residents in their elder mistreatment assessments. The California Medical Training Center has also developed a program to train health care providers to identify, evaluate, and document injuries in collaboration with law enforcement and social services.

The increase in home health nursing services has put a number of nurses on the front lines, well situated to see potential abuse or neglect victims. Nursing training typically includes information on family violence but is also limited on its information about elder mistreatment. A promising nursing specialization, developed along with the field of family violence, is forensic nursing. Similar to the development of a national cadre of sexual assault examiners, these and other nurses are expanding their focus to include evaluation of suspicious and serious unexplained injury. These experts are beginning to be used by adult protective services, law enforcement agencies, and the rest of the criminal justice system on a small scale, particularly for those elderly persons who are not cognitively able to provide testimony about their abuse- and neglect-related injuries. A few nursing schools offer this type of specialized advance practice training. The first masters level program with this specialty has been established at Johns Hopkins University. Research on the effectiveness of forensic nurses in identifying elder mistreatment (in all settings, including the clinic and the courtroom) would be useful.

Another part of the health care system that often provides the first response to elder mistreatment is the emergency medical technician. While some training has been done locally by adult protective services, recently the national organization of emergency medical technicians, in conjunction with the National Center on Elder Abuse, has completed a curriculum for their members on elder mistreatment. Research on emergency medical technicians who are trained and that call in social services (adult protective services) would provide valuable information on this promising new intervention.

The hospital setting may also offer an opportunity to detect mistreatment and to intervene so as to prevent further occurrences. Hospitals and the health care professionals working in hospitals have an obligation to ensure the safest possible discharge for their patients. As methods of detecting mistreatment improve, perhaps through the detection of sentinel events associated with mistreatment, it will be possible to target interventions at hospitalized patients who have been mistreated prior to admission. The panel encourages research on hospital-based interventions to prevent further mistreatment of hospital inpatients after discharge. This research should include hospital emergency departments, where many mistreated elders may be seen but not ultimately admitted to the hospital prior to discharge. Interventions to detect and manage mistreatment in hospital emergency departments should therefore also be evaluated.

Other interventions occur at the organization level. The rules of governing organizations like the Joint Commission on Accreditation of Health Care Organizations as well as rules connecting continued Medicaid funding to long-term care and community residential facilities include requirements for recognizing and responding to cases of elder mistreatment. The primary requirements include having a policy to assess possible victims and adhering to state legal requirements relating to investigation as well as prevention of further mistreatment. Accreditation policies and practices relating to elder mistreatment should be studied on a systematic and ongoing basis.

CRIMINAL JUSTICE INTERVENTIONS

Law enforcement officers respond to and investigate allegations of abuse when they are brought to their attention by some other organization, such as adult protective services, or some other individual. In addition, law enforcement officers are often "first responders" and are the first agency representatives to be called to an environment in which mistreatment is occurring, either to investigate an allegation that a law has been violated or to make a "welfare check." Officers may be the first to realize that an older person is experiencing mistreatment. Officers who recognize the signs of mistreatment and know what community agencies are available to provide assistance can help the victim by bringing in adult protective services, providing referrals to community services, or in other ways. Linking to other agencies is particularly critical when law enforcement officers arrest a caregiver for elder mistreatment and remove him or her from the home; otherwise the victim may be left without needed care.

As discussed by Dyer et al. (this volume), medical examiners and coroners may be called on to determine whether death resulted from or was related to elder mistreatment. Because of their expertise in assessing unnatural injury and death, they may be asked to make similar determinations about suspected victims who are still alive. They may also be the first to discover that abuse has occurred, during an autopsy conducted for some reason other than suspected mistreatment. Medical examiners and coroners can play an important role in fatality review teams that analyze deaths resulting from elder abuse.

A key issue is whether and under what circumstances criminal charges should be filed against alleged perpetrators of mistreatment. Reports from law enforcement, adult protective services, and other practitioners indicate that the number of charges filed in such cases has been increasing. The prosecutorial decisions require complex judgments balancing deterrent and punitive considerations (which focus on the seriousness of the offenders' conduct, including harm and culpability) with protective considerations (which focus on what measures will best ensure the future safety and well-being of the elderly victim).

Prosecutorial response to elder mistreatment is an understudied area that should receive heightened attention by the National Institute of Justice and other funders of criminal justice research.

Victim/witness professionals (sometimes referred to as victim advocates or similar titles) also have a dual role in elder mistreatment intervention. Victim/witness professionals may work in law enforcement agencies, prosecutors' offices, or community services organizations. The timing of their involvement and their role depends to some extent on the entity for which they work. In general, they assist crime victims by providing support and explaining the criminal justice system, accompanying them to court, arranging transportation for proceedings, coordinating respite care if the victim is a caregiver, and helping the victim file for victim compensation funds. It is possible that victim/witness professionals will be the first to recognize that victims are experiencing elder mistreatment. Accordingly, victim/witness professionals need to understand the risk factors for and indicators of mistreatment and to know what services are available for these victims. Elder mistreatment researchers should be aware of the existence of these victim/witness assistance programs, not only as possible targets of research in themselves, but as sources of information in other studies.

PROFESSIONAL SPECIALIZATION AND COLLABORATION

Many professions, advocacy groups, and other organizations are involved in efforts to prevent and respond to elder mistreatment. Although adult protective services is the backbone of the system, community-based interventions draw on the health professions, law enforcement personnel and all participants in the criminal justice system, the bar and other participants in the civil justice system, financial institutions, and many others. Increasingly specialized responses are being developed through targeted training and interdisciplinary collaboration. For example, efforts are under way in many communities to improve the response to elder mistreatment victims by educating criminal justice system participants about the problem, developing specialized investigation and prosecution units, enhancing collaboration, and reforming statutes and policies. Most of these initiatives are of recent origin and have not yet been studied in a systematic way.

Professional Specialization

Professional specialization is a critical feature of an effective social response to any emerging social problem, once the problem has been recognized. In its evolution as a social problem, elder mistreatment is now in this "recognition and specialization" stage. Specialized training of health care professionals, mentioned earlier, continues to be an important challenge (Institute of Medicine, 2001). In addition, the increasing numbers of attorneys specializing in elder law, whether working in private practice or publicly funded legal services programs, can be valuable resources in collaborative efforts to prevent and respond to all forms of elder mistreatment. Prevention is enhanced through adequate counseling about the potential for abuse of common legal planning tools, such as powers of attorney (particularly durable powers of attorney), joint bank accounts, joint property ownership, trusts, and wills (see Hafemeister, this volume). Collaborative efforts between the specialized bar, health care providers (in counseling and vulnerability assessments), adult protective services and law enforcement, when mistreatment is suspected, could produce new ideas about prevention.

Depending on the laws of particular jurisdictions, several legal tools can be used to respond to elder mistreatment when it occurs. To stop physical or sexual abuse, a lawyer might need to obtain a civil order of protection to keep the perpetrator away from the victim or pursue an eviction action against an abusive tenant or adult child living with the victim. To combat financial exploitation, a lawyer might need to void a document or transaction because the victim signed it under duress or due to fraud or undue influence. The lawyer might need to help the victim revoke a power of attorney that is being misused or draft a power of attorney or trust in order to wrest control from a perpetrator. It might be necessary to seek to have a guardian or conservator appointed for an abuse victim in order to reduce or terminate the authority of the abuser. It might also be necessary to defend against the appointment of a guardian or conservator or pursue the appointment of an alternative guardian or conservator when the person seeking appointment is mistreating the older person. Civil lawyers also can pursue actions for damages in order to recover money that has been exploited or to make the victim whole for injuries by the perpetrator, and they can pursue actions against companies employing abusive caregivers for negligent hiring and inadequate supervision.

Research about the use of civil justice interventions and their effectiveness in preventing exploitation and other harm to elders should be jointly sponsored by the National Institute of Justice and the Administration on Aging.

Multidisciplinary Collaboration

One of the few federal responses to elder mistreatment has come from the "aging network." This term refers to a wide array of organizations and services established and funded through the Older Americans Act in part to address elder mistreatment. Title VII of the act supports elder rights programs, including the long-term care ombudsman, legal services, outreach, and elder abuse prevention efforts. The Title VII elder abuse prevention monies fund state units on aging to conduct prevention activities at the state level or to fund area agencies on aging to implement prevention activities at the local level.

Community collaborations have played an increasingly important role in recent years by suggesting interventions when serious elder mistreatment occurs. Some jurisdiction have created multidisciplinary teams (sometimes known as MDTs or M-Teams) composed of professionals and practitioners from health, law enforcement, social services, or others as appropriate, to serve one or both of the following purposes: (1) analysis and collaboration on difficult cases that cannot be resolved through the intervention of a single professional or practitioner and (2) recommendations for and development of systemic improvements in response to problems unearthed through case analysis and experience. Fiduciary abuse specialist teams (sometimes known as financial abuse specialist teams or FASTs) are a distinct type of multidisciplinary team that focuses on fiduciary abuse. As such, they may involve different participants, such as accountants, from a more general team. Fatality review teams (FRTs, also known as death review teams or death investigation review teams) are another specialized form of multidisciplinary team. Their goal is to bring together various disciplines to examine deaths that resulted, or may have resulted, from elder abuse and to determine whether systemic changes in the response to elder abuse victims could prevent similar deaths in the future. Members of fatality review teams may also determine that the circumstances of a death ought to be pursued by a prosecutor; they have been used in the child abuse and domestic violence fields for years, and the elder abuse field is just beginning to establish them.

The Administration on Aging and, more recently, the Department of Justice have funded grant projects and conferences and stimulated efforts to identify and share information about best practices in elder mistreatment interventions. For more than 20 years, the Administration on Aging has funded the National Center on Elder Abuse (NCEA) to develop and disseminate information on elder mistreatment, including adult protective services. The Department of Justice has sponsored some focus groups, a roundtable on forensic issues, a national symposium on elder mistreatment and consumer fraud, and several conferences encouraging law enforcement involvement in mistreatment cases, development of training programs for banking personnel, curricula to educate various professionals about the need for and benefit of collaboration, support of fatality review teams, and the development of recommendations related to forensic issues. The National Center on Elder Abuse recently conducted a national summit, bringing together experts from several professions to develop recommendations for a national agenda on elder mistreatment. Recommendations include a nationwide public awareness campaign, coordination of law enforcement efforts, study of adult protective services, and a federal law on elder mistreatment, among others. All of these efforts are now being pursued in the absence of any evidence regarding the effectiveness of the interventions being proposed and endorsed.

The specialized focus and collaboration reflected in these initiatives is an important step forward, because it increases the likelihood that systemic problems will be identified and that targeted interventions will be implemented. Specialization and interdisciplinary linkages also are more likely to lead to collaboration between practitioners and researchers and therefore to better design and evaluation of new interventions.

The panel strongly encourages government agencies and private sponsors of elder mistreatment programs to give priority to interventions that emphasize specialized professional training and interdisciplinary collaboration. Moreover, in the panel's view, all new initiatives should include sufficient funding for evaluation.

INTERVENTIONS IN RESIDENTIAL CARE FACILITIES

Throughout this report, the panel has focused attention on general issues concerning the definition, identification, and prevention of mistreatment, regardless of setting. Although residential care facilities were not excluded from the panel's view, family living settings have usually been emphasized. This section briefly addresses several specific research priorities pertaining to residential care settings. Current knowledge about mistreatment in nursing homes and other residential care settings is summarized by Hawes (this volume), and a recent report, *Improving the Quality of Long-Term Care*, by the Institute of Medicine (2001) provides a comprehensive review of the broader subject of quality improvement, of which patient safety (including avoidance of mistreatment and harm) is a core component.

Among the most important priorities identified in *Improving the Quality of Long-Term Care* concerns the need for uniform definitions and data elements for characterizing the components, processes, and outcomes of long-term care across different jurisdictions, populations, and settings of care (e.g., nursing homes, assisted living facilities, and home health care). The report envisions national systematic and comprehensive data bearing on the staffing and care provided in the various settings of long-term care. This panel endorses the Institute of Medicine committee's recommendation, while emphasizing that uniform data elements relating to mistreatment (including subjective measures of security) should be included in the outcome measures, and that implementation of this recommendation would facilitate research on the effectiveness of interventions of any kind (whether initiated voluntarily or through regulatory action). Virtually nothing is now known, for example, about the nature and effectiveness of regulatory efforts relating to assisted living facilities and other residential care facilities other than nursing homes (Harrington et al., 2000).

Hawes (this volume) discusses the prevalence and demography of mistreatment among residents of long-term care facilities, as well as discusses the array of government and quasi-government agencies responsible for receiving and investigating complaints of elder mistreatment in nursing homes and other residential care facilities. These agencies include the long-term care ombudsman program, the state agency responsible for licensing nursing homes, the state agency responsible for the operation of the nurse aide registry, Medicaid fraud control units, and professional licensing boards. Adult protective services programs, health care professionals, and participants in the criminal justice and civil justice systems also may be involved in responding to mistreated residents of nursing homes and other long-term care facilities in much the same way that they respond to victims who live in their own homes.

The literature on compliance with, and enforcement of, federal regulations governing nursing homes has been reviewed by the Institute of Medicine (2001) and by Hawes (this volume), and the U.S. General Accounting Office maintains active oversight of regulatory enforcement, calling attention to gaps and weaknesses. For example, a recent report (U.S. General Accounting Office, 2002) called attention to the inconsistent definitions of "abuse" used in various states, the "hidden" nature of many incidents of abuse due to underrecognition and underreporting, and the gaps in employee screening.

Despite the widespread perception that institutional residents are at great risk of elder mistreatment, specific interventions to prevent elder mistreatment in long-term care residential settings have been limited. However, current practices in nursing homes and assisted living facilities, as well as more general research on determinants of quality of care in nursing homes, suggest several avenues for intervention.

Possible interventions to prevent institutional elder mistreatment fall into three general categories: (1) Hiring and supervision of staff: these are steps that the facility can take, either in terms of practice or policies, to reduce the likelihood of elder mistreatment. (2) Staff training and skill development: staff can be trained in concrete techniques to help make them aware of what elder mistreatment is and when and how to prevent it. (3) Response to and treatment of elder mistreatment: victims of elder mistreatment in residential settings may require specialized treatment programs.

Because actual interventions are rare, potentially promising interventions in this area that require testing and evaluation are briefly reviewed.

Hiring and Supervision of Staff

The following are examples of managerial initiatives that may reduce the likelihood of elder mistreatment:

Address hiring practices: the area that has received most attention in nursing home research is staffing. One of the endemic problems over the past decade has been a shortage of qualified staff. According to the Institute of Medicine (2001), "research evidence suggests that both nursing-to-resident staffing levels and the ratio of professional nurses to other nursing personnel are important predictors of high quality in nursing homes." The committee accordingly urged the Center for Medicare and Medicaid Services (CMS) to "give high priority" to research on staffing in nursing homes and the impact of various staffing configurations on outcomes. This panel agrees.

The shortage of workers has led in some cases to lax hiring policies and to a lack of serious screening of employees. Some facilities hire a high proportion of individuals at the certified nursing assistant level who have criminal backgrounds or active substance abuse problems. Interventions that improve facilities' ability to screen employees and determine individuals who are suited for caregiving work would be very useful. State abuse registries may fill some of that need, but research on the problems with state registries and the potential benefits of a federal registry in lieu of, or in addition to, the state registries would be helpful. Tools to assess risk of abusive behavior prior to hiring should be developed.

Improve supervision: a persistent problem in long-term care facilities is inconsistent (or absent) supervision. It is clear that supervisory staff must give a consistent message that caring and responsible staff will be rewarded and that elder mistreatment will not be tolerated. Furthermore, a key component of elder mistreatment prevention is the maintenance of a high index of suspicion on the part of supervisors. In reported cases of nursing home mistreatment, supervisors and administrators sometimes ignore signs and symptoms of elder mistreatment because of a false belief that "it can't happen here." Training and awareness interventions with supervisors in nursing homes, with a focus on detection of elder mistreatment, are likely to be fruitful.

Address burnout: one of the strongest research findings is the positive relationship between staff burnout and abusive behavior (Pillemer and Bachman-Prehn, 1991). There is no question that nursing home staff work under stressful conditions. Job stress and burnout can be addressed both at the structural and at the individual levels. A major cause of burnout is chronic short-staffing that is endemic to long-term care facilities (see Hawes, this volume). Although a discussion of solutions to staffing problems in nursing homes is beyond the scope of this report, there is no question that improving the numbers of staff and decreasing turnover rates would contribute to elder mistreatment prevention. The effects of different staffing models and staffing patterns could be evaluated to determine the effect on prevalence and severity of elder mistreatment (see Hawes, this volume). On the individual level, stress reduction and management programs should be evaluated to determine whether they have potential for preventing elder mistreatment

Staff Training and Skill Development

Several factors have been identified as related to elder mistreatment by staff, which can be addressed through training programs. First, a striking finding from several studies (Pillemer and Moore, 1989; Pillemer and Bachman-Prehn, 1991; Hawes, this volume) is the high degree of interpersonal conflict experienced in nursing home work. For example, the majority of staff reported that they had conflicts at least several times a week over residents' unwillingness to eat, personal hygiene, unwillingness to dress, toileting, and other issues. Many staff reported such conflicts every day (Pillemer and Moore, 1989).

A second area involves problematic behavioral symptoms exhibited by residents, including wandering, yelling, suspiciousness, inability to cooperate with care, and particularly anger and verbal and physical aggression. In nursing homes, one of the most important reasons that mistreatment of residents occurs is a lack of training and ability on the part of staff to deal with aggressive behavior by residents (Hawes et al., 2001).

Both of these areas point to critical training needs for staff. As a method of elder mistreatment prevention, workers in long-term care settings can be shown effective ways of modifying residents' behavior that can defuse these difficult situations before aggressive outcomes occur. Noelker and Bass (1995) pointed out that caregivers also need training by staff to make case management more effective. It cannot be assumed that staff will learn how to manage the interpersonal aspects of resident care on the job, as is typically the case. The provision of a tool kit of techniques and methods of handling these problems has elder mistreatment prevention potential.

The best-known training program that addresses these issues was developed by the Coalition of Advocates for the Rights and Interests of the Elderly (CARIE), entitled Competence With Compassion: An Abuse Prevention Training Program for Long Term Care Staff. This elder mistreatment prevention curriculum is designed for nursing assistants in long-term care facilities. The program has three major objectives: to increase staff awareness of actual elder mistreatment and potentially abusive situations; to equip nursing assistants with appropriate conflict intervention strategies; and thereby to reduce staff-resident conflict and abusive behaviors by staff. Although a randomized, controlled evaluation of this program has not been conducted, project data are promising. Individuals undergoing the training showed improved attitudes toward residents between pretest and posttest. Staff also reported less conflict with residents after the training, as well as reductions in resident aggression toward themselves. This is an indication of the success of the training, since the curriculum addressed how to avoid or defuse conflicts with residents before the resident becomes aggressive.

Most important, self-reported abusive actions by staff declined as a result of the training.

Response to and Treatment of Elder Mistreatment

There is little research or practical guidance regarding effective response to incidents of elder mistreatment in residential settings or to methods of treating victims to ameliorate the negative outcomes of elder mistreatment. As Hawes suggests (this volume), studies of the effectiveness of ombudsman programs (which are primarily responsible for coordinating investigation and response to elder mistreatment cases) would be very useful. Do such programs have an impact on the incidence of elder mistreatment, and do they lead to better outcomes for victims?

It is also possible that the range of victim assistance services offered to family violence victims could be applicable to nursing homes. In some cases of sexual assault, rape crisis services have been provided to nursing home residents (Burgess et al., 2000). Thus far, no formal intervention programs have been created to counsel or provide specialized therapy to elder mistreatment victims in residential settings. Such programs should be developed and evaluated.

Unannounced Long-Term Care Facility Inspection Teams

At least two states, Florida and California, have developed long-term care facility inspection teams (known as Operation Spot Check and Operation Guardian, respectively) that conduct random, unannounced visits of nursing homes and assisted living facilities. The teams are generally composed of representatives from the attorney general's office, law enforcement, the long-term care ombudsman program, and other government enforcement agencies, including code enforcement officers and local or state fire marshals. The unannounced visits supplement the existing annual inspections conducted by state government pursuant to federal law.

It would be valuable to study whether unannounced long-term care facility inspection teams make any difference in the amount or types of abuse and neglect experienced by residents of these facilities. Another researchable question is the impact on staff and management of these unannounced inspections.

URGENT NEED FOR OUTCOME RESEARCH

The need for careful scientific research on the effects of interventions is underscored by the sobering findings of the only published elder mistreatment intervention study using an experimental design. This study, funded by the National Institute of Justice, indicates that households receiving the intervention had an increased risk of subsequent mistreatment (Davis and Medina-Ariza, 2001). The investigators adapted a model they had previously used in a study of the effects of a coordinated team response to family violence (Davis and Taylor, 1997). In the subsequent elder mistreatment study, the target population was persons living in selected public housing units in New York City who reported elder abuse (defined as physical abuse and psychological abuse) incidents to the police. Random assignment for the intervention occurred at two levels. First, 30 of 60 public housing projects were randomly assigned to receive public education about elder abuse (e.g., posters, leaflets, and project staff presentations). Second, in all 60 housing projects, half of the households reporting elder abuse incidents to the police were randomly assigned to receive home visits by a team of a police officer and a domestic violence counselor. The team discussed legal options and police procedures and attempted to link the households to social services. Victims were also encouraged to call the police if repeat incidents occurred. To determine whether abuse continued, police records were checked and victims were interviewed 6 and 12 months after the triggering incident.

Six months after the intervention, households receiving the home visit called the police significantly more often than controls, both in housing projects that received public education and those that did not. This is not surprising, since the home visit was designed to invite such reports. But this expectation was based on the assumption that the intervention would change reporting behavior, not that it would increase incidents of abuse. (If anything, one might have expected the number of actual incidents of abuse to be reduced due to deterrence.) The surprising finding was that that the increased number of calls was accompanied by an increased number of incidents of abuse, as reported by the victims to the research interviewers. That is, when households received both home visits and public education, victims of elder abuse reported significantly higher levels of physical abuse than households that received neither intervention or only one of them. During the period between 6 and 12 months after the intervention, the differences in calls to the police disappeared, but households that received the dual intervention continued to report significantly more incidents of physical abuse to the interviewers.

The researchers have speculated about the possible explanations for this paradoxical finding, including the possibility that the intervention angered the perpetrators. (As they pointed out, however, the perpetrators were not interviewed.) The most pertinent observation from the panel's perspective is that the study raises more questions than it answers. Even well-intentioned interventions may have unexpected, and even harmful, outcomes.

Research on the effects of elder mistreatment interventions is urgently needed. Existing interventions to prevent or ameliorate elder mistreatment should be evaluated, and agencies funding new intervention programs should require and fund a scientifically adequate evaluation as a component of each grant. Specifically:

• Research is needed on reporting practices and on the effects of reporting, taking maximum advantage of the opportunity for comparisons of practices and outcomes in states with and without mandated reporting.

• Research is needed on the effectiveness of adult protective services interventions, ideally in study designs that compare outcomes in cases in which services were provided with those in which eligible recipients declined offered services or other cases in which mistreatment of an equivalent nature has been identified.

• Intervention or prevention research based in existing health care environments that come into contact with mistreated elders, such as hospitals, emergency departments, and emergency response services, should be a priority as it takes advantage of the existing expertise and resources of these services.

• The development of adult protective services/university research teams should be encouraged in order to evaluate existing data, recommend improvements in the collection of data, analyze incident reports, and design the studies of outcomes urged in this report.

8

Research Ethics

It became evident early in the panel's deliberations that investigators are uncertain about the ethical requirements governing research on elder mistreatment. They are particularly concerned about two issues: (1) Under what circumstances is it ethically necessary to exclude elderly persons from participation in research on the ground that they are incapable of giving informed consent? (2) How should investigators respond to evidence of mistreatment elicited during the study, and what should participants be told about this problem in advance?

It also became apparent to the panel that Institutional Review Boards (IRBs) have embraced varying approaches to these problems, and that unduly restrictive IRB positions could impede important advances in the understanding of elder mistreatment. In reviewing proposed research protocols in the current regulatory context, IRBs exercise a great deal of discretion within the general parameters set by the federal research regulations (i.e., the so-called Common Rule) (U.S. Department of Health and Human Services, 2001a) that govern all federally funded research, and the regulations of the U.S. Food and Drug Administration (1999) that govern clinical trials of drugs and devices. To help provide better guidance to investigators and IRBs in preparing and reviewing elder mistreatment research protocols, the panel commissioned a paper by Rebecca Dresser, a leading authority on research ethics. Her paper (this volume) surveys the issues that tend to recur in research on elder mistreatment and offers many helpful suggestions about how to respond to them.

DECISIONAL CAPACITY

As Dresser (this volume) indicates, many of the concerns in elder mistreatment research relate to the assessment of decision-making capacity and the proper responses to situations in which potential participants' decision-making capacity is impaired. Taking into account that elderly persons who are most vulnerable to mistreatment are likely to be decisionally impaired, and that decisional impairment is often embedded in the statutory definition of mistreatment, the opportunity to elicit information from cognitively impaired individuals is essential in almost every study of elder mistreatment. The problem is by no means limited to elder mistreatment research; similar observations could be made about many other types of research focusing on older subjects or on people with mental retardation or schizophrenia. Not surprisingly, ethical issues relating to consent by cognitively impaired subjects and surrogate decision making have come to center stage in recent years and have been addressed in a rapidly developing literature (Berg, 1996; Bonnie, 1997; Dresser, 1999; National Bioethics Advisory Commission, 1998). Although the Dresser paper provides a thorough review of these issues, several points are emphasized here.

First, aging research suggests that most older adults are cognitively intact and should be regarded as presumptively able to make informed, voluntary decisions about research participation; merely being older than age 65 or 75 does not warrant special screening procedures or other protections. Heightened safeguards should be considered when the research involves greater than minimal risk and the study population is especially likely to include persons with decisional impairments or persons who are especially vulnerable to pressure or influence.

Second, a diagnosis of dementia is not congruent with decisional incapacity (Marson et al., 1995). Instead, an assessment of decisional capacity requires a highly contextualized judgment concerning a particular person's ability to perform ethically relevant decision-making tasks in relation to a particular study. Significant advances have recently been made in conceptualizing, operationalizing, and measuring these decision-making abilities. For example, according to one widely used approach, the ethically relevant abilities in making informed decisions about treatment or research participation are understanding of risks and benefits and other ethically relevant information, appreciation of the relevance of that information in one's own situation, reasoning or processing the information logically, and ability to make a stable choice among alternatives (Appelbaum and Grisso, 1988; Grisso and Appelbaum, 1998). Instruments are being developed to help researchers assess and document participants' decision-making abilities, both at the initiation of the study and, if needed, on a continuing basis during the study (Kim et al., 2001; Marson et al., 1995).

Third, it is understood that the decision-making abilities of many older people with dementia or other mental disorders will be impaired to some extent. However, mere impairment does not amount to incapacity. Whether a person's impairment (in understanding, appreciation, or reasoning) is substantial enough to preclude informed consent for a particular study depends on the complexity of the decision-making task for that study, and on its risk-benefit profile (Grisso and Appelbaum, 1998; American Psychiatric Association, 1998; National Bioethics Advisory Commission, 1998). A minimum threshold of capacity must be satisfied for all studies in which the participant is exposed to any risk, but the level of capacity needed above this floor will depend on the characteristics of the particular study. Moreover, impairments that would preclude valid consent in studies with significant risk are ethically immaterial in studies involving less than minimal risk (National Bioethics Advisory Commission, 2001). Similarly, additional safeguards that may be needed to ensure proper consent in studies involving significant risk are not necessary in studies involving lower risk. Risk stratification of this kind is a prominent and essential feature of sensible ethical review.

Fourth, even if an elderly person lacks the capacity to give informed consent for the particular study, his or her participation may be authorized by a surrogate decision maker as long as the subject is adequately protected from harm and the IRB finds that all the other criteria specified in the Common Rule have been met. The Common Rule, however, provides very little guidance to IRBs, within these parameters, about the conditions under which surrogates should be permitted to authorize participation for decisionally incapable subjects in lieu of excluding them from participation altogether (Bonnie, 1997; Dresser, 2001; National Bioethics Advisory Commission, 1998). This lack of guidance has led to inconsistency among IRBs and frustration among investigators. However, recent reports by expert bodies have begun to provide such guidance and to assemble best practices (National Bioethics Advisory Commission, 1998; American Psychiatric Association, 1998). The important point for our purposes is that the Common Rule provides ample flexibility to IRBs to allow important research on elder mistreatment to go forward on the basis of surrogate consent, particularly if it involves less than minimal risk.

Finally, another concern is the availability of a suitable surrogate. The Common Rule refers generally to individuals "authorized under applicable law to consent on behalf of a prospective subject's participation." As Dresser (this volume) notes, however, many states lack clear rules in this area. To the extent that impediments to research arise from ambiguities or constraints in state law governing surrogate decision making, these are generic problems in research that, in the end, depend on clarification of state law. The panel urges states to extend their rules governing surrogate decision making for health care decisions to the context of research (see Hoffman and Schwartz, 1998).

It is possible that the most suitable surrogate would be a family member whose own improper conduct would be exposed by the study. Under these circumstances, involving possible conflicts of interest between the decision maker and the potential research subject, other suitable surrogates should be identified. As Dresser (this volume) notes, analogous problems in child mistreatment research have been addressed in the subpart of the Common Rule prescribing additional protections for children participating in research (U.S. Department of Health and Human Services, 2001a). Overall, it should be emphasized that, in the absence of impediments rooted in state law, the IRBs have a great deal of flexibility in permitting research to go forward with decisionally incapable participants as long as a suitable surrogate authorizes participation and the participants are protected from harm.

PROPER RESPONSES TO EVIDENCE OF MISTREATMENT

Another major area of ethical uncertainty with particular salience in elder mistreatment research concerns ethically permissible responses to evidence of mistreatment that may be elicited during the study (and the associated issue of what potential subjects should be told about this possibility during the consent process). Deciding how the investigator should respond to evidence of mistreatment implicates the investigator's most fundamental ethical duties in human research—the duty to protect participants from harm and the duty to respect their autonomy as persons—and also exposes possible conflicts between the interests of victims of mistreatment (in being protected) and suspected perpetrators of mistreatment (in avoiding possible punitive interventions). Because both the possible perpetrator of mistreatment and the possible victim could be regarded as subjects of (or participants in) the research, the investigator may owe both of them a duty to avoid harm.

If these puzzles were not enough to create ethical complexity, the possibility that state laws may require researchers to disclose evidence of mistreatment to official agencies highlights a possible incongruity between state reporting policies (requiring breaches of confidentiality) and federal research policy (emphasizing the need to protect confidentiality). It can readily be seen why IRBs would be perplexed by these problems (which also arise in research that could elicit evidence of child mistreatment) and why some IRBs might end up embracing policies that effectively preclude otherwise meritorious studies.

Because the goals and methods of elder mistreatment research vary so widely, it is neither possible nor desirable to formulate generally applicable policies or rules about how to resolve these problems. The most sensible approach is to avoid hard-and-fast rules altogether and to permit investigators and IRBs to tailor their responses to the settings and protocols of the particular studies. With this caveat in mind, **the panel recommends that the National Institute on Aging, in collaboration with the Office for Human Research Protections and other sponsors of elder mistreatment research, undertake a consensus project to develop ethical guidelines for responding to evidence of elder mistreatment in various types of research settings** (e.g., telephone surveys, in-person interviews in clinical settings). As part of this process, representative samples or groups of elder persons, caregivers, and other family members should be surveyed to ascertain their attitudes on the relative importance of the competing values at stake and the appropriate responses to the dilemmas regarding disclosure of information bearing on possible mistreatment.

In the absence of more specific guidance emerging from such a consensus process, the panel suggests that investigators undertake to obtain community guidance about some of the ethical difficulties raised by their particular protocols (see Levine, 1986; Melton et al., 1988, Strauss et al., 2001). **Whenever feasible, investigators should consult representative members of the populations being studied (elder persons and caregivers, nursing home residents and staff, etc.) to ascertain their perspectives and preferences regarding the proper responses to evidence of mistreatment (and the related ethical issues raised by the proposed research) and should take this information into account in developing the protocol.**

It appears that the biggest impediment to sensible and consistent resolution of the ethical issues raised by elder mistreatment research is the concern that state law requires researchers to report possible cases of mistreatment to public agencies. Under some circumstances involving clear danger to the elderly subject, researchers may certainly feel ethically bound to take preventive action, and sometimes this may require them to call adult protective services authorities. However, evidence of mistreatment that may be elicited during the interview is often not indicative of current danger, and there are many other ways in which ethically sensitive and caring researchers can respond to such evidence. It should also be recognized that reporting (and triggering an adult protective services investigation) can have disruptive effects on the life of an elderly subject and may not be in his or her best interests. For these reasons, in the panel's view, evidence of mistreatment elicited during research should not trigger a mandatory obligation to report. Whatever may be thought of mandated reporting in ordinary practice settings (see Chapter 7), it is too blunt a response in the research context. Instead, whether the researchers should voluntarily take protective action and, if so, whether such action should include reports to public agencies should be determined by researchers and IRBs in the context of the goals, setting, and methods of the particular study. **Elder mistreatment reporting statutes should be amended to exempt researchers from their mandatory requirements.**

The requirements otherwise imposed by state reporting statutes can be overridden by a certificate of confidentiality issued by the National Institutes of Health (NIH) in accordance with federal law. In the panel's view, **NIH should issue certificates of confidentiality designed to insulate elder mistreatment researchers from any legal obligation to disclose possible cases of mistreatment that otherwise may arise under state law, including tort "duty to protect" obligations as well as reporting statutes. Issuance of these certificates should be predicated on the assumption that IRBs will carefully scrutinize the protocols to ensure that participants' interests are being protected from harm and that, under appropriate circumstances, IRBs will permit investigators to take voluntary steps to protect subjects in danger.** (This point is discussed in greater depth below.)

The panel is confident that the federally issued certificate of confidentiality supersedes otherwise mandatory reporting requirements under state law. Pursuant to §301(d) of the Public Health Service Act, 42 U.S.C. § 241(d):

> The Secretary may authorize persons engaged in biomedical, behavioral, clinical, or other research (including research on mental health, including research on the use and effect of alcohol and other psychoactive drugs) to protect the privacy of individuals who are the subject of such research by withholding from all persons not connected with the conduct of such research the names or other identifying characteristics of such individuals. Persons so authorized to protect the privacy of such individuals may not be compelled in any Federal, State, or local civil, criminal, administrative, legislative, or other proceedings to identify such individuals.

Although some researchers have wondered whether a person is being "compelled" to "identify" their subjects by a statutory reporting obligation for child abuse or elder mistreatment (see Gray et al., 1995), it is clear that a statutory reporting obligation, with penalties for failure to report, is a form of compulsion, and that a report of the perpetrator inevitably identifies the victim. It is also clear that a certificate of confidentiality issued pursuant to this statute will supersede the state's reporting obligation under the supremacy clause of the Constitution (under which federal law is the "supreme law of the land").

Although the issue has never been litigated in federal court, the certificate's authority has been recognized by the highest court of New York in *People v. Newman*, 345 N.Y.S. 2d (1973) (certificate issued pursuant to an equivalent provision in the Comprehensive Drug Abuse Prevention and Control Act of 1970 protected Dr. Newman from a subpoena requiring disclosure of pictures of patients receiving methadone).[1] It should also be noted that regulations issued by the U.S. Department of Health and Human Services (2001b), to which courts would give considerable weight in interpreting the federal statute, do not include state reporting obligations in the list of disclosures permitted by a certificate of confidentiality. Finally, NIH guidelines pertaining to confidentiality certificates include the following provisions:

> **Background:** Confidentiality Certificates are issued by NIH Institutes pursuant to Section 301 (d) of the Public Health Services Act (42 U.S.C. Section 241(d)) to afford special privacy protection to research subjects. A Certificate helps the researcher avoid compelled "involuntary disclosure" (e.g. subpoenas) of identifying information about a research subject. It does not prevent voluntary disclosures such as disclosure to protect the subject or others from serious harm, as in cases of child abuse. Also, a researcher may not rely on a Certificate to withhold data if the subject consents to the disclosure.

> **Informing subjects about certificate:** When a researcher obtains a Confidentiality Certificate, the subjects must be told about the protections afforded by the Certificate, and any exceptions to that protection. This information is usually included in an "informed consent."

> **Need to adapt examples:** Research subjects vary widely in their cultural and educational backgrounds. The language used should cover the basic points—privacy protection means that the subject will not be identified as participating in the study, unless the subject consents, or a disclosure is made to protect the subject or another from serious harm. Researchers may adapt the language to the special needs of their clientele, and to the subject matter of the study.

> Researchers should also review the language about confidentiality which is routinely included in consent forms to be sure that it is consistent with Confidentiality Certificate protections. For example, consent forms sometimes refer to state law reporting requirements. However, *HHS General*

---

[1]There are no cases involving elder reporting obligations. However, the attorney general of Iowa, in Opinion 83-11-3 (1983), concluded that a federal confidentiality certificate superseded Iowa's mandatory state child abuse reporting requirements. The supreme court of Minnesota subsequently ruled that the preemptive effect of the federal law authorizing Health and Human Services to issue confidentiality certificates for alcohol treatment research was itself superseded by a subsequently enacted federal statute requiring states to enact child abuse reporting statutes as a condition of receiving federal funds (*State v. Andring*, 342 N.W. 2d 128, 1984). It should be noted, however, that federal law does not require states to adopt mandatory reporting as a condition of receiving federal funds for elder mistreatment or adult protective services.

> *Counsel advises that such a disclosure would be voluntary, even though (otherwise) required by State law, because the Certificate protects the researcher from the compulsion of that law.* Thus, note that the examples given simply state the circumstances in which disclosures would be made. [emphasis added]

Thus, NIH policy clearly supports the contention that certificates exempt researchers from the obligation to report elder abuse under state reporting statutes.

Assuming that disclosure to public agencies is not mandated by law, the next question is whether the research protocol itself should require or permit such disclosure, and, if so, under what circumstances. In the panel's view, direct disclosure to public authorities should never be required by the protocol, just as it should not be required by law. The better approach is to ask the mistreated person (or the perpetrator, if that person has made the disclosure) whether he or she would like to discuss the problem with a clinician or other service provider and to refer the case if so authorized (or if the person lacks the capacity to make an informed decision). Even if counseling is declined, the person should be given written information regarding available counseling and other services. Further protective action, including reporting to public agencies, should be undertaken only if the researcher (or the consulting clinician) has a substantial basis for believing that the elder person is in immediate danger of serious harm.

These responses require delicate judgment and clinical sensitivity. It is therefore in the principal investigators' interests to train their interviewers carefully and to specify procedures in advance for notifying the principal investigator of disturbing disclosures of past mistreatment and concerns about future danger. These concerns would be most likely to arise in face-to-face interviews. Information elicited in a telephone interview is highly unlikely to be so suggestive of future victimization as to warrant disclosure without consent.

A final question is whether the prospect of referral (without consent) just described (or whatever approach is prescribed in the protocol) should (or must) be disclosed to the prospective participants during the consent process. The proper response probably varies across research contexts. The Common Rule provides that an investigator seeking IRB approval to omit information that ordinarily must be disclosed must establish that participants will be exposed to no more than minimal risk; that waiving or altering informed consent "will not adversely affect the rights and welfare of the subjects;" and that the study would be "impracticable" if the information had to be disclosed. These criteria raise two questions:

First, does the residual possibility that the investigators or others could notify authorities, leading to unwanted intervention, family disruption, or other harm, amount to "more than a minimal risk" of harm to the participant? As Dresser (this volume) suggests, the answer to this question probably turns on whether the research is undertaken in a clinical or social service setting in which the risk (of disclosure, especially under applicable reporting laws) inheres in the clinical or service interaction, not in the research itself. In such instances, the residual possibility that the researcher might disclose evidence of mistreatment does not present a material risk that must be disclosed in order to obtain informed consent. As Dresser observes:

> In applying the Common Rule's minimal risk and consent waiver provisions, the focus should be on whether research participation exposes older persons and caregivers to risks greater than those present in ordinary life and routine medical and social service encounters. For example, consider an interview study of family members caring for older individuals. If the study would expose participants to more detailed scrutiny than they would encounter in their usual interactions with the health care and social services systems, and if investigators planned to report suspected maltreatment to protective services authorities, the study would present more than minimal risk to study participants. The higher risk would exist because study participation would expose family members to reporting risks greater than those present in routine clinical and social services activities. If, however, data would be collected in interviews conducted as part of the ordinary activities of a social services agency, and the agency's ordinary reporting practices would be followed, the research risks would appear not to exceed the minimal risk threshold.

Assuming that the risk is characterized as a minimal one, the second question is whether disclosing it would unduly compromise the scientific integrity of the study by skewing enrollment or the accuracy of responses. Obviously, this question must be addressed in the context of a particular study. However, waiver of the disclosure requirement would seem to be especially warranted in studies aiming to provide accurate estimates of the occurrence of elder mistreatment.

CONCLUSION

In general, it is the panel's view that investigators and IRBs need clearer guidance (without rigid rules) concerning two issues that tend to recur in elder mistreatment research: conditions under which research can properly go forward with participants whose decisional capacity is impaired, and the proper responses to evidence of mistreatment elicited during the course of the study. In the absence of better guidance, IRBs are left setting their own criteria, leading to inconsistencies and confusion—the same IRB often interprets the governing rules differently with each rotation of its chair. Cooperative research between agencies or organizations is also difficult, if not impossible, since different IRBs often take different positions on these issues, including what information must be disclosed to obtain informed consent.

As a first step in this direction, the panel has sought to clarify some of the issues in these two areas and to provide some needed guidance. Eventually, the National Institute on Aging, in collaboration with the Office for Human Research Protections and other federal partners, should take the lead to promote further clarification, thereby helping investigators and IRBs to achieve the proper level of participant protection while enabling important research involving older and vulnerable adults to move forward. In addition, NIH should continue to support research on assessing decisional impairments and the adequacy of participant consent, on the effects of interventions aiming to facilitate and sustain consent by subjects with impairments, and on the nature and consequences of investigator and IRB responses to disclosures of mistreatment during the course of a study.

9

Moving Forward

$\mathbf{K}$nowledge about elder mistreatment will advance only if its importance is recognized by policy makers and funding agencies, if useful theories and methods are successfully extrapolated from relevant disciplines and adjacent fields of research, and if adequate funding is available to support research careers in this field. The first of these conditions is likely to be satisfied as the population ages and mistreatment becomes more evident (a process that can be accelerated by conducting a sound study of national prevalence). The second is most likely to be satisfied if research on elder mistreatment is "located," conceptually and operationally, in the mainstream of research funding. The third will require a concerted effort on the part of agencies that sponsor and regulate research.

FROM THE MARGINS TO THE MAINSTREAM

Recognizing that elder mistreatment crosses categorical boundaries in both health research and social science research, federal funding agencies (e.g., the National Institute on Aging, the Administration on Developmental Disabilities and Rehabilitation Research, and the National Institute of Justice) should work collaboratively to promote research on the abuse (physical and sexual) and financial exploitation of vulnerable adults, including older persons as well as younger adults with disabilities.

Another promising idea is to locate aspects of elder mistreatment research relating to caregiving in the domain of quality assurance in long-term care. According to the prevailing conceptualization of health care quality (easily extended to other human services), patient (or client) safety is one of the four components of quality in services (together with effectiveness, patient-centeredness, and timeliness) (Institute of Medicine, 2001). It is already understood that prevention of mistreatment is a core element of quality assurance in nursing home regulation. However, as noted earlier, 80 percent of vulnerable elderly persons live in community settings, not in nursing homes. Protecting elderly people in these settings, including their own homes, represents a parallel challenge for policy makers and an overlapping agenda for researchers aiming to understand the phenomenology, etiology, and consequences of mistreatment and the interventions that can reduce it. By viewing elder mistreatment through the prism of quality assurance (safety and security) in long-term care, it is possible to draw together the frameworks and methods of researchers studying the needs of, and services provided to, vulnerable elderly people in various long-term care settings, as well as those used by researchers studying power and conflict in human relationships (see Chapter 3).

BUILDING THE INFRASTRUCTURE

Researchers currently in the field indicate that the ability to attract new investigators is hampered by the lack of training funds. Both federal agencies and private foundations should make funds available for both predoctoral and postdoctoral training programs. Career advancement funding should be readily available to investigators who express an interest in pursuing careers in elder mistreatment research. Foundations supporting geriatric education in the professions should pay special attention to those seeking funding or support for careers in elder mistreatment research.

An adequate long-term funding commitment to research on elder mistreatment must be made by relevant federal, state, and private agencies to support research careers and to develop the next generation of investigators in the field.

To help develop the research infrastructure of the field, several steps are needed to remove barriers and create new opportunities:

• The Office for Human Research Protections needs to work with both experts in elder mistreatment and experts on human subjects protection to arrive at useful guidelines concerning research participation.

• Research funding is needed from agencies other than those already in the field. Most research on elder mistreatment has been supported by the National Institute on Aging, the Administration on Aging, and offices within the Department of Justice. Funding agencies with interests in aging or disabled or vulnerable populations, or in health care delivery (especially long-term care) and health/social policy research, should invest in research in this important and understudied domain affecting older adults. For example, the Administration on Developmental Disabilities and Rehabilitation Research, the Centers for Medicare and Medicaid Services, or the Center for Mental Health Services might be interested in supporting research focusing on vulnerable adults who are often served by the adult protective services system. The Agency for Healthcare Research and Quality may be interested in research on reducing elder mistreatment as a measure of quality improvements, not only in nursing homes, but also in the entire range of long-term care settings. In addition, private foundations, such as the American Health Assistance Foundation and the Andrus Foundation, which support research on dementia and Alzheimer's disease, should be encouraged to make elder mistreatment research one of their priority interests.

• Within the grant review system, particularly on the federal level, but within other funding sources as well, ways need to be found to incorporate experts in elder mistreatment into the review structure on a continuing basis. Most review groups include no experts in the field of elder abuse. New fields of interest or those in early stages of scientific development, such as elder mistreatment, are probably disadvantaged in the scientific review process in comparison to mature fields, especially when the review committees are not aware of the poorly developed state of knowledge. This problem can be ameliorated by ensuring that experts in the field participate in the review of relevant applications, either as special consultants or as members of the review groups.

• Persons currently doing research and practicing in the field of elder mistreatment need to disseminate the findings of their research and programmatic efforts in a more systematic and expeditious manner.

CONCLUSION

Systematic implementation of these recommendations will help establish a sound foundation for advancing knowledge on elder mistreatment. A genuine long-term commitment of resources to this important, though understudied, area will also help to recruit a new generation of scientists to the field. By the same token, however, it is clear that, in the absence of the kinds of investment recommended in this report, knowledge and understanding of elder mistreatment will remain thin, even as the population ages and the occurrence of mistreatment increases. A substantial commitment to research is needed to inform and guide a caring society as it aims to cope with the challenges ahead.

References

Administration on Aging
  1997   *Facts on Long-Term Care.* FS-97-4. Washington, DC: U.S. Department of Health and Human Services.
Albertini, R.J.
  1998   Somatic mutations as multipurpose biomarkers. In *Biomarkers: Medical and Workplace Applications,* Mortimer L. Mendelsohn, Lawrence C. Mohr, and John P. Peters, eds. Washington, DC: Joseph Henry Press.
Alecxih, L., J. Corea, D.J. Gross, M.J. Gibson, C.F. Caplan, and N. Brangen
  1997   *Out-of-Pocket Health Spending by Medicare Beneficiaries Age 65 and Older: 1997 Projections.* Washington, DC: American Association of Retired Persons.
American Medical Association
  1992   *Diagnostic and Treatment Guidelines on Elder Abuse and Neglect.* Chicago, IL: American Medical Association.
American Psychiatric Association
  1998   Guidelines for assessing the decision-making capacities of potential research subjects with cognitive impairment. *American Journal of Psychiatry* 155:1649-1650.
Anetzberger, G.
  1987   *The Etiology of Elder Abuse by Adult Offspring.* Springfield, IL: Charles C. Thomas.
Anetzberger, G.J., J.E. Korbin, and C. Austin
  1994   Alcoholism and elder abuse. *Journal of Interpersonal Violence* 9(2):184-193.
Anetzberger, G.J., B.R. Palmigano, M. Sanders, D. Bass, C. Dayton, S. Eckert, and M.R. Schimer
  2000   A model intervention for elder abuse and dementia. *The Gerontologist* 40(4):492-497.
Ansello, E.E.
  1996   Causes and theories. In *Abuse, Neglect and Exploitation of Older Persons: Strategies for Assessment and Intervention,* L.A. Baumhover and S.C. Bell, eds. Baltimore, MD: Health Professions Press.

153

Appelbaum, P., and T. Grisso
    1988   Assessing patients' capacities to consent to treatment. *New England Journal of Medicine* 319:1635-1638.
Berg, J.W.
    1996   Legal and ethical complexities of consent with cognitively impaired research subjects: Proposed guidelines. *Journal of Law, Medicine and Ethics* 24:18-35.
Blenkner, M., M. Bloom, and R. Weber
    1974   *Protective Services for Older People.* Findings from the Benjamin Rose Institute Study. Cleveland, OH: Benjamin Rose Institute.
Bonnie, R.
    1997   Research with cognitively impaired subjects. *Archives of General Psychiatry* 54:105-111.
Bowen, K.
    2000   Child abuse and domestic violence in families of children seen for suspected sexual abuse. *Clinical Pediatrics* 39(1):33-40.
Branch, L.G.
    2001   The Epidemiology of Elder Abuse and Neglect. Unpublished paper presented to the Panel on Elder Abuse and Neglect, Committee on National Statistics, October 1, 2001. Durham, NC: Duke University School of Medicine.
Breckman, R.S., and R.D Adelman
    1988   *Strategies for Helping Victims of Elder Mistreatment.* Newbury Park, CA: Sage Publications.
Bristowe, E., and J.B. Collins
    1989   Family-mediated abuse of non-institutionalized elder men and women living in British Columbia. *Journal of Elder Abuse and Neglect* 1(1):45-54.
Brookmeyer, R., S. Gray, and C. Kawas
    1998   Projections of Alzheimer's disease in the United States and the public health impact of delaying disease onset. *American Journal of Public Health* 88(9):1337-1342.
Burgess, A.W., R.A. Prentky, and E.B. Dowdell
    2000   Sexual predators in nursing homes. *Journal of Psychosocial Nursing* 38:27-35.
Carter L.S., L.A. Weithorn, and R.E. Behrman
    1999   Domestic violence and children: Analysis and recommendations. *The Future of Children* 9(3):4-20.
Clark-Daniels, C.L., R.S. Daniels, and L.A. Baumhover
    1990   Abuse and neglect of the elderly: Are emergency department personnel aware of mandatory reporting laws? *Annals of Emergency Medicine* 19(9):970-977.
Cold, J., A. Petruckevitch, G. Feder, W-S. Chung, J. Richardson, and S. Moorey
    2001   Relation between childhood sexual and physical abuse and risk of revictimisation in women: A cross-sectional study. *Lancet* 358:450-455.
Comijs, H.C., A.M. Pot, H.H Smit, and C. Jonker
    1998   Elder abuse in the community: Prevalence and consequences. *Journal of the American Geriatrics Society* 46:885-888.
Compton, S.A., P. Flanagan, and W. Gregg
    1997   Elder abuse in people with dementia in Northern Ireland: Prevalence and predictors in cases referred to a psychiatry of old age service. *International Journal of Geriatric Psychiatry* 12(6):632-635.
Cooney, C., and A. Mortimer
    1995   Elder abuse and dementia: A pilot study. *International Journal of Social Psychiatry* 41(4):276-283.

Corder, L.
  2001   Survey Design Issues: Development of Elder Abuse Estimates. Unpublished pa-
          per presented to the Panel on Elder Abuse and Neglect, Committee on National
          Statistics, October 1, 2001. Durham, NC: Center for Demographic Studies,
          Duke University.
Coyne, A.C., W.E. Reichman, and L.J. Berbig
  1993   The relationship between dementia and elder abuse. *American Journal of Psy-
          chiatry* 150(4):643-646.
Davidson, J.L.
  1979   Elder abuse. In *The Battered Elder Syndrome: An Exploratory Study*, M.R.
          Block and J.D. Sinnott, eds. College Park, MD: Center on Aging, University of
          Maryland.
Davis R., and J. Medina-Ariza
  2001   *Results from an Elder Abuse Prevention Experiment in New York City.* Re-
          search in Brief. Washington DC: National Institute of Justice.
Davis, R., and B.G. Taylor
  1997   A proactive response to family violence: The results of a randomized experiment.
          Criminology 35(2): 307-333.
Dolan R., and B. Blakely
  1989   Elder abuse and neglect: A study of adult protective service workers in the United
          States. *Journal of Elder Abuse and Neglect* I:31-49.
Dresser, R.
  1996   Mentally disabled research subjects: The enduring policy issues. *Journal of the
          American Medical Association* 276:67-72.
  1999   Research involving persons with mental disabilities: A review of policy issues and
          proposals. In National Bioethics Advisory Commission, *Research Involving Per-
          sons with Mental Disorders That May Affect Decisionmaking Capacity* vol. 2
          Bethesda, MD: National Bioethics Advisory Commission.
  2001   Dementia research: Ethics and policy for the twenty-first century. *Georgia Law
          Review* 35:661-690.
Dube S.R., R.F. Anda, V.J. Felitti, D.P. Chapman, D.F. Williamson, and W.H. Giles
  2001   Child abuse, household dysfunction, and the risk of attempted suicide throughout
          the life span. *Journal of the American Medical Association* 286:3089-3096.
Dyer, C.B., M.S. Gleason, K.P. Murphy, V.N. Pavlik, B. Portal, T. Regar, and D.J. Hyman
  1999   Treating elder neglect: Collaboration between a geriatrics assessment team and
          adult protective services. *Southern Medical Journal* 92(2):242-244.
Eberhardt, M.S., D.D. Ingram, D.M. Makuc, et al.
  2001   *Urban and Rural Health Chartbook.* Hyattsville, MD: National Center for
          Health Statistics.
Edleson, J.L.
  2000   Studying the co-occurrence of child maltreatment and woman battering in fami-
          lies. In *Intimate Violence in the Lives of Children: The Future of Research,
          Intervention, and Social Policy*, S.A. Graham-Bermann and J.L. Edleson, eds.
          Washington, DC: American Psychological Association.
Engels, G.L.
  1977   The need for a new medical model: A challenge for bio-medicine. *Science*
          196:129-136.
Ensel, W.M., and N. Lin
  2000   Age, the stress process, and physical distress: The role of distal stressors. *Journal
          of Aging and Health* 12(2):136-168.

Fiegener, J.J., M. Fiegener, and J. Meszaros
    1989   Policy implications of a statewide survey on elder abuse. *Journal of Elder Abuse and Neglect* 1(2):39-58.
Fisher B.S., F.T. Cullen, and M.G. Turner
    2000   *The Sexual Victimization of College Women.* National Institute of Justice, NCJ 182369. Washington, DC: U.S. Department of Justice.
Freedman V.A., and L.G. Martin
    1999   The role of education in explaining and forecasting trends in functional limitations among older Americans. *Demography* 36(4): 461-473.
Fulmer, T., and B. Gurland
    1996   Restriction as elder mistreatment: Differences between caregiver and elder perceptions. *Journal of Mental Health and Aging* 2:89-98.
Fulmer, T., and T. Wetle
    1986   Elder abuse screening and intervention. *Nurse Practitioner* 11(5):33-38.
Fulmer, T., and T.A. O'Malley
    1987   *Inadequate Care of the Elderly: A Health Care Perspective on Abuse and Neglect.* New York: Springer.
Gordis, L.
    1996   *Epidemiology.* Philadelphia: W.B. Saunders.
Grafstrom, M., A. Nordberg, and B. Winblad
    1993   Abuse is in the eye of the beholder. *Scandinavian Journal of Social Medicine* 21(4):247-255.
Gray, J., P.M. Lyons, and G.B. Melton
    1995   *Ethical and Legal Issues in AIDS Research.* Baltimore, MD: Johns Hopkins University Press.
Greenberg, J.R., M. McKibben, and J.A. Raymond
    1990   Dependent adult children and elder abuse. *Journal of Elder Abuse and Neglect* 2:73-86.
Grisso, T., and P. Appelbaum
    1998   *Assessing Competence to Consent to Treatment: A Guide for Physicians and Other Health Professionals.* New York: Oxford University Press.
Hajjar, I., and E. Duthie, Jr.
    2001   Prevalence of elder abuse in the United States: A comparative report between the national and Wisconsin data. *Wisconsin Medical Journal* 100(6):22-26.
Harrell, R., C.H. Torongo, J. McLaughlin, V.N. Pavlik, D.J. Hyman, and C.B. Dyer
    2002   How geriatricians identify elder abuse and neglect. *American Journal of Medical Science* 323(1):34-38.
Harrington, C., M. LaPlante, R.J. Newcomer, B. Bedney, S. Shostak, P. Summers, J. Weinberg, and I. Basnett
    2000   A review of Federal Statutes and Regulations for Personal Care and Home and Community-Based Services: A Final report. Unpublished paper. San Francisco: University of California, Department of Social and Behavioral Sciences.
Hawes, C., M. Rose, and C.D. Phillips
    1999   *A National Study of Assisted Living for the Frail Elderly: Results of a National Survey of Facilities.* Beachwood, OH: Myers Research Institute.
Hawes, C., D. Blevins, and L. Shanley
    2001   *Preventing Abuse and Neglect in Nursing Homes: The Role of the Nurse Aide Registries.* Report to the Centers for Medicare and Medicaid Services (formerly HCFA) from the School of Rural Public Health. College Station, TX: Texas A&M University System Health Science Center.

Henderson, S.
1998   Epidemiology of dementia. *Annals de Medicine Interne* (Paris) 149(4):181-186.
Hetzel, L., and A. Smith
2001   *The 65 Years and Over Population: 2000.* Report No. C2KBR/01-10. Economic and Statistic Administration, Bureau of the Census. Washington, DC: U.S. Department of Commerce.
Hickey, T., and R.L. Douglass
1981   Mistreatment of the elderly in the domestic setting: An exploratory study. *American Journal of Public Health* 71(5):500-507.
Himes, C.L., A.K. Jordan, and J.I. Farkas
1996   Factors influencing parental caregiving by adult women: Variations in care intensity and duration. *Research on Aging* 18:349-370.
Hoffman, D., and J. Schwartz
1998   Proxy consent to participation of the decisionally impaired in medical research—Maryland's policy initiative. *Journal of Health Care Law and Policy* 1:123-153.
Homer, A.C., and C. Gilleard
1990   Abuse of elderly people by their caregivers. *British Medical Journal* 301(6765): 1359-1362.
House, J.S., D. Umberson, and K.R. Landis
1988   Structures and processes of social support. *Annual Review of Sociology* 14:293-318.
Hwalek, M.A., M.C. Sengstock, and R. Lawrence
1984   Assessing the Probability of Abuse of the Elderly. Paper presented at the 37th Annual Scientific Meeting of the Gerontological Society of America, San Antonio, TX.
Hwalek, M.A., and M.C. Sengstock
1986   Hwalek-Sengstock Elder Abuse Screening Test-Revised. *Journal of Applied Gerontology* 5(2):153-173.
Institute of Medicine
1996   *Nursing Staff in Hospitals and Nursing Homes: Is It Adequate?* Committee on the Adequacy of Nursing Staff in Hospitals and Nursing Homes. G.S. Wunderlich, F.A. Sloan, and C.K. Davis, eds. Washington, DC: National Academy Press.
1997   *The Hidden Epidemic: Confronting Sexually Transmitted Diseases.* Thomas R. Eng and William T. Butler, eds. Committee on Prevention and Control of Sexually Transmitted Diseases, Institute of Medicine. Washington, DC: National Academy Press.
1999   *Reducing the Burden of Injury: Advancing Prevention and Treatment.* Committee on Injury Prevention and Control. Richard J. Bonnie, Carolyn E. Fulco, and Catharyn T. Liverman, eds. Washington, DC: National Academy Press.
2001   *Improving the Quality of Long-Term Care.* Committee on Improving Long-Term Care, Division of Health Care Services. Gooloo S. Wunderlich and Peter O. Kohler, eds. Washington, DC: National Academy Press.
Jones J.S., J.P. Veenstra, J.P. Seamon, and J. Krohmer
1997   Elder mistreatment: National survey of emergency physicians. *Annals of Emergency Medicine* 30(4):473-479.
Kelman C., and L. Smith
2000   It's time: Record linkage—the vision and the reality. *Australian and New Zealand Journal of Public Health* 24(1):100-101.

Kempe, C., F. Silverman, B. Steele, W. Droegemueller, and H. Silver
    1962   The battered-child syndrome. *Journal of the American Medical Association*
            181:17-24.
Kim, S., E.D. Caine, G.W. Currier, A. Leibovici, and J.M. Ryan
    2001   Assessing the competence of persons with Alzheimer's disease in providing in-
            formed consent for participation in research. *American Journal of Psychiatry*
            158:712-717.
Kivela, S.L., P. Kongas-Saviaro, E. Kesti, K. Pahkala, and M.L. Ijas
    1992   Abuse in old age: Epidemiological data from Finland. *Journal of Elder Abuse
            and Neglect* 4(3):1-18.
Lachs, M.S., L. Berkman, T. Fulmer, and R. Horwitz
    1994   A prospective community-based pilot study of risk factors for the investigation of
            elder mistreatment. *Journal of the American Geriatrics Society* 42(2):169-173.
Lachs, M.S., and K. Pillemer
    1995   Abuse and neglect of elderly persons. *New England Journal of Medicine*
            333(7):437.
Lachs, M.S., C. Williams, S. O'Brien, L. Hurst, and R. Horwitz
    1996   Older adults. An 11-year longitudinal study of adult protective service use. *Ar-
            chives of Internal Medicine* 156(4):449-453.
    1997a   Risk factors for reported elder abuse and neglect: A nine-year observational
            cohort study. *The Gerontologist* 37(4):469-474.
Lachs, M.S., C.S. Williams, S. O'Brien, L. Hurst, A. Kossack, A. Siegal, and M.E. Tinetti
    1997b   ED use by older victims of family violence. *Annals of Emergency Medicine*
            30(4):448-454.
Langlois, N.E.I., and G.A. Gresham
    1991   The ageing of bruises: A review and study of the colour changes with time.
            Forensic Science International 50:227-238.
Laumann, E.O., J. Gagnon, R.T. Michael, and S. Michaels
    1994   *The Social Organization of Sexuality: Sexual Practices in the United States.*
            Chicago: University of Chicago Press.
Laumann, E.O., and Y. Youm
    2001   Racial/ethnic group differences in the prevalence of sexually transmitted diseases
            in the United States: A network approach. In *Sex, Love, and Health in America:
            Private Choices and Public Policies*, Edward O. Laumann and Robert T. Michael,
            eds. Chicago: University of Chicago Press.
Levine, R.
    1986   Ethics and regulations of clinical research. Baltimore, MD: Urban and
            Schwarzenberg.
Lin, N., X. Ye, and W.M. Ensel
    1999   Social support and depressed mood: A structural analysis. *Journal of Health and
            Social Behavior* 40:344-359.
Mahay, J., E.O. Laumann, and S. Michaels
    2001   Race, gender, and class in sexual scripts. In *Sex, Love, and Health: Private
            Choices and Public Policies*, Edward O. Laumann and Robert T. Michael, eds.
            Chicago: University of Chicago Press.
Malone, M.L., N. Rozario, M. Gavinski, and J. Goodwin
    1991   The epidemiology of skin tears in the institutionalized elderly. *Journal of the
            American Geriatric Society* 39:591-595.
Marson, D., K. Ingram, H. Cody, and L. Harrell
    1995   Assessing the competency of patients with Alzheimer's disease under different
            legal standards: A prototype instrument. *Archives of Neurology* 52:949-954.

Manton K.G., L. Corder, and E. Stallard
  1997   Chronic disability trends in elderly United States populations: 1982-1994. *Proceedings of the National Academy of Sciences of the United States of America* 94(6):2593-2598.
Melton, G.B.
  2002   Chronic neglect of family violence: More than a decade of reports to guide U.S. policy. Paper presented to the Center for Child and Family Policy, Duke University, May 15, 2002.
Melton, G., and F. Barry, eds.
  1994   *Protecting Children from Abuse and Neglect.* New York: Guilford Press.
Melton, G.B., J. Petrila, N.G. Poythress, and C. Slobogin
  1997   *Psychological Evaluations for the Courts: A Handbook for Mental Health Professionals and Lawyers* 2nd ed. New York: Guilford.
Melton, G., R. Levine, G. Koocher, R. Rosenthal, and W. Thompson
  1988   Community consultation in socially sensitive research: Lessons from clinical trials of treatments for AIDS. *American Psychology* 43:573-581.
Melton, G., and A.B. Andrews
  2000   Building systems for safety in the family: The U.S experience. New Global Development. *Journal of International and Comparative Social Welfare* 16:24-25.
Melton, G., R. Thompson, and M. Small
  2001   *Toward a Child-Centered Neighborhood-Based Child Protection System.* Westport, CT: Praeger Press.
Moody, L., A. Voss, and C.A. Lengacher
  2000   Assessing abuse among the elderly living in public housing. *Journal of Nursing Measurement* 8(1):61-70.
Myers, J.E.B.
  1993   The competence of young children to testify in legal proceedings. *Behavioral Science and the Law* 11:121.
National Association of Adult Protective Services Administrators
  2002   Adult Protective Services Ethical Principles and Best Practice Guidelines. Available at: http://www.elderabusecenter.org/publication/ethics.pdf. [July 8, 2002].
National Bioethics Advisory Commission
  1998   *Research Involving Persons with Mental Disorders That May Impair Decisionmaking Capacity* vol. 1. Bethesda, MD: National Bioethics Advisory Commission.
  2001   *Ethical and Policy Issues in Research Involving Human Participants: Report and Recommendations.* Bethesda, MD: National Bioethics Advisory Commission.
National Center on Elder Abuse
  1998   The National Elder Abuse Incidence Study, Final Report. Prepared for the Administration on Aging in collaboration with Westat, Inc.
National Institute of Justice
  2000   Elder Justice: Medical Forensic Issues Concerning Abuse and Neglect. Summary of a Roundtable, October 18, 2000, Washington, DC.
National Research Council
  1988   *The Aging Population in the Twenty-First Century. Statistics for Health Policy.* Committee on National Statistics. Dorothy M. Gilford, ed. Commission on Behavioral and Social Sciences and Education. Washington, DC: National Academy Press.
  1993   *Understanding and Preventing Violence.* Panel on the Understanding and Control of Violent Behavior. Albert J. Reiss, Jr., and Jeffrey A. Roth, eds. Commission on Behavioral and Social Sciences and Education. Washington, DC: National Academy Press.

1996   *Understanding Violence Against Women.* Panel on Research on Violence Against Women. Nancy A. Crowell and Ann W. Burgess, eds. Commission on Behavioral and Social Sciences and Education. Washington, DC: National Academy Press.

2000a   *Improving Access to and Confidentiality of Research Data: Report of a Workshop.* Committee on National Statistics, Christopher Mackie and Norman Bradburn, eds. Division of Behavioral and Social Sciences and Education. Washington, DC: National Academy Press.

2000b   *Cells and Surveys: Should Biological Measures Be Included in Social Science Research?* Committee on Population. Caleb E. Finch, James W. Vaupel, and Kevin Kinsella, eds. Division of Behavioral and Social Sciences and Education. Washington, DC: National Academy Press.

2001   *Confronting Chronic Neglect: The Education and Training of Health Professionals on Family Violence.* Committee on the Training Needs of Health Professionals to Respond to Family Violence. Felicia Cohn, Marla E. Salmon, and John D. Stobo, eds. Washington, DC: National Academy Press.

National Research Council and the Institute of Medicine
1998   *Understanding Child Abuse and Neglect.* Panel on Research on Child Abuse and Neglect, Commission on Behavioral and Social Sciences and Education. Washington, DC: National Academy Press.

Nelson, B.
1984   *Making an Issue of Child Abuse.* Chicago: University of Chicago Press.

Newberger, E.
1998   Child abuse. In *Public Health and Preventive Medicine*, R.B. Wallace, editor. Stamford, CT: Appleton and Lange.

Nielsen C., and R.S. Lang
1999   Principles of screening. *Medical Clinics of North America* 83(6):1323-1337.

Noelker L.S., and D.M. Bass
1995   Service use by caregivers of elderly receiving case management. *Journal of Case Management* 4:156-161.

Ogg, J.
1993   Researching elder abuse in Britain. *Journal of Elder Abuse and Neglect* 5(2): 37-54.

Ogg, J., and G.C.J. Bennett
1992   Elder abuse in Britain. *British Medical Journal* 305:998-999.

Paveza G.J., D. Cohen, C. Eisdorfer, S. Freels, T. Semla, W. Ashford, P. Gorelick, R. Hirschman, D. Luchins, and P. Levy
1992   Severe family violence and Alzheimer's disease: Prevalence and risk factors. *The Gerontologist* 32:493-497.

Pavlik, V.N., D.J. Hyman, N.A. Festa, and C.B. Dyer
2001   Quantifying the problem of abuse and neglect in adults: Analysis of a statewide database. *Journal of the American Geriatrics Society* 49(1):45-48.

Peddle, N., and C.T. Wang
2001   *Current Trends in Child Abuse Prevention Reporting and Fatalities: The 1999 Fifty State Survey.* Chicago: Prevent Child Abuse America.

Pelton, L.
1994   The role of material factors in child abuse and neglect. In *Protecting Children from Abuse and Neglect*, Gary Melton and Frank Barry, eds. New York: Guilford Press.

Pepper, C., and M.R. Okar
  1981   *Elder Abuse: An Examination of a Hidden Problem.* Pub. No. 97-277. Wash-
          ington, DC: U.S. Government Printing Office.
Phillips, L.R.
  1983   Abuse and neglect of the frail elderly at home: An exploration of theoretical
          relationships. *Journal of Advanced Nursing* 8:379-392.
Pillemer, K.A.
  1985   The dangers of dependency: New findings on domestic violence against the
          elderly. *Social Problems* 33(2):146-158.
  1986   Risk factors in elder abuse: Results from a case-control study. In *Elder Abuse:
          Conflict in the Family,* K.A. Pillemer and R.S. Wolf, eds. Dover, DE: Auburn
          House Publishing Company.
  1988   Maltreatment of patients in nursing homes: Overview and research agenda. *Jour-
          nal of Health and Social Behavior* 29(September):227-238.
  2001   Critical Research Needs in the Study of Elder Abuse. Unpublished paper pre-
          sented to the Panel on Elder Abuse and Neglect, Washington, DC, May 24, 2000.
          Ithaca, NY: Department of Human Development, Cornell University.
Pillemer, K., and R. Bachman-Prehn
  1991   Helping and hurting: Predictors of maltreatment of patients in nursing homes.
          Research on Aging 13:74-95.
Pillemer, K.A., and D. Finkelhor
  1988   The prevalence of elder abuse: A random sample survey. *The Gerontologist*
          28(1):51-57.
  1989   Causes of elder abuse: Caregiver stress versus problem relatives. *American Jour-
          nal of Orthopsychiatry* 59:179-187.
Pillemer, K., and B. Hudson
  1993   A model abuse prevention program for nursing assistants. *The Gerontologist*
          33:128-131.
Pillemer, K., and D.W. Moore
  1989   Abuse of patients in nursing homes: Findings from a survey of staff. *The Geron-
          tologist* 29:314-320.
Pillemer, K., and J.J. Suitor
  1992   Violence and violent feelings: What causes them among family givers? *Journal of
          Gerontology* 47:S165-S172.
Platt, A.M.
  1969   *The Child Savers.* Chicago: University of Chicago Press.
Podnieks, E.
  1992   National Survey on Abuse of the Elderly in Canada. *Journal of Elder Abuse and
          Neglect* 41(1/2):5-58.
Population Projections Program
  2000   Population Projections of the United States by Age, Sex, Race, Hispanic Origin,
          and Nativity: 1999 to 2100. [Available at: http://ftp.census.gov/population/
          projections/nation/detail/np-d5-cd.txt.]
Quayhagen, M., M.P. Quayhagen, T.L. Patterson, M. Irwin, R. L. Hauger, and I. Grant
  1997   Coping with dementia: Family caregiver burnout and abuse. *Journal of Mental
          Health and Aging* 3:357-364.
Reay, A.M., and K.D. Browne
  2001   Risk factors for caregivers who physically abuse or neglect their elderly depen-
          dents. *Aging and Mental Health* 5(1):56-62.

Reis, M., D. Nahmiash, and R. Schrier
  1993   The Brief Abuse Screen for the Elderly. Paper presented at the 22nd Annual
          Scientific and Educational Meeting of the Canadian Association on Gerontology,
          Montreal, Quebec, Canada.
Reis, M., and D. Nahmiash
  1995   Validation of the caregiver abuse screen (CASE). *Canadian Journal of Aging*
          14:45-60.
  1998   Validation of the indicators of abuse (IOA) screen. *The Gerontologist* 38(4):471-
          480.
Rice, D.P., H.M. Fillit, W. Max, D.S. Kropman, J.R. Lloyd, and S. Duttagupta
  2001   Prevalence, costs, and treatment of Alzheimer's disease and related dementia: A
          managed care perspective. *American Journal of Managed Care* 7(8):809-818.
Rich, J.S., and H.C. Sox
  2000   Screening in the elderly: Principles and practice. *Hospital Practice* (Office Edi-
          tion) 35(10):45-48, 53-56.
Sandefur, R., and E.O. Laumann
  1998   A paradigm for social capital. *Rationality and Society* (November) 10:481-501.
Saywitz, K.J., G.S. Goodman, and T.D. Lyon
  2002   Interviewing children in and out of court: Current research and practice implica-
          tions. In *The APSAC Handbook on Child Maltreatment* 2nd ed., J.E.B. Myers,
          L. Berliner, J. Briere, C.T. Hendrix, C. Jenny, and T.A. Reid, eds. Thousand
          Oaks, CA: Sage Publications.
Schechter, S., and J.L. Edleson
  1999   *Effective Intervention in Domestic Violence and Child Maltreatment: Guidelines
          for Policy and Practice.* Reno, NV: National Council of Juvenile and Family
          Court Judges.
Schiamberg, L.B., and D. Gans
  1999   Elder abuse by adult children: An applied ecological framework for understand-
          ing contextual risk factors and the intergenerational character of the quality of
          life. *International Journal of Aging and Human Development* 50:329-359.
Schoeni R.F., V.A. Freedman, and R.B. Wallace
  2001   Persistent, consistent, widespread, and robust? Another look at recent trends in
          old-age disability. *Journals of Gerontology Series B-Psychological Sciences &
          Social Sciences* 56(4):S206-218.
Schulz R., and S.R. Beach
  1999   Caregiving as a risk factor for mortality: The Caregiver Health Effects Study.
          Journal of the American Medical Association 282(23):2215-2219.
Simon, W., and J.H. Gagnon
  1987   A sexual scripts approach. In *Theories of Human Sexuality,* W.T. O'Donohue
          and J.H. Greer, eds. New York: Plenum.
Spitzer, R.L.
  1983   Psychiatric diagnosis: Are clinicians still necessary? *Comprehensive Psychiatry*
          24:399-411.
Stark, E., and A.H. Flitcraft
  1998   Woman battering. In *Public Health and Preventive Medicine,* R.B. Wallace, ed.
          Stamford, CT: Appleton and Lange.
Steinmetz, S.K.
  1988   *Duty Bound: Elder Abuse and Family Care.* Newbury Park, CA: Sage Publica-
          tions.

Stone, R.I.
  2000   *Long-Term Care for the Elderly With Disabilities: Current Policy, Emerging Trends, and Implications for the Twenty-First Century.* New York: Milbank Memorial Fund.
Straus, M.A.
  1978   The Conflict Tactic Scale. Reprinted in *Handbook of Family Measurement Techniques*, J. Touliatos, B. Perlmutter, and M. Straus, eds. Newbury Park, CA: Sage Publications.
Straus, M.A., and R.J Gelles
  1990   *Physical Violence in American Families.* New Brunswick, NJ: Transaction Publishers.
  1992   National Family Violence Survey: Wife battering and violence outside the family. *Journal of Interpersonal Violence* 7:462-470.
Strauss, R.P., S. Sengputa, S.C. Quinn, J. Goeppinger, C. Spaulding, S.M. Kegeles, and G. Millett
  2001   The role of community advisory boards: Involving communities in the informed consent process. *American Journal of Public Health* (12)91:1938-1943.
Thomas, C.
  2000   First national study of elder abuse and neglect: Contrast with results from other studies. *Journal of Elder Abuse and Neglect* 12(1):1-14.
Timmreck, T.C.
  1998   *An Introduction to Epidemiology.* Boston: Jones & Bartlett Publishers.
Tornstam, L.
  1989   Abuse of the elderly in Denmark and Sweden: Results from a population study. *Journal of Elder Abuse and Neglect* 1(1):35-44.
U.S. Advisory Board on Child Abuse and Neglect
  1990   *Child Abuse and Neglect: Critical First Steps in Response to a National Emergency.* Washington, DC: U.S. Department of Health and Human Services.
  1993   *The Continuing Child Protection Emergency: A Challenge to the Nation.* Washington, DC: U.S. Department of Health and Human Services.
U.S. Department of Health, Education, and Welfare
  1966   State letter No. 925. Subject: Four Model Demonstration Projects...Services to Older Adults in the Public Welfare Program. Cited in District of Columbia, 1967, *Protective Services for Adults: Report on Protective Services Prepared for the D.C. Interdepartmental Committee on Aging*, Washington, DC.
U.S. Department of Health and Human Services
  2001a Federal policy for the protection of human subjects (Common Rule). *Code of Federal Regulations* 45:§46.
  2001b Protection of identity—Research subjects. *Code of Federal Regulations* 42:§2a.
U.S. Food and Drug Administration
  1999   Protection of human subjects. *Code of Federal Regulations* 21:Parts 50 and 56.
U.S. General Accounting Office
  2002   *Nursing Homes: More Can Be Done to Protect Residents from Abuse*, GAO-02-312. Washington, DC: U.S. Government Printing Office.
Weisberg, D.
  1984   The discovery of sexual abuse. *University of California (Davis) Law Review* 18:1-57.
Williamson, G.M., and D.R. Shaffer
  2001   Caregiver loss and quality of care provided: Pre-illness relationship makes a difference. In *Loss and Trauma: General and Close Relationship Perspectives*, J.H. Harvey and E.D. Miller, eds. Philadelphia: Brunner/Mazel.

Wisconsin Department of Health and Family Services
   2001   Adult Protective Services Modernization Project Report. Available at: http://
           www.dhfs.state.wi.us/aps/.
Wolf, R.
   1997a   Elder abuse and neglect: Causes and consequences. *Journal of Geriatric Psychia-
           try* 30(1):153-174.
   1997b   *Factors Affecting the Rate of Elder Abuse Reporting to a State Protective Services
           Program.* Washington, DC: National Committee for the Prevention of Elder
           Abuse.
   1999   A Research Agenda on Abuse of Older Persons and Adults with Disabilities.
           Available at: http://www.preventelderabuse.org/professionals/r_agenda.html.
Wolf, R.S., M. Godkin, and K.A. Pillemer
   1984   *Elder Abuse and Neglect: Findings from Three Model Projects.* Worcester, MA:
           University of Massachusetts Medical Center, University Center on Aging.
Wolf, R.S., and K. Pillemer
   1989   *Helping Elderly Victims: The Reality of Elder Abuse.* New York: Columbia
           University Press.
Wolf, R.S., and D. Li
   1999   Factors affecting the rate of elder abuse reporting to a state protective services
           program. *The Gerontologist* 39(2):222-228.
Wolf, R.S., C.P. Strugnell, and M.A. Godkin
   1982   *Preliminary Findings from Three Model Projects on Elderly Abuse, Center on
           Aging.* Worcester, MA: University of Massachusetts Medical Center.

APPENDIX
A
Elder Mistreatment
Measures and Studies

TABLE A-1 Elder Mistreatment Measures

Measure	Summary	Characteristics	Properties
Pathophysiological signs and symptoms Fulmer (1984) Lachs and Fulmer (1993) Dyer et al. (2000) Haviland and O'Brien (1989) O'Brien (1986)	Uses items such as unexplained bruising, dehydration, urine burns, fractures.	Subjective and objective clinical observations as documented by health care clinicians.	Poor sensitivity and specificity.
Conflict Tactic Scale Straus (1978)	Perception of upsetting and injurious circumstances in a person's life.	19-item self-report, e.g., "Has anyone threatened you with a knife or gun?"	Chronbach's alpha reliability: 0.88. Content validity 0.80. Available in Spanish.
Elder Assessment Instrument Fulmer (1984)	Provides information to clinicians to better inform judgments about risk of elder mistreatment.	40-item screening tool with both subjective and objective items to determine if an older person should be referred for suspected elder mistreatment.	Content validity 0.83. Interrater agreement 0.84. Available in Spanish.
The QUALCARE Scale Phillips et al. (1990a, 1990b)	Assessment of six areas: physical, medical management, psychosocial, environmental, human rights, and financial.	53-item observational rating scale designed to quantify and qualify family caregiving.	Extensive psychometrics reported: Interrater agreement range: 0.79-0.88. Chronbach's alpha: 0.81-0.95 on 6 subscales.
Hwalek-Sengstock Elder Abuse Screening Test Neale et al. (1991)	Assessment of physical, financial, psychological, and neglectful situations.	15-item assessment screen for detecting suspected elder abuse and neglect.	Discriminant function analysis: 9 items identified 94% of cases. Three conceptual domains: violation of personal rights, characteristics of vulnerability, and potentially abusive situations.

TABLE A-1 Continued

Measure	Summary	Characteristics	Properties
Fulmer Restriction Scale Fulmer and Gurland (1996)	Assessment of physical, psychological, and financial restriction of older adults.	34-item scale designed to elicit information regarding unnecessary restriction of the older adult.	Chronbach's alpha: 0.78. Interrater agreement: 0.93. Available in Spanish.
Indicators of Abuse Screen Reis and Nahmiash (1998)	Developed specifically for use by social service agency practitioners likely to visit the older adult in the home.	29-item set of indicators for use by social service agency practitioners to identify elder mistreatment.	Discriminant function analysis: 29 items identified 96.3% of cases. Factor analysis: no reliable pattern of variable clusters.
Adult Protective Service Reports	Intake forms used to document calls of suspected elder mistreatment from public hot lines and state agencies.	No specific format.	No psychometrics available.

VASS (Vulnerability to Abuse Scale)
Schofield, M.J. & Mishra, G.D. (2003). Gerontologist 43(1), 110-120.
ask for list of other screens

TABLE A-2 Elder Mistreatment Studies

Study	Methods	Selected Findings
Childs et al. (2000)	Design: Descriptive Measure: (1) SVWS; (2) EAA BIS-R Sample: Nonrandom: 422 young and 201 middle-aged adults Theory: N/A	Middle-aged respondents viewed psychological behavior more harshly than younger respondent.s Both middle-aged women and young men were less tolerant of middle-aged perpetrators. Data support relativistic nature of elder abuse.
Coyne et al. (1993)	Design: Descriptive survey Measure: Demographics; Zarit Burden interview; Zung Self-Rating Depression Scale Sample: 1,000 caregivers who called a telephone help line for dementia; 342 respondents	Mean age of caregiver 56.1; 54.5% were adult children caring for parents; 37.1% caring for spouses; 8.4% cared for other relatives. 11.9% reported they had been physically abusive toward dementia patients. Abusers had been providing care for more years; patients functioned at a lower level; caregivers had higher burden and depression scores.
Dyer et al. (2000)	Design: Case-control study Intervention: Comprehensive geriatric assessment Measure: Standard geriatric assessment tools Sample: 47 older persons referred for neglect and 97 referred for other reasons	45 cases of abuse or neglect identified. 37 were self-neglect. Elder mistreatment cases were more likely to be white and male. Higher prevalence of depression and dementia.
Ertem et al. (2000)	Design: Descriptive Method: Meta-analysis Sample: 10 studies	10 studies: 4 cohort, 1 cross-sectional, and 5 case- control. The RR of maltreatment in children of abused parents were significantly increased in 4 studies (RR 4.75-37.8). In 3 other studies the RR was less than 2. Significant validity issues.

TABLE A-2 Continued

Study	Methods	Selected Findings
Fulmer and Gurland (1996)	Design: Descriptive Measure: CTS, FRS and NMAP Survey, Beck Depression Scale, BDBS Sample: 125 elder-caregiver dyads; 51 dyads with cognitive impairment and 74 dyads with no cognitive impairment; mean age of the elder 78 years Theory: Risk and vulnerability	Cognitive impairment risk factor for elder mistreatment. CTS higher for CI patients. FRS higher for CI patients. CI patients more dependent. CI patients had higher BDBS. CI patients had higher Zarit Burden scores.
Fulmer et al. (1999)	Design: Descriptive Method: Analysis of a probability sample of ADHC clients in New York State. Social workers served as informants. Sample: 9 sites drawn through random sampling	Prevalence of elder mistreatment 12.3%. Apprehensive behavior was highest reported behavior; with this item removed, prevalence 3.6%. Social workers noted concern regarding elders who appeared frightened in the presence of their home caregiver.
Fulmer et al. (2000)	Design: Descriptive Measure: EAI, MMSE Sample: 180 emergency department patients over the age of 70 with MMSE of 18 or greater	36 patients eligible for study. 7 patients screened positive for neglect. Nurses were able to screen for elder neglect with greater than 70% accuracy; true positive 71%, false positive 7%.
Huber et al. (2001)	Design: Descriptive Method: Analysis of cross-sectional 6-state ombudsman database Sample: 23,787 complaints	5 most frequent complaints were (1) loss of dignity and respect; (2) accidents; (3) physical abuse; (4) call lights unanswered; (5) poor personal hygiene. Race and gender differences noted.
Hudson (1991)	Design: Descriptive Measure: 3-round Delphi survey Sample: 63 elder mistreatment experts	Agreement on a 5-level taxonomy. 11 theoretical definitions proposed by panel.

TABLE A-2 Continued

Study	Methods	Selected Findings
Hwalek et al. (1996)	Design: Descriptive Method: Database analysis Measure: Risk of Future Abuse instrument Sample: State of Illinois Abuse, Neglect and Exploitation Tracking System; 2,577 cases from October 1989 to December 1991. 552 substantiated reports used for this study	73% of victims were women. Mean age 77 (60-99). Caucasian 73%; widowed 54%; living at home 76%. Caregiver substance abuse more likely to involve physical or emotional abuse.
Jogerst et al. (2000)	Design: Descriptive Method: Analysis of county-level data between 1984 and 1993 to test association between county characteristics and rates of elder abuse Sample: 99 counties in Iowa Analysis: univariate correlational analysis and stagewise linear regression	Community characteristics that had a positive association with rates of reported or substantiated elder mistreatment were: (1) population density; (2) children in poverty; (3) reported child abuse.
Jones et al. (1997)	Design: Descriptive Method: Random sample survey Sample: 3,000 members of the American College of Emergency Physicians; 705 completed surveys (response rate 24%)	52% of respondents described elder mistreatment as prevalent but less than spouse or child abuse. Respondents evaluated a mean of 4 ± 8 suspected cases of elder mistreatment in the last 12 months; 50% were reported.
Lachs et al. (1994)	Design: Prospective cohort study Method: Case matching with adult protective services database Sample: 329 elders investigated in 1985 and 1986 Analysis: Relative risk calculations	68 (2.4%) of database cohort members received ombudsman investigation. Risk factors for elder mistreatment investigation using logistic regression included requiring assistance with feeding OR 3.5, being a minority elder OR 2.3, over age 75 at cohort inception OR 1.9, and poor social networks OR 1.7.

TABLE A-2 Continued

Study	Methods	Selected Findings
Lachs et al. (1997a)	Design: Prospective cohort study Method: Case matching with adult protective services database Sample: 184 cohort members Analysis: Pooled logistic regression	47 cohort members were seen for elder mistreatment (prevalence 1.6%). Age, race, poverty, functional disability, and cognitive impairment were identified as risk factors for reported elder mistreatment, with ORs reported. The onset of new cognitive impairment was also associated with abuse and neglect. The influence of race and poverty is likely to be overestimated due to reporting bias.
Lachs et al. (1997b)	Design: Prospective cohort study Method: 7-year longitudinal database with identification of 182 victims of elder abuse Sample: 114 elders seen in 2 emergency departments	114 individuals accounted for 628 visits (median 3, range 1-46). 30.6% resulted in hospital admission. 66% had at least one visit that resulted in an injury-related chief complaint.
Lachs et al. (1998)	Design: Prospective cohort study Measure: mortality among elders for whom protective services were used to corroborate mistreatment and elderly persons for whom protective services were used for self-neglect Sample: 176 adult protective services elders	Cohort members seen for elder mistreatment at any time during follow up had poorer survival (9%) than others. Reported and corroborated elder mistreatment and self-neglect are associated with shorter survival after adjusting for other factors associated with increased mortality in older adults.

TABLE A-2 Continued

Study	Methods	Selected Findings
Moody et al. (2000)	Design: Descriptive Measure: H-S/EAST Sample: 100 black, Hispanic, and white elders living in public housing	Principal components FA of 15-item instrument supported the 3-factor structure for a total of 10 items explaining 38% of the variance. Discriminant function analysis showed that 6 items were as effective as the 9-item model in classifying cases as abused (71.4%).
National Center on Elder Abuse at the American Public Human Services Association [formerly American Public Welfare Association] in collaboration with Westat, Inc. (1998)	Design: Descriptive study Method: Incidence study using sentinel agency reports Sample: 20 counties in 15 states: nationally representative sample	551,000 elder mistreatment cases in 1996. Female elders are abused at higher rates than males. The oldest elders (80 years and older) are abused and neglected at 2-3 times their proportion in the elderly population. In almost 90% of elder mistreatment cases, the perpetrator is a family member and 2/3 are adult children or spouses. Victims of self-neglect are usually depressed, confused, or extremely frail.
O'Malley et al. (1984)	Design: Descriptive Measure: Case analysis using OARS Sample: 24 cases from primary care clinic	Cases divided into three categories: (1) extremely impaired who receive care from individuals responsible for abuse and neglect (N = 4); (2) impaired elders who receive inadequate or intermittent care (N = 9); (3) involved independent elders whose only care needs resulted from threats or violence from relatives (N = 11).

TABLE A-2 Continued

STudy	Methods	Selected Findings
Paveza et al. (1992)	Design: Descriptive Measure: CTS Sample: Purposive sample from Alzheimer's disease registry: 184 patients	Severe family violence as measured by the CTS was a significant problem: overall prevalence 17.4%. 15.8% of patients had been violent since diagnosis. 5.4% of caregivers reported being violent toward the patient. Violence by the Alzheimer's disease patient against the caregiver was serious problem.
Pavlik et al. (2001)	Design: Descriptive Method: Analysis of Texas Department of Protective and Regulatory Services, Adult Protective Services Sample: 62,258 allegations of elder mistreatment in 1997	Neglect accounted for 80% of allegations. The incidence of being reported to adult protective services increased sharply after age 65. Prevalence was 1,310 over 100,000 > 65 years of age.
Phillips and Rempusheski (1985)	Design: Descriptive Method: Interviews with grounded theory analysis Sample: 29 health care providers (16 nurses and 13 social workers)	4-stage model describing decisions of health care providers about elder abuse. Model identifies 3 types of decisions: diagnostic, value, and intervention Complexity of decision processes is revealed via 5 pathways.
Phillips et al. (1990a)	Design: Adaptation of the QUALPACS Method: Instrument development Sample: Piloted with 8 data collectors (4 in each of 2 sites) who interviewed 4 elder-caregiver dyads. A total of 29 elder-caregiver dyads were interviewed	QUALCARE Scale contains six subscales and 53 items. Included in 6 subscales: environmental, physical, medical maintenance, psychological, human rights, and financial.

TABLE A-2 Continued

Study	Methods	Selected Findings
Phillips et al. (1990b)	Design: Descriptive correlational study Measure: QUALCARE Sample: Convenient sample of 249 elder-caregiver dyads	Interrater reliability for 55 observations ranged from 79% to 88%. Internal consistency: alpha = .097. Conceptual structure: confirmatory factor analysis indicated 6 significant factors accounting for 64.4% of the variance. Criterion validity: all correlations between criteria variables and QUALCARE were in correct direction and $p \leq 0.05$ level. Construct validity: 8 of 9 correlations in the predicted direction.
Pillemer and Finkelhor (1988)	Design: Descriptive Method: Stratified random sample survey Sample: 2,020 community-dwelling elders in metropolitan Boston	63 elder persons were maltreated. Rate of 32 per 1,000. 95% confidence interval of 25-39 per 1,000. No minority differences or age differences. Those in poor health were 3 to 4 times likely to be abused. Males were more likely to be abused than females.
Pillemer and Finkelhor (1989)	Design: Descriptive Method: Case control Sample: 46 abuse or neglect victims and 215 random controls	Factors associated with elder mistreatment included abuser factors of deviance, dependence on victim, and life stress. Victim factors included court help, disability, dependence on abuser, and conflictual relationship (spouse only).

TABLE A-2 Continued

Study	Methods	Selected Findings
Pillemer and Moore (1989)	Design: Descriptive Measure: CTS Sample: 577 nursing personnel from 31 nursing homes in New Hampshire	36% of the sample had seen at least one incident of physical abuse in the preceding year. Most frequent abuse observed was excessive restraint. Second most frequent type was physical abuse. 81% observed at least one psychologically abusive incident in the preceding year. 10% of respondents reported committing physical abuse. 40% of respondents reported committing psychological abuse.
Pillemer and Suitor (1992)	Design: Descriptive Method: Analysis of quantitative and qualitative data Sample: 236 family caregivers for dementia victims	Characteristics predictive of violent feelings in caregivers included physical aggression by elder, disruptive behaviors, and a shared living situation. Structural relationship and caregiver age were related to actual violence; spouses were more likely to be violent than other relatives, as were older individuals. Violence by elder was positively related to caregiver violence.
Rosenblatt et al. (1996)	Design: Descriptive Method: Analysis of State of Michigan records of reported cases of suspected elder abuse 1989–1993 Sample: 27,371 cases of possible elder mistreatment	17,238 of cases were older than age 65. Physicians reported only 2% of cases. Physician reporting rates did not increase over a 5-year period.

TABLE A-2 Continued

Study	Methods	Selected Findings
Shaw (1998)	Design: Descriptive Method: Grounded theory Sample: 21 semistructured interviews conducted with six abuse investigators and 15 nursing home staff	The two types of abusive nursing home staff were identified as reactive and sadistic.
Wolf (1986)	Design: Descriptive Method: Analysis of cases from an elder mistreatment intervention project Sample: 59 elder mistreatment cases compared with 49 cases randomly selected from a nonabuse caseload	Victims and nonabuse clients were similar in age, sex, and health status. Caretakers for both groups were similar in age and health status. More perpetrators were males. A majority of elder mistreatment cases resided with family members versus nonabused persons living alone. Victims and perpetrators had more psychological and emotional health problems. Abused elders did not appear to be more dependent.
Wolf and Pillemer (1997)	Design: Descriptive Measure: ADLs, IADLs, CTS Sample: 73 older women: 22 victimized by husbands and 51 victimized by adult children	Wives more likely to be dependent on husbands for IADLs. Adult children more likely to be dependent on mothers for housing and finances. Husbands more likely to use physical violence against wives than adult children

TABLE A-2 Continued

Study	Methods	Selected Findings
		against mothers.
Wolf and Li (1999)	Design: Descriptive Measure: DV was number of reports per 1,000 persons age 60 years and older during 1994 Sample: 27 geographical areas in Massachusetts	Rate of reports varied from a low of 2.41 per 1,000 through 9.31 per 1,000. Higher rates of reporting were associated with lower socioeconomic status, more community training, higher agency service rating scores, lower community agency relationship score.

SOURCE: Adapted from Fulmer (2002).

REFERENCES

Childs, H.W., B. Hayslip, Jr, L.M. Radika, and J.A. Reinberg
   2000   Young and middle-aged adults' perceptions of elder abuse. *The Gerontologist* 40(1):75-85.
Coyne, A.C., W.E. Reichman, and L.J. Berbig
   1993   The Relationship Between Dementia and Abuse. *American Journal of Psychiatry* 150(4):643-646.
Dyer, C.B., V.N. Pavlik, K.P. Murphy, and D.J. Hyman
   2000   The high prevalence of depression and dementia in elder abuse or neglect. *Journal of the American Geriatrics Society* 48(2):205-208.
Ertem, I.O., J.M. Leventhal, and S. Dobbs
   2000   Intergenerational continuity of child physical abuse: How good is the evidence? *Lancet* 356(9232):814-9.
Fulmer, T.
   1984   Elder abuse assessment tool. *Dimensions of Critical Care Nursing* 3(4):216-220.
   2002   Elder mistreatment. In *Annual Review of Nursing Research: Focus on Geriatric Nursing*, vol. 20. P. Archbold and B. Stewart, eds. New York: Springer.
Fulmer, T., and V.M. Cahill
   1984   Assessing elder abuse: A study. *Journal of Gerontological Nursing* 10(12):16-20.
Fulmer, T., and B. Gurland
   1996   Restriction as elder mistreatment: Differences between caregiver and elder perceptions. *Journal of Mental Health and Aging* 2:89-98.
Fulmer, T., G. Paveza, I. Abraham, and S. Fairchild
   2000   Elder neglect assessment in the emergency department. *Journal of Emergency Nursing* 26(5):436-443.
Fulmer, T., M. Ramirez, S. Fairchild, D. Holmes, M.J. Koren, and J. Teresi
   1999   Prevalence of elder mistreatment as reported by social workers in a probability sample of adult day health care clients. *Journal of Elder Abuse and Neglect* 11(3):25-36.
Haviland, S., and J. O'Brien
   1989   Physical abuse and neglect of the elderly: Assessment and intervention. *Orthopedic Nursing* 8(4):11-19.
Huber, R., K. Borders, F.E. Netting, and H.W. Nelson
   2001   Data from long-term care ombudsman programs in six states: The implications of collecting resident demographics. *The Gerontologist* 41(1):61-68.
Hudson, M.F.
   1991   Elder mistreatment: A taxonomy with definitions by Delphi. *Journal of Elder Abuse and Neglect* 3(2):1-20.
Hwalek, M., A. Neale, C. Goodrich, and K. Quinn
   1996   The association of elder abuse and substance abuse in the Illinois Elder Abuse System. *The Gerontologist* 36(5):694-700.
Jogerst, G.J., J.D. Dawson, A. J. Hartz, J.W. Ely, and L.A. Schweitzer
   2000   Community characteristics associated with elder abuse. *Journal of the American Geriatrics Society* 48(5):513-518.
Jones, J.S., T.R. Veenstra, J.P. Seamon, and J. Krohmer
   1997   Elder mistreatment: National survey of emergency physicians. *Annals of Emergency Medicine* 30(4):473-479.

Lachs, M.S., L. Berkman, T. Fulmer, and R. Horwitz
   1994   A prospective community-based pilot study of risk factors for the investigation of elder mistreatment. *Journal of the American Geriatrics Society* 42(2):169-73.
Lachs, M.S., and T. Fulmer
   1993   Recognizing elder abuse and neglect. *Clinical Geriatric Medicine* 9(3):665-81.
Lachs, M.S., C. Williams, S. O'Brien, L. Hurst, and R.I. Horwitz
   1997a   Risk factors for reported elder abuse and neglect: A nine-year observational cohort study. *The Gerontologist* 37(4):469-474.
Lachs, M.S., C.S.Williams, S. O'Brien, L. Hurst, A. Kossack, A. A. Siegal, and M.E. Tinetti
   1997b   ED use by older victims of family violence. *Annals of Emergency Medicine* 30(4):448-454.
Lachs, M. S., C.S. Williams, S. O'Brien, K.A. Pillemer, and M.E. Charlson
   1998   The mortality of elder mistreatment. *Journal of the American Medical Association* 280(5):428-432.
Moody, L. E., A. Voss, and C.A. Lengacher
   2000   Assessing abuse among the elderly living in public housing. *Journal of Nursing Measurement* 8(1):61-70.
The National Center on Elder Abuse
   1998   *The National Elder Abuse Incidence Study Final Report*: Washington, DC: National Center on Elder Abuse.
Neale, A., M. Hwalek, R. Scott, M. Sengstock, and C. Stahl
   1991   Validation of the Hwalek-Sengstock Elder Abuse Screening Test. *Journal of Applied Gerontology* 10(4):406-418.
O'Brien, J. G.
   1986   Elder abuse and the physician. *Michigan Medical Journal* 85(11):618, 620.
O'Malley, T.A., H.C. O'Malley, D.E. Everitt, and D. Sarson
   1984   Categories of family-mediated abuse and neglect of elderly persons. *Journal of the American Geriatrics Society* 32(5):362-9.
Paveza, G.J., D. Cohen, C. Eisdorfer S. Freels, T. Semla, J.W. Ashford, P. Gorelick, R. Hirschman, D.J. Luchins, and P. Levy
   1992   Severe family violence and Alzheimer's disease: Prevalence and risk factors. *The Gerontologist* 32(4):493-497.
Pavlik, V.N., D.J.Hyman, N.A. Festa, and C. Bitondo Dyer
   2001   Quantifying the problem of abuse and neglect in adults—analysis of a statewide database. *Journal of the American Geriatrics Society* 49(1):45-48.
Phillips, L.R., E.F. Morrison, and Y.M. Chae
   1990a   The QUALCARE Scale: Developing an instrument to measure quality of home care. *International Journal of Nursing Studies* 27(1), 61-75.
   1990b   The QUALCARE Scale: Testing of a measurement instrument for clinical practice. *International Journal of Nursing Studies* 27(1):77-91.
Phillips, L.R., and V.F. Rempusheski
   1985   A decision-making model for diagnosing and intervening in elder abuse and neglect. *Nursing Research* 34(3):134-139.
Pillemer, K.A., and D. Finkelhor
   1988   The prevalence of elder abuse: A random sample survey. *The Gerontologist*, 28(1):51-57.
Pillemer, K.A., and D. Finkelhor
   1989   Causes of elder abuse: Caregiver stress versus problem relatives. *American Journal of Orthopsychiatry* 59(2):179-187.

Pillemer, K.A., and D.W. Moore
    1989   Abuse of patients in nursing homes: Findings from a survey of staff. *The Geron-tologist* 29(3):314-320.
Pillemer, K. A., and J.J. Suitor
    1992   Violence and violent feelings: What causes them among family caregivers? *Journal of Gerontological Nursing* 47(4):S165-S172.
Reis, M., and D. Nahmiash
    1998   Validation of the indicators of abuse (IOA) screen. *The Gerontologist* 38(4):471-480.
Rosenblatt, D. E., K.H. Cho, and P.W. Durance
    1996   Reporting mistreatment of older adults: The role of physicians. *Journal of the American Geriatrics Society* 44(1):65-70.
Shaw, M.M.C.
    1998   Nursing home resident abuse by staff: Exploring the dynamics. *Journal of Elder Abuse and Neglect* 9(4):1-21.
Straus, M..A.
    1978   The Conflict Tactic Scale. Reprinted in *Handbook of Family Measurement Techniques,* J. Touliatos, B. Perlmutter, and M. Straus, editors. Newbury Park, CA: Sage.
Tatara, T
    1993   Understanding the nature and scope of domestic elder abuse with the use of state aggregate data: Summaries of key findings of a national survey of state APS and aging agencies. *Journal of Elder Abuse and Neglect* 5:35-57.
Wolf, R.S.
    1986   Major findings from three model projects on elderly abuse. In *Elder Abuse: Conflict in the Family*, K.A. Pillemer and R.S. Wolf, eds. Dover MA: Auburn House Publishing.
Wolf, R.S., and D. Li
    1999   Factors affecting the rate of elder abuse reporting to a state protective services program. *The Gerontologist* 39(2):222-228.
Wolf, R.S., and K.A. Pillemer
    1997   The older battered woman: wives and mothers compared. *Journal of Mental Health & Aging* 3(3):325-336.

Analysis of Elder Abuse and Neglect Definitions Under State Law

Lora Flattum Hamp

ALABAMA: Code of Ala. § 38-9-2 (2001)

"**Abuse**" means the infliction of physical pain, injury, willful deprivation by a caregiver or other person of services necessary to maintain mental and physical health.

> *Defined separately: Emotional abuse* is the willful or reckless infliction of emotional or mental anguish or the use of a physical or chemical restraint, medication or isolation as punishment or as a substitute for treatment or care of any protected person. *Sexual abuse* includes any conduct that is a crime as defined in § 13A-6-60 to § 13A-6-70 of the Code of Alabama.

"**Neglect**" means the failure of a caregiver to provide food, shelter, clothing, medical services, or health care for the person unable to care for self; or the failure of person to provide these needs for self as result of mental or physical inability.

"**Exploitation**" means expenditure, diminution, use of property, assets, or resources of protected person without the express voluntary consent of that person or that person's legally authorized representative.

"**Adult in need of protective services**" means a person 18 years of age or older whose behavior indicates that he or she is mentally incapable of adequately caring for himself or herself and his or her interests without serious consequences to himself or herself or others, or who, because of physical or mental impairment, is unable to protect himself or herself from abuse, neglect, exploitation, sexual abuse, or emotional abuse by others, and who has no guardian, relative, or other appropriate person able, willing, and available to assume the kind and degree of protection and supervision required under the circumstances.

"Caregiver" means an individual who has the responsibility for care of a protected person as a result of family relationship or who has assumed the responsibility for care of the person voluntarily by contract or as a result of the ties of friendship.

ALASKA: Alaska Stat. § 47.24.900 (2001)

"Abuse" means willful, intentional, reckless, nonaccidental, and nontherapeutic infliction of physical pain injury or mental distress or sexual assault.

"Neglect" means the intentional failure by a caregiver to provide essential care or services necessary to maintain the physical and mental health of the vulnerable adult. Self-neglect includes an act or omission by a vulnerable adult that results or could result in the deprivation of essential services necessary to maintain minimal mental, emotional, or physical health and safety.

"Exploitation" means the unjust or improper use of another person or another person's resources for one's own profit or advantage.

"Vulnerable adult" means a person 18 years of age or older who, because of physical or mental impairment, is unable to meet person's own needs or to seek help without assistance.

"Caregiver" means a person providing care to a vulnerable adult as a result of family relationship; or who has assumed responsibility for the care of a vulnerable adult voluntarily, by contract, or by court order; or an employee of an out-of-home care facility who provides care to one or more vulnerable adults.

ARIZONA: A.R.S. § 46-451 (2000); A.R.S. § 13-3623 (2001)

"**Abuse**" under § 46-451 and § 13-3623 means the intentional infliction of physical harm; injury caused by negligent acts or omissions; unreasonable confinement; sexual abuse or sexual assault.

> *Defined separately under § 13-3623*: *Emotional abuse* means a pattern of ridiculing or demeaning a vulnerable adult, making derogatory remarks to a vulnerable adult, verbally harassing a vulnerable adult, or threatening to inflict physical or emotional harm on a vulnerable adult. *Physical injury* means the impairment of physical condition and includes any skin bruising, pressure sores, bleeding, failure to thrive, malnutrition, dehydration, burns, fracture of any bone, subdural hematoma, soft tissue swelling, injury to any internal organ, or any physical condition that imperils health or welfare.

"**Neglect**" under § 46-451 means a pattern of conduct without the person's informed consent resulting in deprivation of food, water, medication, medical services, shelter, cooling, heating, or other services necessary to maintain minimum physical or mental health.

"**Exploitation**" under § 46-451 means the illegal or improper use of an incapacitated or vulnerable adult or his resources for another's profit or advantage.

"**Vulnerable adult**" under § 46-451 and § 13-3623 means an individual who is 18 years of age or older who is unable to protect himself from abuse, neglect, or exploitation by others because of a physical or mental impairment.

ARKANSAS: A.C.A. § 5-28-101 (2001)

"**Abuse**" means any intentional or unnecessary physical act which inflicts pain on or causes injury to endangered or impaired adult, including sexual abuse; or any intentional or demeaning act which subjects an endangered or impaired adult to ridicule; or psychological injury in manner likely to provoke fear or harm.

Defined separately: *Sexual abuse* means deviate sexual activity, sexual contact, or sexual intercourse, as those terms are defined in § 5-14-101, with another person who is not the actor's spouse and who is incapable of consent because he or she is mentally defective, mentally incapacitated, or physically helpless, as those terms are defined in § 5-14-101.

"**Neglect**" means acts or omissions by an endangered adult; for example, self-neglect or intentional acts or omissions by a caregiver responsible for the care and supervision of an endangered or impaired adult constituting: (a) Negligently failing to provide necessary treatment, rehabilitation, care, food, clothing, shelter, supervision, or medical services to an endangered or impaired adult; (b) Negligently failing to report health problems or changes in health problems or changes in the health condition of an endangered or impaired adult to the appropriate medical personnel; or (c) Negligently failing to carry out a prescribed treatment plan.

"**Exploitation**" means the illegal use or management of endangered or impaired adult's funds, assets, or property, or the use of an endangered or impaired adult's person, power of attorney, or guardianship for the profit or advantage of himself, herself, or another.

"**Endangered adult**" means an adult 18 years of age or older who is found to be in a situation or condition which poses an imminent risk of death or serious bodily harm to that person and who demonstrates a lack of capacity to comprehend the nature and consequences of remaining in that situation or condition; or a resident 18 years of age or older of a long-term care facility which is required to be licensed under § 20-10-224, who is found to be in a situation or condition which poses imminent risk of death or serious bodily harm to the person and who demonstrates the lack of capacity to comprehend the nature and consequences of remaining in that situation or condition. "**Impaired adult**" means a person 18 years or older who, as a result of mental or physical impairment, is unable to protect himself or herself from abuse, sexual abuse, neglect, or exploitation, and as a consequence thereof is endangered.

"**Caregiver**" means a related or unrelated person, owner, agent, high managerial agent of a public or private organization, or public or private organization that has responsibility for protection, care, or custody of an endangered or impaired adult as a result of assuming the responsibility voluntarily, by contract, through employment, or by order of the court.

CALIFORNIA: Cal. Wel. & Inst. Code §§ 15610.07, 15610.30, 15610.57 (2001); Cal. Pen. Code § 368 (2001)

"**Abuse of an elder or dependent adult**" under § 15610.07 includes physical abuse, neglect, financial abuse, abandonment, isolation, abduction, or other treatment with resulting physical harm or pain or mental suffering; the deprivation by a care custodian of goods or services that are necessary to avoid physical harm or mental suffering.

"**Abuse**" under Cal. Pen. Code § 368 occurs when any person who, under circumstances or conditions likely to produce great bodily harm or death, willfully causes or permits any elder or dependent adult, with knowledge that he or she is an elder or a dependent adult, to suffer, or inflicts thereon unjustifiable physical pain or mental suffering, or having the care or custody of any elder or dependent adult, willfully causes or permits the person or health of the elder or dependent adult to be injured, or willfully causes or permits the elder or dependent adult to be placed in a situation in which his or her person or health is endangered.

"**Neglect**" under § 15610.17 includes (1) negligent failure of any person having the care or custody of elder of a dependent adult to exercise that degree of care that a reasonable person in a like position would exercise; (2) negligent failure of person themselves to exercise that degree of care that a reasonable person in a like position would exercise.

"**Financial abuse**" under § 15610.30 occurs when a person or entity does any of the following: (1) Takes, secretes, appropriates, or retains real or personal property of an elder or dependent adult to a wrongful use or with intent to defraud, or both; (2) assists in taking, secreting, appropriating, or retaining real or personal property of an elder or dependent adult to a wrongful use or with intent to defraud, or both.

"**Elder**" under Cal. Pen. Code § 368 means any person residing in this state, 65 years of age or older.

"**Dependent adult**" under Cal. Pen. Code § 368 means any person residing in this state, between the ages of 18 and 64 years, who has physical or mental limitations that restrict his or her ability to carry out normal activities or to protect his or her rights including, but not limited to, persons who have physical or developmental disabilities or whose physical or mental abilities have diminished because of age; includes any person between the ages of 18 and 64 who is admitted as an inpatient to a 24-hour health facility, as defined in Sections 1250, 1250.2, and 1250.3 of the Health and Safety Code.

"**Caretaker**" under Cal. Pen. Code § 368 means any person who has the care, custody, or control of, or who stands in a position of trust with, an elder or a dependent adult.

COLORADO: C.R.S. §§ 18-6.5-102, 26-3.1-101 (2001)

"**Mistreatment**" under § 26-3.1-101 means an act or omission which threatens health, safety, or welfare of an at-risk adult...or which exposes the adult to a situation or condition that poses an imminent risk of death, serious bodily injury or bodily injury to the adult. Includes but is not limited to (a) Abuse which occurs: (I) Where there is infliction of physical pain or injury, as demonstrated by, but not limited to, substantial or multiple skin bruising, bleeding, malnutrition, dehydration, burns, bone fractures, poisoning, subdural hematoma, soft tissue swelling, or suffocation; (II) Where unreasonable confinement or restraint is imposed; or (III) Where there is subjection to nonconsensual sexual conduct or contact classified as a crime under the "Colorado Criminal Code" title 18, C.R.S; (b) Caretaker neglect which occurs when adequate food, clothing, shelter, psychological care, physical care, medical care, or supervision is not secured for the at-risk adult or is not provided by a caretaker in a timely manner and with the degree of care that a reasonable person in the same situation would exercise; except that the withholding of artificial nourishment in accordance with the "Colorado Medical Treatment Decision Act," article 18 of title 15, C.R.S., shall not be considered as abuse; (c) Exploitation which is the illegal or improper use of an at-risk adult for another person's advantage.

"**Caretaker neglect**" under § 26-3.1-101 and § 18-6.5-102 occurs when adequate food, clothing, shelter, psychological care, physical care, medical care, or supervision is not secured for the at-risk adult or is not provided by a caretaker in a timely manner and with degree of care that a reasonable person in the same situation would exercise. Self-neglect (defined separately): act or failure to act whereby an at-risk adult substantially endangers the adult's health, safety, welfare, or life by not seeking or obtaining services necessary to meet the adult's essential human needs. Choice of lifestyle or living arrangements shall not, by itself, be evidence of self-neglect:

"**Exploitation**" under § 26-3.1-101 means the illegal or improper use of an at-risk adult for another person's advantage.

"**At-risk adult**" under § 26-3.1-101 means an individual 18 years of age or older who is susceptible to mistreatment ...or self-neglect as such term is defined because individual is unable to perform or obtain services necessary for individual's health, safety, or welfare or lacks sufficient understanding or capacity to make or communicate responsible decisions concerning the individual's person or affairs. "**At-risk adult**" under § 18-6.5-102 means any person who is 60 years of age or older or any person who is 18 years of age or older and is a person with a disability.

"**Caretaker**" under § 26-3.1-101 means a person who is responsible for care of at-risk adult as a result of family or legal relationship or who has assumed responsibility for the care of an at-risk adult.

CONNECTICUT: Conn. Gen. Stat. § 17b-450 (2001)

"**Abuse**" includes, but is not limited to, willful infliction of physical pain, injury, or mental anguish, or the willful deprivation by a caretaker of services which are necessary to maintain physical or mental health.

"**Neglect**" refers to an elderly person who is either living alone and not able to provide for oneself the services which are necessary to maintain physical and mental health or is not receiving the said necessary services from the responsible caretaker.

"**Exploitation**" refers to the act or process of taking advantage of an elderly person by another person or caretaker whether for monetary, personal, or other benefit, gain, or profit.

"**Elderly person**" means a resident of Connecticut who is 60 years of age or older.

"**Caretaker**" means a person who has the responsibility for the care of an elderly person as a result of a family relationship or who has assumed the responsibility for the care of the elderly voluntarily, by contract, or by order of a court of competent jurisdiction.

DELAWARE: 31 Del. C. § 3902 (2000); 16 De. C. § 1131 (2000)

"**Abuse**" under § 3902 includes physical abuse by unnecessarily inflicting pain or injury on an infirm adult; or a pattern of emotional abuse, which includes, but is not limited to, ridiculing or demeaning an infirm adult, making derogatory remarks to an infirm adult, or cursing or threatening to inflict physical or emotional harm on an infirm adult.

> INSTITUTIONAL ABUSE: "**Abuse**" under § 1131 includes (a) physical abuse by unnecessarily inflicting pain or injury to a patient or resident. This includes, but is not limited to hitting, kicking, . . . sexual molestation; (b) emotional abuse which includes, but is not limited to, ridiculing or demeaning a patient or resident, making derogatory remarks to a patient or resident, or cursing directed toward

patient or resident, or threatening to inflict physical or emotional harm on a patient. Mistreatment shall include the inappropriate use of meds, isolation, or physical or chemical restraints on or of a patient or resident.

"Neglect" under § 3902 includes (a) lack of attention by a caregiver to physical needs of an infirm adult including but not limited to toileting, bathing, meals, and safety; (b) failure by a caregiver to carry out a treatment plan prescribed by a health care professional for an infirm adult; or (c) intentional and permanent abandonment or desertion in any place of an infirm adult by a caregiver who does not make reasonable efforts to ensure that essential services, as defined in this section, will be provided for said infirm adult.

> INSTITUTIONAL NEGLECT: "Neglect" under § 1131 means (a) lack of attention to physical needs of the patient or resident including, but not limited to toileting, bathing, meals, and safety; (b) failure to report patient or resident health problems or changes in health problems or changes in health condition to an immediate supervisor or nurse; (c) failure to carry out a prescribed treatment plan for a patient or resident; (d) a knowing failure to provide adequate staffing which results in a medical emergency to any patient or resident where there has been documented history of at least 2 prior cited instances of such inadequate staffing within the past 2 years in violation of minimum maintenance of staffing levels as required by statute or regulations promulgated by the Department, all so as to evidence a willful pattern of such neglect.

"Exploitation" under both § 3902 and § 1131: Illegal or improper use or abuse of an infirm person, the infirm person's resources or the infirm person's rights, by another person, whether for profit or other advantage.

"Infirm adult" under § 3902: Any person 18 years of age or over who, because of physical or mental disability, is substantially impaired in the ability to provide adequately for the person's own care and custody.

"Caregiver" under § 3902 means any adult who has assumed the permanent or temporary care, custody, or responsibility for the supervision of an infirm adult.

DISTRICT OF COLUMBIA: D.C. Code § 6-2501 (2001)

"Abuse" means intentional or reckless infliction of serious physical pain or injury; use or threatened use of violence to force participation in sexual conduct; repeated intentional imposition of unreasonable confinement, resulting in severe mental distress; repeated use of threats or violence, resulting in shock or an intense, expressed fear for one's life or of serious physical injury; or intentional or deliberately indifferent deprivation of essential food, shelter, or health care in violation of a caregiver's responsibilities, when that deprivation constitutes a serious threat to one's life or physical health.

"Neglect" includes (a) the repeated, careless infliction of serious physical pain or injury; (b) the repeated failure of a caregiver to take reasonable steps, within the purview of his or her responsibilities, to protect against acts of abuse; (c) the repeated, careless imposition of unreasonable confinement, resulting in severe mental distress; or (d) the careless deprivation of essential food, shelter, or health care in violation of a caregiver's responsibilities, when that deprivation constitutes a serious threat to one's life or physical health.

"Exploitation" means the unlawful appropriation or use of another's property for one's own benefit or that of a third person.

"Adult in need of protective services" means an individual aged 18 or older who is: highly vulnerable to abuse, neglect, or exploitation, because of a physical or mental impairment; being or has recently been abused, neglected, or exploited by another; and likely to continue being abused, neglected, or exploited by others because he or she has no one willing and able to provide adequate protection.

"Caregiver" means a person that, by law, contract, court order, or voluntary action, is charged with or has assumed the responsibility for an adult's essential food, shelter, or health care needs.

FLORIDA: Fla. Stat. § 415.102 (2000); Fla. Stat. § 825.102 (2001)

"Abuse" under § 415.102: Willful act or threatened act that causes or is likely to cause significant impairment to a vulnerable adult's physical, mental, or emotional health. Abuse includes acts and omissions.

Defined separately: *Sexual abuse* defined separately: means acts of a sexual nature committed in the presence of a vulnerable adult without that person's informed consent. Sexual abuse includes, but is not limited to, the acts defined in § 794.011(1)(h), fondling, exposure of a vulnerable adult's sexual organs, or the use of a vulnerable adult to solicit for or engage in prostitution or sexual performance. Sexual abuse does not include any act intended for a valid medical purpose or any act that may reasonably be construed to be normal caregiving action or appropriate display of affection.

"Abuse" under § 825.102: (a) Intentional infliction of physical or psychological injury upon an elderly person or disabled adult; (b) An intentional act that could reasonably be expected to result in physical or psychological injury to an elderly person or disabled adult; or (c) Active encouragement of any person to commit an act that results or could reasonably be expected to result in physical or psychological injury to an elderly person or disabled adult.

"Neglect" under § 415.102 and § 825.102: Failure or omission on the part of the caregiver to provide the care, supervision, and services necessary to maintain the physical and mental health of the vulnerable adult, including, but not limited to, food, clothing, medicine, shelter, supervision, and medical services, that a prudent person would consider essential for the well-being of a vulnerable adult. The term "neglect" also means the failure of a caregiver to make a reasonable effort to protect a vulnerable adult from abuse, neglect, or exploitation by others. "Neglect" is repeated conduct or a single incident of carelessness which produces or could reasonably be expected to result in serious physical or psychological injury or a substantial risk of death.

"Exploitation" under § 415.102 occurs when a person who: 1. Stands in a position of trust and confidence with a vulnerable adult and knowingly, by deception or intimidation, obtains or uses, or endeavors to obtain or use, a vulnerable adult's funds, assets, or property with the intent to temporarily or permanently deprive a vulnerable adult of the use, benefit, or possession of the funds, assets, or property for the benefit of someone other than the vulnerable adult; or 2. Knows or should know that the vulnerable adult lacks the capacity to consent, and obtains or uses, or endeavors to obtain or use, the vulnerable adult's funds, assets, or property with the intent to temporarily or permanently deprive the vulnerable adult of the use, benefit, or possession of the funds, assets, or property for the benefit of someone other than the vulnerable adult; "Exploitation" may include, but is not limited to: 1. Breaches of fiduciary relationships, such as the misuse of a power of attorney or the abuse of guardianship duties, resulting in the unauthorized appropriation, sale, or transfer of property; 2. Unauthorized taking of personal assets; 3. Misappropriation, misuse, or transfer of moneys belonging to a vulnerable adult from a personal or joint account; or 4. Intentional or negligent failure to effectively use a vulnerable adult's income and assets for the necessities required for that person's support and maintenance.

"**Vulnerable adult**" under § 415.102 means a person 18 years of age or older whose ability to perform the normal activities of daily living or to provide for his or her own care or protection is impaired due to a mental, emotional, physical, or developmental disability or dysfunctioning, or brain damage, or the infirmities of aging.

"**Caregiver**" under § 415.102 means a person who has been entrusted with or has assumed the responsibility for frequent and regular care of or services to a vulnerable adult on a temporary or permanent basis and who has a commitment, agreement, or understanding with that person or that person's guardian that a caregiver role exists. "Caregiver" includes, but is not limited to, relatives, household members, guardians, neighbors, and employees and volunteers of facilities as defined in subsection (8). For the purpose of departmental investigative jurisdiction, the term "caregiver" does not include law enforcement officers or employees of municipal or county detention facilities or the Department of Corrections while acting in an official capacity.

GEORGIA: O.C.G.A. §§ 30-5-3, 31-8-81 (2000)

"**Abuse**" under § 30-5-3 means willful infliction of physical pain, physical injury, mental anguish, unreasonable confinement, or the willful deprivation of essential services to a disabled adult or elder person.

INSTITUTIONAL ABUSE "**Abuse**" under § 31-8-81 means any intentional or grossly negligent act or series of acts or intentional or grossly negligent omission to act which causes injury to a resident, including, but not limited to, assault or battery, failure to provide treatment or care, or sexual harassment of the resident.

"**Neglect**" under § 30-5-3 means absence or omission of essential services to the degree that it harms or threatens with harm the physical or emotional health of a disabled adult or elder person.

"**Exploitation**" under § 30-5-3 means illegal or improper use of a disabled adult or elder person or that person's resources for another's profit or advantage.

"**Elder person**" under § 30-5-3 means a person 65 years of age or older who is not a resident of a long-term care facility as defined in Article 4 of Chapter 8 of Title 31.

"**Caretaker**" under § 30-5-3 means a person who has the responsibility for the care of a disabled adult or elder person as a result of family relationship, contract, voluntary assumption of that responsibility, or by operation of law.

HAWAII: HRS § 346-222 (2000)

"**Abuse**" means actual or imminent physical injury, psychological abuse or neglect, sexual abuse, financial exploitation, negligent treatment, or maltreatment as further defined in this chapter.

"**Neglect**" includes the failure to exercise that degree of care toward a dependent adult which a reasonable person with the responsibility of a caregiver would exercise, including, but not limited to, failure to: (A) Assist in personal hygiene; (B) Provide necessary food, shelter, and clothing; (C) Provide necessary health care, access to health care, or prescribed medication; (D) Protect a dependent adult from health and safety hazards.

"**Financial and economic exploitation**" means the wrongful or negligent taking, withholding, misappropriation, or use of a dependent adult's money, real property, or personal property; includes but is not limited to: (A) Breaches of fiduciary relationships such as the misuse of a power of attorney or the abuse of guardianship privileges, resulting in the unauthorized appropriation, sale, or transfer of property; (B) The unauthorized taking of personal assets; (C) The misappropriation, misuse, or transfer of moneys belonging to the dependent adult from a personal or joint account; or (D) The intentional or negligent failure to effectively use a dependent adult's income and assets for the necessities required for the person's support and maintenance. The exploitation may involve coercion, manipulation, threats, intimidation, misrepresentation, or exertion of undue influence. Protect against acts of abuse by third parties.

"**Dependent adult**" means any adult who, because of mental or physical impairment is dependent upon another person, a care organization, or a care facility for personal health, safety, or welfare.

IDAHO: Idaho Code §§ 18-1505, 39-5302 (2000)

"**Abuse**" under § 39-5302 and § 18-1505 means intentional or negligent infliction of physical pain, injury, or mental injury.

"**Neglect**" under § 39-5302 includes self-neglect and means the failure of a caretaker to provide food, clothing, shelter, or medical care reasonably necessary to sustain the life and health of a vulnerable adult, or the failure of a vulnerable adult to provide those services for himself.

"**Neglect**" under § 18-1505 means failure of a caretaker to provide food, clothing, shelter, or medical care to a vulnerable adult, in such a manner as to jeopardize the life, health and safety of the vulnerable adult.

"**Exploitation**" under § 39-5302 and § 18-1505 means an action which may include, but is not limited to, the misuse of a vulnerable adult's funds, property, or resources by another person for profit or advantage.

"**Vulnerable adult**" under § 39-5302 and § 18-1505 means a person 18 years of age or older who is unable to protect himself from abuse, neglect ,or exploitation due to physical or mental impairment which affects the person's judgment or behavior to the extent that he lacks sufficient understanding or capacity to make or communicate or implement decisions regarding his person.

"**Caretaker**" under § 39-5302 and § 18-1505 means any individual or institution that is responsible by relationship, contract, or court order to provide food, shelter, or clothing, medical or other life-sustaining necessities to a vulnerable adult.

ILLINOIS: 320 ILCS 20/2 (2001); 320 ILCS 15/2 (2001); 210 ILCS 30/3 (2001); 210 ILCS 45/1-103 (2001); 720 ILCS 5/12-19 (2001)

"**Abuse**" under 320 ILCS 20/2 means causing any physical, mental, or sexual injury to an eligible adult, including exploitation of such adult's financial resources.

"**Abuse**" under 320 ILCS 15/2 means intentionally or knowingly causing any physical injury or exploiting the resources of an elderly individual.

INSTITUTIONAL ABUSE: "**Abuse**" under 210 ILCS 30/3 means any physical injury, sexual abuse, or mental injury inflicted on a resident other than by accidental means.

"**Abuse**" under 210 ILCS 45/1-103 means any physical or mental injury or sexual assault inflicted on a resident other than by accidental means in a facility.

"**Abuse**" under 720 ILCS 5/12-19 means intentionally or knowingly causing any physical or mental injury or committing any sexual offense set forth in this Code.

"**Neglect**" under 320 ILCS 20/2 means another individual's failure to provide an eligible adult with or willful withholding from an eligible adult the necessities of life including, but not limited to, food, clothing, shelter, or medical care. This subsection does not create any new affirmative duty to provide support to eligible adults. Nothing in this Act shall be construed to mean that an eligible adult is a victim of neglect because of health care services provided or not provided by licensed health care professionals.

INSTITUTIONAL NEGLECT: "**Neglect**" under 210 ILCS 30/3, 210 ILCS 45/1-117, and 720 ILCS 5/12-19 means a failure in a long-term care facility to provide adequate medical or personal care or maintenance, which failure results in physical or mental injury to a resident or in the deterioration of a resident's physical or mental condition.

"**Gross Neglect**" under 720 ILCS 5/12-19 means recklessly failing to provide adequate medical or personal care or maintenance, which failure results in physical or mental injury or the deterioration of a physical or mental condition.

"**Eligible adult**" under 320 ILCS 20/2 means a person 60 years of age or older who resides in a domestic living situation and is, or is alleged to be, abused, neglected, or financially exploited by another individual.

"**Elderly Individual**" under 320 ILCS 15/2 means a person 60 years of age or older.

"**Resident**" under 210 ILCS 30/3 means a person residing in and receiving personal care from a long-term care facility, or residing in a mental health facility or developmental disability facility as defined in the Mental Health and Developmental Disabilities Code.

"**Caregiver**" under 320 ILCS 20/2 means a person who either as a result of a family relationship, voluntarily, or in exchange for compensation has assumed responsibility for all or a portion of the care of an eligible adult who needs assistance with activities of daily living.

INDIANA· Burns Ind. Code Ann. § 12-10-3-2 (2000); Burns Ind. Code Ann. § 35-46-1-12 (2001)

"**Exploitation of endangered adult**" under § 35-46-1-12 occurs when a person who recklessly, knowingly, or intentionally exerts unauthorized use of personal services or the property of an endangered adult for the person's own profit or advantage or for the profit or advantage of another person.

"**Endangered adult**" under § 12-10-3-2 means an individual who is: (1) at least 18 years of age; (2) incapable by reason of mental illness, mental retardation, dementia, habitual drunkenness, excessive use of drugs, or other physical or mental incapacity of managing or directing the management of the individual's property or providing or directing the provision of self-care; and (3) harmed or threatened with harm as a result of: (A) neglect; (B) battery; or (C) exploitation of the individual's personal services or property.

IOWA· Iowa Code §§ 235B.2, 726.7, 726.8 (2001)

"**Dependent adult abuse**" under § 235B.2 means: (1) Any of the following as a result of the willful or negligent acts or omissions of a caretaker: (a) Physical injury to, or injury which is at a variance with the history given of the injury, or unreasonable confinement, unreasonable punishment, or assault of a dependent adult. (b) The commission of a sexual offense under chapter 709 or section 726.2 with or against a dependent adult. (c) Exploitation of a dependent adult which means the act or process of taking unfair advantage of a dependent adult or the adult's physical or financial resources for one's own personal or pecuniary profit, without the informed consent of the dependent adult, including theft, by the use of undue influence, harassment, duress, deception, false representation, or false pretenses. (d) The deprivation of the minimum food, shelter, clothing, supervision, physical or mental health care, or other care necessary to maintain a dependent adult's life or health. (2) The deprivation of the minimum food, shelter, clothing, supervision, physical or mental health care, and other care necessary to maintain a dependent adult's life or health as a result of the acts or omissions of the dependent adult. (3) Sexual exploitation of a dependent adult who is a resident of a health care facility, as defined in section 135C.1, by a caretaker providing services to or employed by the health care facility, whether within the health care facility or at a location outside of the health care facility.

> *Defined separately: Sexual exploitation* means any consensual or nonconsensual sexual conduct with a dependent adult for the purpose of arousing or satisfying the sexual desires of the caretaker or dependent adult, which includes but is not limited to kissing; touching of the clothed or unclothed inner thigh, breast, groin, buttock, anus, pubes, or genitals; or a sex act, as defined in section 702.17. Sexual exploitation does not include touching which is part of a necessary examination, treatment, or care by a caretaker acting within the scope of the practice or employment of the caretaker; the exchange of a brief touch or hug between the dependent adult and a caretaker for the purpose of reassurance, comfort, or casual friendship; or touching between spouses.

"**Neglect**" under § 235B.2 is defined within "abuse" definition.

"**Wanton neglect or nonsupport of a dependent adult**" under § 726.8 occurs when a caretaker knowingly acts in a manner likely to be injurious to the physical, mental, or emotional welfare of a dependent adult.

> INSTITUTIONAL NEGLECT: "**Wanton neglect of a resident of a health care facility**" under § 726.7 occurs when a person knowingly acts in a manner likely to be injurious to the physical or mental welfare of a resident of a health care facility as defined in § 135C.1.

"**Exploitation**" under § 235B.2 is defined within "abuse" definition.

"**Dependent adult**" means a person 18 years of age or older who is unable to protect the person's own interests or unable to adequately perform or obtain services necessary to meet essential human needs, as a result of a physical or mental condition which requires assistance from another, or as defined by departmental rule.

"**Caretaker**" means a related or nonrelated person who has the responsibility for the protection, care, or custody of a dependent adult as a result of assuming the responsibility voluntarily, by contract, through employment, or by order of the court.

KANSAS: K.S.A. §§ 39-1401, 39-1430 (2000)

"**Abuse**" under § 39-1430 and § 39-1401 means any act or failure to act performed intentionally or recklessly that causes or is likely to cause harm to an adult, including: (1) Infliction of physical or mental injury; (2) any sexual act with an adult when the adult does not consent or when the other person knows or should know that the adult is incapable of resisting or declining consent to the sexual act due to mental deficiency or disease or due to fear of retribution or hardship; (3) unreasonable use of a physical restraint, isolation, or medication that harms or is likely to harm an adult; (4) unreasonable use of a physical or chemical restraint, medication, or isolation as punishment, for convenience, in conflict with a physician's orders or as a substitute for treatment, except where such conduct or physical restraint is in furtherance of the health and safety of the adult; (5) a threat or menacing conduct directed toward an adult that results or might reasonably be expected to result in fear or emotional or mental distress to an adult; (6) fiduciary abuse; or (7) omission or deprivation by a caretaker or another person of goods or services which are necessary to avoid physical or mental harm or illness.

"**Neglect**" under § 39-1430 and § 39-1401 means the failure or omission by one's self, caretaker, or another person to provide goods or services which are reasonably necessary to ensure safety and well-being and to avoid physical or mental harm or illness.

"**Exploitation**" under § 39-1430 and § 39-1401 means misappropriation of an adult's property or intentionally taking unfair advantage of an adult's physical or financial resources for another individual's personal or financial advantage by the use of undue influence, coercion, harassment, duress, deception, false representation or false pretense by a caretaker or another person. (e) "Fiduciary abuse" means a situation in which any person who is the caretaker of, or who stands in a position of trust to, an adult, takes, secretes, or appropriates their money or property, to any use or purpose not in the due and lawful execution of such person's trust.

"**Adult**" under § 39-1430 means an individual 18 years of age or older alleged to be unable to protect their own interest and who is harmed or threatened with harm through action or inaction by either another individual or through their own action or inaction when (1) such person is residing in such person's own home, the home of a family member or the home of a friend, (2) such person resides in an adult family home as defined in K.S.A. § 39-1501 and amendments thereto, or (3) such person is receiving services through a provider of community services and affiliates thereof operated or funded by the department of social and rehabilitation services or the department on aging or a residential facility licensed pursuant to K.S.A. § 75-3307b and amendments thereto. Such term shall not include persons to whom K.S.A. § 39-1401 et seq. and amendments thereto apply.

"Resident" under § 39-1401 means (1) Any resident, as defined by K.S.A. § 39-923 and amendments thereto; or (2) any individual kept, cared for, treated, boarded or otherwise accommodated in a medical care facility; or (3) any individual, kept, cared for, treated, boarded or otherwise accommodated in a state psychiatric hospital or state institution for the mentally retarded.

"Caretaker" under § 39-1430 means a person who has assumed the responsibility for an adult's care or financial management or both.

"Caretaker" under § 39-1401 means a person or institution who has assumed the responsibility for the care of the resident voluntarily, by contract or by order of a court of competent jurisdiction.

KENTUCKY: KRS §§ 209.020, 508.090 (2001)

"Abuse" under § 209.020 means the infliction of physical pain, mental injury, or injury of an adult.

"Abuse" under § 508.090 means the infliction of physical pain, injury, or mental injury, or the deprivation of services by a person which are necessary to maintain the health and welfare of a person, or a situation in which an adult, living alone, is unable to provide or obtain for himself the services which are necessary to maintain his health or welfare.

"Neglect" under § 209.020 means a situation in which an adult is unable to perform or obtain for himself the services which are necessary to maintain his health or welfare, or the deprivation of services by a caretaker which are necessary to maintain the health and welfare of an adult, or a situation in which a person deprives his spouse of reasonable services to maintain health and welfare.

"**Exploitation**" under § 209.020 means the improper use of an adult or an adult's resources by a caretaker or other person for the profit or advantage of the caretaker or other person.

"**Adult**" under § 209.020 means: (a) A person 18 years of age or older, who, because of mental or physical dysfunctioning, is unable to manage his own resources or carry out the activity of daily living or protect himself from neglect, or a hazardous or abusive situation without assistance from others, and who may be in need of protective services; or (b) a person without regard to age who is the victim of abuse and neglect inflicted by a spouse.

"**Caretaker**" under § 209.020 means an individual or institution who has the responsibility for the care of the adult as a result of family relationship, or who has assumed the responsibility for the care of the adult person voluntarily, or by contract, or agreement.

LOUISIANA: La. R.S. §§ 14:403.2, 46:61 (2001)

"**Abuse**" under La. R.S. § 14:403.2 is the infliction of physical or mental injury on an adult by other parties, including but not limited to such means as sexual abuse, abandonment, isolation, exploitation, or extortion of funds or other things of value, to such an extent that his health, self-determination, or emotional well-being is endangered.

> *Defined separately: Abandonment* is the desertion or willful forsaking of an adult by anyone having care or custody of that person under circumstances in which a reasonable person would continue to provide care and custody. *Isolation* includes: (a) Intentional acts committed for the purpose of preventing, and which do serve to prevent, an adult from having contact with family, friends, or concerned persons. This shall not be construed to affect a legal restraining order. (b) Intentional acts committed to prevent an adult from receiving his mail or telephone calls. (c) Intentional acts of physical or chemical restraint of an adult committed for the purpose of preventing contact with visitors, family, friends, or other concerned persons. (d) Intentional acts which restrict, place, or confine an adult in a restricted area for the purposes of social deprivation or preventing contact with family, friends, visitors, or other concerned persons. However, medical isolation prescribed by a licensed physician caring for the adult shall not be included in this definition.

"**Elderly abuse**" under § 46:61 means abuse of any person 60 years of age or older and shall include the abuse of any infirm person residing in a state licensed facility.

"**Neglect**" under § 14:403.2 is the failure, by a caregiver responsible for an adult's care or by other parties, to provide the proper or necessary support or medical, surgical, or any other care necessary for his well-being. No adult who is being provided treatment in accordance with a recognized religious method of healing in lieu of medical treatment shall for that reason alone be considered to be neglected or abused.

"**Exploitation**" under § 14:403.2 is the illegal or improper use or management of an aged person's or disabled adult's funds, assets, or property, or the use of an aged person's or disabled adult's power of attorney or guardianship for one's own profit or advantage.

"**Adult**" under § 14:403.2 is any person 60 years of age or older, any disabled person 18 years of age or older, or an emancipated minor.

"**Caregiver**" under § 14:403.2 is any person or persons, either temporarily or permanently, responsible for the care of an aged person or a physically or mentally disabled adult. Caregiver includes but is not limited to adult children, parents, relatives, neighbors, day care personnel, adult foster home sponsors, personnel of public and private institutions and facilities, adult congregate living facilities, and nursing homes which have voluntarily assumed the care of an aged person, or disabled adult, have assumed voluntary residence with an aged person or disabled adult, or have assumed voluntary use or tutelage of an aged or disabled person's assets, funds, or property, and specifically shall include city, parish, or state law enforcement agencies.

MAINE: 22 M.R.S. § 3472 (2000)

"**Abuse**" means the infliction of injury, unreasonable confinement, intimidation, or cruel punishment with resulting physical harm or pain or mental anguish; sexual abuse or exploitation; or the willful deprivation of essential needs.

> *Defined separately: Sexual abuse or exploitation* means contact or interaction of a sexual nature involving an incapacitated or dependent adult without that adult's consent.

"**Neglect**" means a threat to an adult's health or welfare by physical or mental injury or impairment, deprivation of essential needs or lack of protection from these.

"**Exploitation**" means the illegal or improper use of an incapacitated or dependent adult or his resources for another's profit or advantage.

"**Dependent adult**" means any adult who is wholly or partially dependent upon one or more other persons for care or support, either emotional or physical, and who would be in danger if that care or support were withdrawn.

"**Caretaker**" means any individual or institution who has or assumes the responsibility for the care of an adult.

MARYLAND: Md. Family Law Code Ann. § 14-101 (2001); Md. Ann. Code Art. 27, § 35D (2001); Md. Health General Code Ann. § 19-347 (2001)

"**Abuse**" under § 14-101 means the sustaining of any physical injury by a vulnerable adult as a result of cruel or inhumane treatment or as a result of a malicious act by any person.

"**Abuse**" under Art. 27, § 35D means (i) the sustaining of any physical pain or injury by a vulnerable adult as a result of cruel or inhumane treatment or as a result of a malicious act by a caregiver, a parent, or other person who has permanent or temporary care or custody or responsibility for the supervision of a vulnerable adult, or by any household or family member under circumstances that indicate that the vulnerable adult's health or welfare is harmed or threatened. (ii) Abuse" includes the sexual abuse of a vulnerable adult. (iii) "Abuse" does not include the performance of an accepted medical or behavioral procedure ordered by a health care provider acting within the scope of the health care provider's practice.

INSTITUTIONAL ABUSE: "**Abuse**" under § 19-347 means the nontherapeutic infliction of physical pain or injury, or any persistent course of conduct intended to produce or resulting in mental or emotional distress; "Abuse" does not include the performance of an accepted medical procedure that a physician orders.

"**Neglect**" under § 14-101 means the willful deprivation of a vulnerable adult of adequate food, clothing, essential medical treatment or rehabilitative therapy, shelter, or supervision.

"**Neglect**" under Art. 27, § 35D means intentional failure to provide necessary assistance and resources for the physical needs of the vulnerable adult, including food, clothing, toileting, essential medical treatment, shelter, or supervision.

"**Exploitation**" under § 14-101 means any action which involves the misuse of a vulnerable adult's funds, property, or person.

"**Vulnerable adult**" under § 14-101 and Art. 27, § 35D means an adult who lacks the physical or mental capacity to provide for the adult's daily needs.

"**Caregiver**" under Art. 27, § 35D means a person under a duty to care for a vulnerable adult because of a contractual undertaking to provide care.

MASSACHUSETTS: Mass. Ann. Laws Ch. 19A § 14 (2001); Mass. Ann. Laws Ch. 111 § 72F (2001)

"**Abuse**" under Ch. 19A § 14 means an act or omission which results in serious physical or emotional injury to an elderly person or financial exploitation of an elderly person; provided, however, that no person shall be considered to be abused or neglected for the sole reason that such person is being furnished or relies upon treatment in accordance with the tenets and teachings of a church or religious denomination by a duly accredited practitioner thereof.

> INSTITUTIONAL ABUSE: "**Abuse**" under Ch. 111 § 72F means the willful infliction of injury, unreasonable confinement, intimidation, including verbal or mental abuse, or punishment with resulting physical harm, pain, or mental anguish or assault and battery; provided, however, that verbal or mental abuse shall require a knowing and willful act directed at a specific person.

> INSTITUTIONAL NEGLECT: "**Neglect**" under Ch. 111 § 72F means failure to provide goods and services necessary to avoid physical harm, mental anguish, or mental illness.

"**Financial exploitation**" under Ch. 19A § 14 means an act or omission by another person, which causes a substantial monetary or property loss to an elderly person, or causes a substantial monetary or property gain to the other person, which gain would otherwise benefit the elderly person but for the act or omission of such other person; provided, however, that such an act or omission shall not be construed as financial exploitation if the elderly person has knowingly consented to such act or omission unless such consent is a consequence of misrepresentation, undue influence, coercion or threat of force by such other person; and, provided further, that financial exploitation shall not be construed to interfere with or prohibit a bona fide gift by an elderly person or to apply to any act or practice in the conduct of any trade or commerce declared unlawful by section two of chapter ninety-three A.

"**Elderly person**" under Ch. 19A § 14 means an individual who is 60 years of age or over.

"**Resident**" under Ch. 111 § 72F means an individual who resides in a long-term care facility licensed under section 71.

"**Caretaker**" under Ch. 19A § 14 means the person responsible for the care of an elderly person, which responsibility may arise as the result of a family relationship, or by a voluntary or contractual duty undertaken on behalf of an elderly person, or may arise by a fiduciary duty imposed by law.

MICHIGAN: MCLS §§ 400.11, 400.586k, 750.145n (2001)

"**Abuse**" under § 400.11 means harm or threatened harm to an adult's health or welfare caused by another person. Abuse includes, but is not limited to, nonaccidental physical or mental injury, sexual abuse, or maltreatment.

"**Abuse of older persons**" under § 400.586k includes the following types of abuse involving an older person: physical abuse, emotional or social abuse, financial abuse, or environmental abuse.

"**Vulnerable adult abuse**" under MCLS § 750.145n: (1) A caregiver is guilty of vulnerable adult abuse in the first degree if the caregiver intentionally causes serious physical harm or serious mental harm to a vulnerable adult. (2) A caregiver or other person with authority over the vulnerable adult is guilty of vulnerable adult abuse in the second degree if the reckless act or reckless failure to act of the caregiver or other person with authority over the vulnerable adult causes serious physical harm or serious mental harm to a vulnerable adult. (3) A caregiver is guilty of vulnerable adult abuse in the third degree if the caregiver intentionally causes physical harm to a vulnerable adult. (4) A caregiver or other person with authority over the vulnerable adult is guilty of vulnerable adult abuse in the fourth degree if the reckless act or reckless failure to act of the caregiver or other person with authority over a vulnerable adult causes physical harm to a vulnerable adult.

"Neglect" under § 400.11 means harm to an adult's health or welfare caused by the inability of the adult to respond to a harmful situation or by the conduct of a person who assumes responsibility for a significant aspect of the adult's health or welfare. Neglect includes the failure to provide adequate food, clothing, shelter, or medical care. A person shall not be considered to be abused, neglected, or in need of emergency or protective services for the sole reason that the person is receiving or relying upon treatment by spiritual means through prayer alone in accordance with the tenets and practices of a recognized church or religious denomination, and this act shall not require any medical care or treatment in contravention of the stated or implied objection of that person.

"Exploitation" under § 400.11 means an action that involves the misuse of an adult's funds, property, or personal dignity by another person.

"Adult in need of protective services" or "adult" under § 400.11 means a vulnerable person not less than 18 years of age who is suspected of being or believed to be abused, neglected, or exploited. "Vulnerable" means a condition in which an adult is unable to protect himself or herself from abuse, neglect, or exploitation because of a mental or physical impairment or because of advanced age.

"Vulnerable adult" under § 750.145 means 1 or more of the following: (i) An individual age 18 or over who, because of age, developmental disability, mental illness, or physical disability requires supervision or personal care or lacks the personal and social skills required to live independently. (ii) An adult as defined in section 3(1)(b) of the adult foster care facility licensing act, MCL 400.703. (iii) An adult as defined in section 11(b) of the social welfare act, MCL 400.11.

"Caregiver" under § 750.145 means an individual who directly cares for or has physical custody of a vulnerable adult.

MINNESOTA: Minn. Stat. § 626.5572 (2000)

"**Abuse**" means: (a) An act against a vulnerable adult that constitutes a violation of, an attempt to violate, or aiding and abetting a violation of: (1) assault in the first through fifth degrees as defined in sections 609.221 to 609.224; (2) the use of drugs to injure or facilitate crime as defined in section 609.235; (3) the solicitation, inducement, and promotion of prostitution as defined in section 609.322; and (4) criminal sexual conduct in the first through fifth degrees as defined in sections 609.342 to 609.3451. A violation includes any action that meets the elements of the crime, regardless of whether there is a criminal proceeding or conviction. (b) Conduct which is not an accident or therapeutic conduct as defined in this section, which produces or could reasonably be expected to produce physical pain or injury or emotional distress including, but not limited to, the following: (1) hitting, slapping, kicking, pinching, biting, or corporal punishment of a vulnerable adult; (2) use of repeated or malicious oral, written, or gestured language toward a vulnerable adult or the treatment of a vulnerable adult which would be considered by a reasonable person to be disparaging, derogatory, humiliating, harassing, or threatening; (3) use of any aversive or deprivation procedure, unreasonable confinement, or involuntary seclusion, including the forced separation of the vulnerable adult from other persons against the will of the vulnerable adult or the legal representative of the vulnerable adult; and (4) use of any aversive or deprivation procedures for persons with developmental disabilities or related conditions not authorized under section 245.825. (c) Any sexual contact or penetration as defined in section 609.341, between a facility staff person or a person providing services in the facility and a resident, patient, or client of that facility. (d) The act of forcing, compelling, coercing, or enticing a vulnerable adult against the vulnerable adult's will to perform services for the advantage of another. (e) For purposes of this section, a vulnerable adult is not abused for the sole reason that the vulnerable adult or a person with authority to make health care decisions for the vulnerable adult under sections 144.651, 144A.44, chapter 145B, 145C or 252A, or section 253B.03 or 525.539 to 525.6199, refuses consent or withdraws consent, consistent with that authority and within the boundary of reasonable medical practice, to any therapeutic conduct, including any care, service, or procedure to diagnose, maintain, or treat the physical or mental condition of the vulnerable adult or, where permitted under law, to provide nutrition and hydration parenterally or through intubation. This paragraph does not enlarge or diminish rights otherwise held under law by: (1) a vulnerable adult or a person acting on behalf of a vulnerable adult, including an involved family member, to consent to or refuse consent for therapeutic conduct; or (2) a caregiver to offer or provide or refuse to offer or provide therapeutic conduct. (f) For purposes of this section, a vulnerable adult is not abused for the sole reason that the vulnerable adult, a person with authority to make health care decisions for the vulnerable adult, or a caregiver in good faith selects and depends upon spiritual means or prayer for treatment or care of disease or remedial care of the vulnerable adult in lieu of medical care, provided that this is consistent with the prior practice or belief of the vulnerable adult or with the expressed intentions of the vulnerable adult. (g) For purposes of this section, a vulnerable adult is not abused for the sole reason that the vulnerable adult, who is not impaired in judgment or capacity by mental or emotional dysfunction or undue influence, engages in consensual sexual contact with: (1) a person, including a facility staff person, when a consensual sexual personal relationship existed prior to the caregiving relationship; or (2) a personal care attendant, regardless of whether the consensual sexual personal relationship existed prior to the caregiving relationship.

"**Neglect**" means (a) The failure or omission by a caregiver to supply a vulnerable adult with care or services, including but not limited to, food, clothing, shelter, health care, or supervision which is: (1) reasonable and necessary to obtain or maintain the vulnerable adult's physical or mental health or safety, considering the physical and mental capacity or dysfunction of the vulnerable adult; and (2) which is not the result of an accident or therapeutic conduct. (b) The absence or likelihood of absence of care or services, including but not limited to, food, clothing, shelter, health care, or supervision necessary to maintain the physical and mental health of the vulnerable adult which a reasonable person would deem essential to obtain or maintain the vulnerable adult's health, safety, or comfort considering the physical or mental capacity or dysfunction of the vulnerable adult.

"**Financial exploitation**" means: (a) In breach of a fiduciary obligation recognized elsewhere in law, including pertinent regulations, contractual obligations, documented consent by a competent person, or the obligations of a responsible party under section 144.6501, a person: (1) engages in unauthorized expenditure of funds entrusted to the actor by the vulnerable adult which results or is likely to result in detriment to the vulnerable adult; or (2) fails to use the financial resources of the vulnerable adult to provide food, clothing, shelter, health care, therapeutic conduct or supervision for the vulnerable adult, and the failure results or is likely to result in detriment to the vulnerable adult. (b) In the absence of legal authority a person: (1) willfully uses, withholds, or disposes of funds or property of a vulnerable adult; (2) obtains for the actor or another the performance of services by a third person for the wrongful profit or advantage of the actor or another to the detriment of the vulnerable adult; (3) acquires possession or control of, or an interest in, funds or property of a vulnerable adult through the use of undue influence, harassment, duress, deception, or fraud; or (4) forces, compels, coerces, or entices a vulnerable adult against the vulnerable adult's will to perform services for the profit or advantage of another. (c) Nothing in this definition requires a facility or caregiver to provide financial management or supervise financial management for a vulnerable adult except as otherwise required by law.

"**Vulnerable adult**" means any person 18 years of age or older who: (1) is a resident or inpatient of a facility; (2) receives services at or from a facility required to be licensed to serve adults under sections 245A.01 to 245A.15, except that a person receiving outpatient services for treatment of chemical dependency or mental illness, or one who is committed as a sexual psychopathic personality or as a sexually dangerous person under chapter 253B, is not considered a vulnerable adult unless the person meets the requirements of clause (4); (3) receives services from a home care provider required to be licensed under section 144A.46; or from a person or organization that exclusively offers, provides, or arranges for personal care assistant services under the medical assistance program as authorized under sections 256B.04, subdivision 16, 256B.0625, subdivision 19a, and 256B.0627; or (4) regardless of residence or whether any type of service is received, possesses a physical or mental infirmity or other physical, mental, or emotional dysfunction: (i) that impairs the individual's ability to provide adequately for the individual's own care without assistance, including the provision of food, shelter, clothing, health care, or supervision; and (ii) because of the dysfunction or infirmity and the need for assistance, the individual has an impaired ability to protect the individual from maltreatment.

"**Caregiver**" means an individual or facility who has responsibility for the care of a vulnerable adult as a result of a family relationship, or who has assumed responsibility for all or a portion of the care of a vulnerable adult voluntarily, by contract, or by agreement.

MISSISSIPPI: Miss. Code Ann. § 43-47-5 (2001)

"**Abuse**" shall mean the willful or nonaccidental infliction of physical pain, injury, or mental anguish on a vulnerable adult, the unreasonable confinement of a vulnerable adult, or the willful deprivation by a caretaker of services which are necessary to maintain the mental and physical health of a vulnerable adult. "Abuse" shall include sexual abuse. "Abuse" shall not mean conduct which is a part of the treatment and care of, and in furtherance of the health and safety of a patient or resident of a care facility. "Abuse" includes, but is not limited to, a single incident.

"**Neglect**" shall mean either the inability of a vulnerable adult who is living alone to provide for himself the food, clothing, shelter, health care or other services which are necessary to maintain his mental and physical health, or failure of a caretaker to supply the vulnerable adult with the food, clothing, shelter, health care, supervision or other services which a reasonably prudent person would do to maintain the vulnerable adult's mental and physical health. "Neglect" includes, but is not limited to, a single incident.

"**Exploitation**" shall mean the illegal or improper use of a vulnerable adult or his resources for another's profit or advantage with or without the consent of the vulnerable adult. "Exploitation" includes, but is not limited to, a single incident.

"**Vulnerable adult**" shall mean a person 18 years of age or older or any minor whose ability to perform the normal activities of daily living or to provide for his or her own care or protection is impaired due to a mental, emotional, physical, or developmental disability or dysfunction, or brain damage or the infirmities of aging. The term "vulnerable adult" shall also include all residents or patients, regardless of age, in a care facility for the purposes of Sections 43-47-19 and 43-47-37 only. The department shall not be prohibited from investigating, and shall have the authority and responsibility to fully investigate, in accordance with the provisions of this chapter, any allegation of abuse, neglect, and/or exploitation regarding a patient in a care facility, if the alleged abuse, neglect, and/or exploitation occurred at a private residence.

"**Caretaker**" shall mean an individual, corporation, partnership, or other organization which has assumed the responsibility for the care of a vulnerable adult, but shall not include the Division of Medicaid, a licensed hospital, or a licensed nursing home within the state.

MISSOURI: § 660.250 R.S. Mo. (2000); § 565.180 R.S. Mo. (2000); § 565.182 R.S. Mo. (2000); § 565.184 R.S. Mo. (2000); § 198.006 R.S.Mo. (2000)

"**Abuse**" under § 660.250 means the infliction of physical, sexual, or emotional injury or harm including financial exploitation by any person, firm, or corporation.

"**Elder abuse**" under § 565.180 occurs when a person attempts to kill, knowingly causes or attempts to cause serious physical injury, as defined in § 565.002, to any person 60 years of age or older or an eligible adult as defined in § 660.250. It occurs under § 565.182 when a person (1) Knowingly causes, attempts to cause physical injury to any person 60 years of age or older or an eligible adult, as defined in § 660.250 by means of a deadly weapon or dangerous instrument; or (2) Recklessly and purposely causes serious physical injury, as defined in § 565.002, to a person 60 years of age or older or an eligible adult as defined in § 660.250. It occurs under § 565.184 when a person (1) Knowingly causes or attempts to cause physical contact with any person 60 years of age or older or an eligible adult as defined in § 660.250, knowing the other person will regard the contact as harmful or provocative; or (2) Purposely engages in conduct involving more than one incident that causes grave emotional distress to a person 60 years of age or older or an eligible adult, as defined in § 660.250. The course of conduct shall be such as would cause a reasonable person age 60 years of age or older or an eligible adult, as defined in § 660.250, to suffer substantial emotional distress; or (3) Purposely or knowingly places a person 60 years of age or older or an eligible adult, as defined in § 660.250 in apprehension of immediate physical injury; or (4) Intentionally fails to provide care, goods or services to a person 60 years of age or older or an eligible adult, as defined in § 660.250. The cause of the conduct shall be such as would cause a reasonable person age 60 or older or an eligible adult, as defined in § 660.250, to suffer physical or emotional distress; or (5) Knowingly acts or knowingly fails to act in a manner which results in a grave risk to the life, body, or health of a person 60 years of age or older or an eligible adult, as defined in § 660.250.

INSTITUTIONAL ABUSE: "**Abuse**" under § 198.006 means the infliction of physical, sexual, or emotional injury or harm.

"**Neglect**" under § 660.250 means the failure to provide services to an eligible adult by any person, firm or corporation with a legal or contractual duty to do so, when such failure presents either an imminent danger to the health, safety, or welfare of the client or a substantial probability that death or serious physical harm would result.

INSTITUTIONAL NEGLECT: "**Neglect**" under § 198.006 means the failure to provide, by those responsible for the care, custody, and control of a resident in a facility, the services which are reasonable and necessary to maintain the physical and mental health of the resident, when such failure presents either an imminent danger to the health, safety, or welfare of the resident or a substantial probability that death or serious physical harm would result.

"**Eligible adult**" under § 660.250 means a person 60 years of age or older or an adult with a handicap, as defined in § 660.053, between the ages of 18 and 59 who is unable to protect his own interests or adequately perform or obtain services which are necessary to meet his essential human needs.

"**Resident**" under § 198.006 means a person who by reason of aging, illness, disease, or physical or mental infirmity receives or requires care and services furnished by a facility and who resides or boards in or otherwise kept, cared for, treated or accommodated in such facility for a period exceeding 24 consecutive hours.

MONTANA: Mont. Code Anno. § 52-3-803 (2001)

"**Abuse**" means: (a) the infliction of physical or mental injury; or (b) the deprivation of food, shelter, clothing, or services necessary to maintain the physical or mental health of an older person or a person with a developmental disability without lawful authority. A declaration made pursuant to 50-9-103 constitutes lawful authority.

> *Defined separately*: *Sexual abuse* means the commission of sexual assault, sexual intercourse without consent, indecent exposure, deviate sexual conduct, or incest.

"**Neglect**" means the failure of a person who has assumed legal responsibility or a contractual obligation for caring for an older person or a person with a developmental disability or who has voluntarily assumed responsibility for the person's care, including an employee of a public or private residential institution, facility, home, or agency, to provide food, shelter, clothing, or services necessary to maintain the physical or mental health of the older person or the person with a developmental disability.

"**Exploitation**" means: (a) the unreasonable use of an older person or a person with a developmental disability or of a power of attorney, conservatorship, or guardianship with regard to an older person or a person with a developmental disability to obtain control of or to divert to the advantage of another the ownership, use, benefit, or possession of the person's money, assets, or property by means of deception, duress, menace, fraud, undue influence, or intimidation with the intent or result of permanently depriving the older person or person with a developmental disability of the ownership, use, benefit, or possession of the person's money, assets, or property; (b) an act taken by a person who has the trust and confidence of an older person or a person with a developmental disability to obtain control of or to divert to the advantage of another the ownership, use, benefit, or possession of the person's money, assets, or property by means of deception, duress, menace, fraud, undue influence, or intimidation with the intent or result of permanently depriving the older person or person with a developmental disability of the ownership, use, or benefit of the person's money, assets, or property.

"**Older person**" means a person who is at least 60 years of age. For purposes of prosecution under 52-3-825(2), the person 60 years of age or older must be unable to provide personal protection from abuse, sexual abuse, neglect, or exploitation because of a mental or physical impairment or because of frailties or dependencies brought about by advanced age. "Person with a developmental disability" means a person 18 years of age or older who has a developmental disability.

NEBRASKA: R.R.S. Neb. §§ 28-351, 28-353, 28-355, 28-358, 28-371 (2001)

"**Abuse**" means any knowing, intentional, or negligent act or omission on the part of a caregiver, a vulnerable adult, or any other person which results in physical injury, unreasonable confinement, cruel punishment, sexual abuse, exploitation, or denial of essential services to a vulnerable adult.

"**Denial of essential services**" under § 28-355 shall mean that essential services are denied or neglected to such an extent that there is actual physical injury to a vulnerable adult or imminent danger of the vulnerable adult suffering physical injury or death.

"**Exploitation**" under § 28-358 shall mean the taking of property of a vulnerable adult by means of undue influence, breach of a fiduciary relationship, deception, or extortion or by any unlawful means.

"**Vulnerable adult**" under § 28-371 shall mean any person 18 years of age or older who has a substantial mental or functional impairment or for whom a guardian has been appointed under the Nebraska Probate Code.

"**Caregiver**" under § 28-353 shall mean any person or entity which has assumed the responsibility for the care of a vulnerable adult voluntarily, by express or implied contract, or by order of a court of competent jurisdiction.

NEVADA: Nev. Rev. Stat. Ann. §§ 41.1395, 200.5092 (2001)

"Abuse" under § 41.1395 means willful and unjustified: (1) Infliction of pain, injury or mental anguish; or (2) Deprivation of food, shelter, clothing or services which are necessary to maintain the physical or mental health of an older person or a vulnerable person.

"Abuse" under § 200.5092 means willful and unjustified: (a) Infliction of pain, injury or mental anguish on an older person; or (b) Deprivation of food, shelter, clothing, or services which are necessary to maintain the physical or mental health of an older person.

"Neglect" under § 41.1395 means the failure of a person who has assumed legal responsibility or a contractual obligation for caring for an older person or a vulnerable person, or who has voluntarily assumed responsibility for his care, to provide food, shelter, clothing, or services within the scope of his responsibility or obligation, which are necessary to maintain the physical or mental health of the older person or vulnerable person. For the purposes of this paragraph, a person voluntarily assumes responsibility to provide care for an older or vulnerable person only to the extent that he has expressly acknowledged his responsibility to provide such care.

"Neglect" under § 200.5092 means the failure of: (a) A person who has assumed legal responsibility or a contractual obligation for caring for an older person or who has voluntarily assumed responsibility for his care to provide food, shelter, clothing, or services which are necessary to maintain the physical or mental health of the older person; or (b) An older person to provide for his own needs because of inability to do so.

"Exploitation" under § 41.1395 and § 200.5092 means any act taken by a person who has the trust and confidence of an older person or a vulnerable person or any use of the power of attorney or guardianship of an older person or a vulnerable person to obtain control, through deception, intimidation, or undue influence, over the money, assets or property of the older person or vulnerable person with the intention of permanently depriving the older person or vulnerable person of the ownership, use, benefit, or possession of his money, assets, or property. As used in this paragraph, "undue influence" does not include the normal influence that one member of a family has over another.

"Older person" under § 41.1395 and § 200.5092 means a person who is 60 years of age or older. "Vulnerable person" means a person who: (1) Has a physical or mental impairment that substantially limits one or more of the major life activities of the person; and (2) Has a medical or psychological record of the impairment or is otherwise regarded as having the impairment.

NEW HAMPSHIRE: RSA 161-F:43 (2000)

"**Abuse**" means any act or omission by a person which is not accidental and harms or threatens to harm an incapacitated adult's physical, mental, or emotional health or safety. The term abuse includes the following: (a) "Emotional abuse" means the misuse of power, authority, or both, verbal harassment, or unreasonable confinement which results or could result in the mental anguish or emotional distress of an incapacitated adult. (b) "Physical abuse" means the use of physical force which results or could result in physical injury to an incapacitated adult. (c) "Sexual abuse" means contact or interaction of a sexual nature involving an incapacitated adult who is being used without his or her informed consent.

"**Neglect**" means an act of omission which results or could result in the deprivation of essential services necessary to maintain the minimum mental, emotional, or physical health and safety of an incapacitated adult. "Self-neglect" is defined separately at §161-F:43(VII).

"**Exploitation**" means the illegal use of an incapacitated adult's person or property for another person's profit or advantage, or the breach of a fiduciary relationship through the use of a person or a person's property for any purpose not in the proper and lawful execution of a trust, including, but not limited to, situations where a person obtains money, property, or services from an incapacitated adult through the use of undue influence, harassment, duress, deception, or fraud.

"**Adult**" means any person who is 18 years of age or older who is thought to manifest a degree of incapacity by reason of limited mental or physical function which may result in harm or hazard to himself or others or who is a person unable to manage his estate.

NEW JERSEY: N.J. Stat. §§ 52:27D-407, 30:1A-3 (2001)

"**Abuse**" under § 52:27D-407 means the willful infliction of physical pain, injury, or mental anguish, unreasonable confinement, or the willful deprivation of services which are necessary to maintain a person's physical and mental health.

INSTITUTIONAL ABUSE: "**Abuse**" under § 30:1A-3 means the willful infliction of physical pain, injury, or mental anguish; unreasonable confinement; or, the willful deprivation of services which are necessary to maintain a person's physical and mental health.

"**Neglect**" under § 52:27D-407 means an act or failure to act by a vulnerable adult or his caretaker which results in the inadequate provision of care or services necessary to maintain the physical and mental health of the vulnerable adult, and which places the vulnerable adult in a situation which can result in serious injury or which is life-threatening.

"**Exploitation**" under § 52:27D-407 means the act or process of illegally or improperly using a person or his resources for another person's profit or advantage.

INSTITUTIONAL EXPLOITATION: "**Exploitation**" under § 30:1A-3 means the act or process of using a person or his resources for another person's profit or advantage.

"**Vulnerable adult**" under § 52:27D-407 means a person 18 years of age or older who resides in a community setting and who, because of a physical or mental illness, disability, or deficiency, lacks sufficient understanding or capacity to make, communicate, or carry out decisions concerning his well-being and is the subject of abuse, neglect ,or exploitation. A person shall not be deemed to be the subject of abuse, neglect, or exploitation or in need of protective services for the sole reason that the person is being furnished nonmedical remedial treatment by spiritual means through prayer alone or in accordance with a recognized religious method of healing in lieu of medical treatment, and in accordance with the tenets and practices of the person's established religious tradition.

"**Caretaker**" under § 52:27D-407 means a person who has assumed the responsibility for the care of a vulnerable adult as a result of family relationship or who has assumed responsibility for the care of a vulnerable adult voluntarily, by contract, or by order of a court of competent jurisdiction, whether or not they reside together.

NEW MEXICO: N.M. Stat. Ann. §§ 27-7-16, 30-47-3 (2001)

"**Abuse**" under § 27-7-16 means: (1) knowingly, intentionally or negligently and without justifiable cause inflicting physical pain, injury, or mental anguish; or (2) the intentional deprivation by a caretaker or other person of services necessary to maintain the mental and physical health of an adult;

INSTITUTIONAL ABUSE: "**Abuse**" under § 30-47-3 means any act or failure to act performed intentionally, knowingly or recklessly that causes or is likely to cause harm to a resident, including: (1) physical contact that harms or is likely to harm a resident of a care facility; (2) inappropriate use of a physical restraint, isolation, or medication that harms or is likely to harm a resident; (3) inappropriate use of a physical or chemical restraint, medication, or isolation as punishment or in conflict with a physician's order; (4) medically inappropriate conduct that causes or is likely to cause physical harm to a resident; (5) medically inappropriate conduct that causes or is likely to cause great psychological harm to a resident;(6) an unlawful act, a threat, or menacing conduct directed toward a resident that results and might reasonably be expected to result in fear or emotional or mental distress to a resident.

"**Neglect**" under § 27-7-16 means failure of the caretaker of an adult to provide basic needs such as clothing, food, shelter, supervision, and care for the physical and mental health for that adult or failure by an adult to provide such basic needs for himself.

INSTITUTIONAL NEGLECT: "**Neglect**" under § 30-47-3 means, subject to the resident's right to refuse treatment and subject to the caregiver's right to exercise sound medical discretion, the grossly negligent: (1) failure to provide any treatment, service, care, medication, or item that is necessary to maintain the health or safety of a resident; (2) failure to take any reasonable precaution that is necessary to prevent damage to the health or safety of a resident; or (3) failure to carry out a duty to supervise properly or control the provision of any treatment, care, good, service, or medication necessary to maintain the health or safety of a resident.

"**Exploitation**" under § 27-7-16 means an unjust or improper use of an adult's money or property for another person's profit or advantage, pecuniary or otherwise.

"**Adult**" under § 27-7-16 means a person 18 years of age or older.

"**Caretaker**" under § 27-7-16 means an individual or institution that has assumed the responsibility for the care of an adult.

NEW YORK: NY CLS Soc. Serv. § 473 (2001); NY CLS Penal §§ 260.30, 260.32, 260.34 (2001)

"**Physical abuse**" means the nonaccidental use of force that results in bodily injury, pain or impairment, including but not limited to, being slapped, burned, cut, bruised, or improperly physically restrained. (b) "Sexual abuse" means nonconsensual sexual contact of any kind, including but not limited to, forcing sexual contact or forcing sex with a third party. (c) "Emotional abuse" means willful infliction of mental or emotional anguish by threat, humiliation, intimidation, or other abusive conduct, including but not limited to, frightening or isolating an adult.

"**Endangering the welfare of a vulnerable elderly person**" occurs under NY CLS Penal § 260.32 when, being a caregiver for a vulnerable elderly person: 1. With intent to cause physical injury to such person, he or she causes such injury to such person; or 2. He or she recklessly causes physical injury to such person; or 3. With criminal negligence, he or she causes physical injury to such person by means of a deadly weapon or a dangerous instrument; or 4. He or she subjects such person to sexual contact without the latter's consent. "Endangering the welfare of a vulnerable elderly person" under NY CLS Penal § 260.34 occurs when, being a caregiver for a vulnerable elderly person: 1. With intent to cause physical injury to such person, he or she causes serious physical injury to such person; or 2. He or she recklessly causes serious physical injury to such person.

"**Active neglect**" under NY CLS Soc. Serv. § 473 means willful failure by the caregiver to fulfill the care-taking functions and responsibilities assumed by the caregiver, including but not limited to, abandonment, willful deprivation of food, water, heat, clean clothing and bedding, eyeglasses or dentures, or health-related services. "Passive neglect" under NY CLS Soc. Serv. § 473 means nonwillful failure of a caregiver to fulfill care-taking functions and responsibilities assumed by the caregiver, including but not limited to, abandonment or denial of food or health-related services because of inadequate caregiver knowledge, infirmity, or disputing the value of prescribed services. "Self-neglect" defined separately.

"**Financial exploitation**" means improper use of an adult's funds, property, or resources by another individual, including but not limited to, fraud, false pretenses, embezzlement, conspiracy, forgery, falsifying records, coerced property transfers, or denial of access to assets.

"**Vulnerable elderly person**" under NY CLS Penal § 260.30 means a person 60 years of age or older who is suffering from a disease or infirmity associated with advanced age and manifested by demonstrable physical, mental, or emotional dysfunction to the extent that the person is incapable of adequately providing for his or her own health or personal care.

"**Caregiver**" under NY CLS § 260.30 means a person who (i) assumes responsibility for the care of a vulnerable elderly person pursuant to a court order; or (ii) receives monetary or other valuable consideration for providing care for a vulnerable elderly person.

NORTH CAROLINA: N.C. Gen. Stat. §§ 14-32.3, 108A-101, 131D-2 (2000)

"**Abuse**" under § 108A-101 means the willful infliction of physical pain, injury ,or mental anguish, unreasonable confinement, or the willful deprivation by a caretaker of services which are necessary to maintain mental and physical health.

"**Abuse**" under § 14-32.3 occurs when a person is a caretaker of a disabled or elder adult who is residing in a domestic setting and, with malice aforethought, knowingly and willfully: (i) assaults, (ii) fails to provide medical or hygienic care, or (iii) confines or restrains the disabled or elder adult in a place or under a condition that is cruel or unsafe, and as a result of the act or failure to act the disabled or elder adult suffers mental or physical injury.

> INSTITUTIONAL ABUSE: "**Abuse**" under § 131D-2 means the willful or grossly negligent infliction of physical pain, injury, or mental anguish, unreasonable confinement, or the willful or grossly negligent deprivation by the administrator or staff of an adult care home of services which are necessary to maintain mental and physical health.

"**Neglect**" under § 108A-101 refers to a disabled adult who is either living alone and not able to provide for himself the services which are necessary to maintain his mental or physical health or is not receiving services from his caretaker. A person is not receiving services from his caretaker if, among other things and not by way of limitation, he is a resident of one of the State-owned hospitals for the mentally ill, centers for the mentally retarded or North Carolina Special Care Center he is, in the opinion of the professional staff of that hospital or center, mentally incompetent to give his consent to medical treatment, he has no legal guardian appointed pursuant to Chapter 35A, or guardian as defined in G.S. 122C-3(15), and he needs medical treatment. "**Neglect**" occurs under § 14-32.3 when a person is a caretaker of a disabled or elder adult who is residing in a domestic setting and, wantonly, recklessly, or with gross carelessness: (i) fails to provide medical or hygienic care, or (ii) confines or restrains the disabled or elder adult in a place or under a condition that is unsafe, and as a result of the act or failure to act the disabled or elder adult suffers mental or physical injury.

> INSTITUTIONAL NEGLECT: **"Neglect"** under § 131D-2 means the failure to provide the services necessary to maintain a resident's physical or mental health.

"Exploitation" under § 108A-101 means the illegal or improper use of a disabled adult or his resources for another's profit or advantage. "Exploitation" under § 14-32.3 occurs when a person is a caretaker of a disabled or elder adult who is residing in a domestic setting, and knowingly, willfully, and with the intent to permanently deprive the owner of property or money: (i) makes a false representation, (ii) abuses a position of trust or fiduciary duty, or (iii) coerces, commands, or threatens, and, as a result of the act, the disabled or elder adult gives or loses possession and control of property or money.

> INSTITUTIONAL EXPLOITATION: *"Exploitation"* under § 131D-2 means the illegal or improper use of an aged or disabled resident or his resources for another's profit or advantage.

"Disabled adult" under § 108A-101 shall mean any person 18 years of age or over or any lawfully emancipated minor who is present in the State of North Carolina and who is physically or mentally incapacitated due to mental retardation, cerebral palsy, epilepsy, or autism; organic brain damage caused by advanced age or other physical degeneration in connection therewith; or due to conditions incurred at any age which are the result of accident, organic brain damage, mental or physical illness, or continued consumption or absorption of substances.

"Disabled adult" under § 14-32.3 means a person 18 years of age or older or a lawfully emancipated minor who is present in the State of North Carolina and who is physically or mentally incapacitated as defined in G.S. 108A-101(d).

"Elder adult" under § 14-32.3 means a person 60 years of age or older who is not able to provide for the social, medical, psychiatric, psychological, financial, or legal services necessary to safeguard the person's rights and resources and to maintain the person's physical and mental well-being.

"Resident" under § 131D-2 means a person living in an assisted living residence for the purpose of obtaining access to housing and services provided or made available by housing management.

"**Caretaker**" under § 108A-101 and § 14-32.3 shall mean an individual who has the responsibility for the care of the disabled adult as a result of family relationship or who has assumed the responsibility for the care of the disabled adult voluntarily or by contract.

NORTH DAKOTA: N.D. Cent. Code § 50-25.2-01 (2001)

"**Abuse**" means any willful act or omission of a caregiver or any other person, which results in physical injury, mental anguish, unreasonable confinement, sexual abuse or exploitation, or financial exploitation to or of a vulnerable adult.

"**Neglect**" means the failure of a caregiver to provide essential services necessary to maintain the physical and mental health of a vulnerable adult, or the inability or lack of desire of the vulnerable adult to provide essential services necessary to maintain and safeguard the vulnerable adult's own physical and mental health.

"**Financial exploitation**" means the taking or misuse of property or resources of a vulnerable adult by means of undue influence, breach of a fiduciary relationship, deception, harassment, criminal coercion, theft, or other unlawful or improper means.

"**Vulnerable adult**" means an adult who has a substantial mental or func tional impairment.

"**Caregiver**" means any person who has assumed the legal responsibility or a contractual obligation for the care of a vulnerable adult or has voluntarily assumed responsibility for the care of a vulnerable adult. The term includes a facility operated by any public or private agency, organization, or institution which provides services to, and has assumed responsibility for the care of, a vulnerable adult.

OHIO: ORC Ann. §§ 2903.33, 3721.21, 3722.12, 5101.60 (2001)

"**Abuse**" under § 5101.60 means the infliction upon an adult by self or others of injury, unreasonable confinement, intimidation, or cruel punishment with resulting physical harm, pain, or mental anguish.

"**Abuse**" under § 2903.33 means knowingly causing physical harm or recklessly causing serious physical harm to a person by physical contact with the person or by the inappropriate use of a physical or chemical restraint, medication, or isolation on the person.

> INSTITUTIONAL ABUSE: "**Abuse**" under § 3721.21 means knowingly causing physical harm or recklessly causing serious physical harm to a resident by physical contact with the resident or by use of physical or chemical restraint, medication, or isolation as punishment, for staff convenience, excessively, as a substitute for treatment, or in amounts that preclude habilitation and treatment.

> "**Abuse**" under § 3722.12 means the unreasonable confinement or intimidation of a resident, or the infliction of injury or cruel punishment upon a resident, resulting in physical harm, pain, or mental anguish.

"**Neglect**" under § 5101.60 means the failure of an adult to provide for self the goods or services necessary to avoid physical harm, mental anguish, or mental illness or the failure of a caretaker to provide such goods or services.

"**Gross neglect**" under § 2903.33 means knowingly failing to provide a person with any treatment, care, goods, or service that is necessary to maintain the health or safety of the person when the failure results in physical harm or serious physical harm to the person. "Neglect" means recklessly failing to provide a person with any treatment, care, goods, or service that is necessary to maintain the health or safety of the person when the failure results in serious physical harm to the person.

> INSTITUTIONAL NEGLECT: "**Neglect**" under § 3721.21 means recklessly failing to provide a resident with any treatment, care, goods, or service necessary to maintain the health or safety of the resident when the failure results in serious physical harm to the resident. "**Neglect**" does not include allowing a resident, at the resident's option, to receive only treatment by spiritual means through prayer in accordance with the tenets of a recognized religious denomination.

"**Neglect**" under § 3722.12 means failure to provide a resident with goods or services necessary to prevent physical harm, mental anguish, or mental illness.

"**Exploitation**" under § 5101.60 means the unlawful or improper act of a caretaker using an adult or an adult's resources for monetary or personal benefit, profit, or gain.

INSTITUTIONAL MISAPPROPRIATION: "**Misappropriation**" under § 3721.21 means depriving, defrauding, or otherwise obtaining the real or personal property of a resident by any means prohibited by the Revised Code, including violations of Chapter 2911 or 2913 of the Revised Code.

"**Exploitation**" under § 3722.12 means the unlawful or improper utilization of an adult resident or his resources for personal or monetary benefit, profit, or gain.

"**Adult**" under § 5101.60 means any person 60 years of age or older within this state who is handicapped by the infirmities of aging or who has a physical or mental impairment which prevents the person from providing for the person's own care or protection, and who resides in an independent living arrangement. An "independent living arrangement" is a domicile of a person's own choosing, including, but not limited to, a private home, apartment, trailer, or rooming house. Except as otherwise provided in this division, "independent living arrangement" includes a community alternative home licensed pursuant to § 3724.03 of the Revised Code but does not include other institutions or facilities licensed by the state, or facilities in which a person resides as a result of voluntary, civil, or criminal commitment. "Independent living arrangement" does include adult care facilities licensed pursuant to Chapter 3722 of the Revised Code.

"**Caretaker**" under § 5101.60 means the person assuming the responsibility for the care of an adult on a voluntary basis, by contract, through receipt of payment for care, as a result of a family relationship, or by order of a court of competent jurisdiction.

OKLAHOMA: 43A Okl. St. § 10-103 (2000); 63 Okl. St. § 1-1902 (2000); 63 Okl. St. § 1-820 (2000)

"**Abuse**" under § 10-103 means the intentional infliction of physical pain, injury, sexual abuse, or mental anguish or the deprivation of food, clothing, shelter, or medical care to a vulnerable adult by a caretaker or other person responsible for providing these services.

INSITUTIONAL ABUSE: "**Abuse**" under § 1-1902 and § 1-820 means the willful infliction of injury, unreasonable confinement, intimidation or punishment, with resulting physical harm, impairment or mental anguish.

"**Neglect**" under § 10-103 means the failure to provide protection for a vulnerable adult who is unable to protect the person's own interest; or the failure to provide adequate shelter or clothing; or the harming or threatening with harm through action or inaction by either another individual or through the person's own action or inaction because of a lack of awareness, incompetence, or incapacity, which has resulted or may result in physical or mental injury.

INSTITUTIONAL NEGLECT: "**Neglect**" under § 1-1902 and § 1-820 means failure to provide goods and/or services necessary to avoid physical harm, mental anguish, or mental illness.

"**Exploitation**" or "exploit" under § 10-103 means an unjust or improper use of the resources of a vulnerable adult for the profit or advantage, pecuniary or otherwise, of a person other than the vulnerable adult through the use of undue influence, coercion, harassment, duress, deception, false representation or false pretense.

"**Vulnerable adult**" under § 10-103 means an individual who is an incapacitated person or who, because of physical or mental disability, incapacity, or other disability, is substantially impaired in the ability to provide adequately for the care or custody of self, or is unable to manage his or her property and financial affairs effectively, or to meet essential requirements for mental or physical health or safety, or to protect self from abuse, neglect, or exploitation without assistance from others.

"**Resident**" under § 1-1902 means a person residing in a facility due to illness, physical or mental infirmity, or advanced age.

"**Caretaker**" under § 10-103 means a person who has: a. the responsibility for the care of the person or financial management of the resources of the vulnerable adult as a result of a family relationship, b. assumed the responsibility for the care of the vulnerable adult voluntarily, by contract, or as a result of the ties of friendship, or c. been appointed a guardian, limited guardian, or conservator pursuant to the Oklahoma Guardianship and Conservatorship Act.

OREGON: ORS §§ 124.005, 441.630 (1999)

"Abuse" under § 124.005 means one or more of the following: (a) Any physical injury caused by other than accidental means, or that appears to be at variance with the explanation given of the injury. (b) Neglect that leads to physical harm through withholding of services necessary to maintain health and well-being. (c) Abandonment, including desertion or willful forsaking of an elderly or disabled person or the withdrawal or neglect of duties and obligations owed an elderly or disabled person by a caregiver or other person. (d) Willful infliction of physical pain or injury. (e) Use of derogatory or inappropriate names, phrases, or profanity, ridicule, harassment, coercion, threats, cursing, intimidation or inappropriate sexual comments of such a nature as to threaten significant physical or emotional harm to the elderly or disabled person. (f) Causing any sweepstakes promotion to be mailed to an elderly, disabled, or incapacitated person who had received sweepstakes promotional material in the United States mail, spent more than $500 in the preceding year on any sweepstakes promotions, or any combination of sweepstakes promotions from the same service, regardless of the identities of the originators of the sweepstakes promotion and who represented to the court that the person felt the need for the court's assistance to prevent the person from incurring further expense.

INSTITUTIONAL ABUSE: "Abuse" under § 441.630 means: (a) Any physical injury to a resident of a long-term care facility which has been caused by other than accidental means. (b) Failure to provide basic care or services, which failure results in physical harm or unreasonable discomfort or serious loss of human dignity. (c) Sexual contact with a resident caused by an employee, agent, or other resident of a long-term care facility by force, threat, duress ,or coercion. (d) Illegal or improper use of a resident's resources for the personal profit or gain of another person. (e) Verbal or mental abuse as prohibited by federal law. (f) Corporal punishment. (g) Involuntary seclusion for convenience or discipline.

"Elderly person" under § 124.005 means any person 65 years of age or older who is not subject to the provisions of ORS 441.640 to 441.665.

PENNSYLVANIA: 35 P.S. § 10225.103 (2001); 63 P.S. § 672 (2001)

"Abuse" under § 10225.103 and § 672 means the occurrence of one or more of the following acts: (1) The infliction of injury, unreasonable confinement, intimidation or punishment with resulting physical harm, pain, or mental anguish. (2) The willful deprivation by a caretaker of goods or services which are necessary to maintain physical or mental health. (3) Sexual harassment, rape or abuse, as defined in the act of October 7, 1976 (P.L. 1090, No. 218), known as the Protection From Abuse Act. No older adult shall be found to be abused solely on the grounds of environmental factors which are beyond the control of the older adult or the caretaker, such as inadequate housing, furnishings, income, clothing, or medical care.

"Neglect" under § 10225.103 means the failure to provide for oneself or the failure of a caretaker to provide goods or services essential to avoid a clear and serious threat to physical or mental health. No older adult who does not consent to the provision of protective services shall be found to be neglected solely on the grounds of environmental factors which are beyond the control of the older adult or the caretaker, such as inadequate housing, furnishings, income, clothing, or medical care.

"Exploitation" under § 10225.103 means an act or course of conduct by a caretaker or other person against an older adult or an older adult's resources, without the informed consent of the older adult or with consent obtained through misrepresentation, coercion, or threats of force, that results in monetary, personal or other benefit, gain or profit for the perpetrator or monetary or personal loss to the older adult.

"Older adult" under § 10225.103 means a person within the jurisdiction of the Commonwealth who is 60 years of age or older. "Older adult in need of protective services" means an incapacitated older adult who is unable to perform or obtain services that are necessary to maintain physical or mental health, for whom there is no responsible caretaker and who is at imminent risk of danger to his person or property.

"Caretaker" under § 10225.103 means an individual or institution that has assumed the responsibility for the provision of care needed to maintain the physical or mental health of an older adult. This responsibility may arise voluntarily, by contract, by receipt of payment for care, as a result of family relationship, or by order of a court of competent jurisdiction. It is not the intent of this act to impose responsibility on any individual if such responsibility would not otherwise exist in law.

RHODE ISLAND: R.I. Gen. Laws §§ 23-17.8-1, 42-66-4.1 (2001)

"**Abuse**" under § 42-66-4.1 means the subjection of an elderly person to the willful infliction of physical pain, or willful deprivation of services by a caretaker or other person with a duty of care for the elderly person. Abuse also includes neglect, abandonment, and exploitation.

INSTITUTIONAL ABUSE: "**Abuse**" under § 23-17.8-1 means: (i) Any assault as defined in chapter 5 of title 11, including, but not limited to, hitting, kicking, pinching, slapping, or the pulling of hair, provided, however, unless such is required as an element of the offense charged, it shall not be necessary to prove that the patient or resident was injured thereby, or; (ii) Any assault as defined in chapter 37 of title 11, or; (iii) Any offense under chapter 10 of title 11, or; (iv) Any conduct which harms or is likely to physically harm the patient or resident except where the conduct is a part of the care and treatment, and in furtherance of the health and safety of the patient or resident, or (v) Intentionally engaging in a pattern of harassing conduct which causes or is likely to cause emotional or psychological harm to the patient or resident, including but not limited to, ridiculing or demeaning a patient or resident, making derogatory remarks to a patient or resident or cursing directed towards a patient or resident, or threatening to inflict physical or emotional harm on a patient or resident.

"**Mistreatment**" under § 23-17.8-1 means the inappropriate use of medications, isolation, or use of physical or chemical restraints (1) as punishment, (2) for staff convenience, (3) as a substitute for treatment or care, (4) in conflict with a physician's order, (5) or in quantities which inhibit effective care or treatment, which harms or is likely to harm the patient or resident.

"**Neglect**" under § 42-66-4.1 means the willful refusal to provide services necessary to maintain physical and mental health on the part of a caretaker or other person with a duty of care.

INSTITUTIONAL NEGLECT: "**Neglect**" under § 23-17.8-1 means the intentional failure to provide treatment, care, goods, and services necessary to maintain the health and safety of the patient or resident, or the intentional failure to carry out a plan of treatment or care prescribed by the physician of the patient or resident, or the intentional failure to report patient or resident health problems or changes in health problems or changes in health conditions to an immediate supervisor or nurse, or the intentional lack of attention to the physical needs of a patient or resident including, but not limited to toileting, bathing, meals, and safety. Provided, however, no person shall be considered to be neglected for the sole reason that he or she relies on or is being furnished treatment in accordance with the tenets and teachings of a well recognized church or denomination by a duly accredited practitioner thereof.

"**Exploitation**" under § 42-66-4.1 means an act or process of taking pecuniary advantage of an elderly person by use of undue influence, harassment, duress, deception, false representation, or false pretenses.

SOUTH CAROLINA: S.C. Code Ann. § 43-35-10 (2000)

"**Abuse**" means physical abuse or psychological abuse. "Physical abuse" means intentionally inflicting or allowing to be inflicted physical injury on a vulnerable adult by an act or failure to act. Physical abuse includes, but is not limited to, slapping, hitting, kicking, biting, choking, pinching, burning, actual or attempted sexual battery as defined in Section 16-3-651, use of medication outside the standards of reasonable medical practice for the purpose of controlling behavior, and unreasonable confinement. Physical abuse also includes the use of a restrictive or physically intrusive procedure to control behavior for the purpose of punishment except that a therapeutic procedure prescribed by a licensed physician or other qualified professional or that is part of a written plan of care by a licensed physician or other qualified professional is not considered physical abuse. Physical abuse does not include altercations or acts of assault between vulnerable adults. "Psychological abuse" means deliberately subjecting a vulnerable adult to threats or harassment or other forms of intimidating behavior causing fear, humiliation, degradation, agitation, confusion, or other forms of serious emotional distress.

"**Neglect**" means the failure or omission of a caregiver to provide the care, goods, or services necessary to maintain the health or safety of a vulnerable adult including, but not limited to, food, clothing, medicine, shelter, supervision, and medical services. Neglect may be repeated conduct or a single incident which has produced or can be proven to result in serious physical or psychological harm or substantial risk of death. Noncompliance with regulatory standards alone does not constitute neglect. Neglect includes the inability of a vulnerable adult, in the absence of a caretaker, to provide for his or her own health or safety which produces or could reasonably be expected to produce serious physical or psychological harm or substantial risk of death.

"**Exploitation**" means: (a) causing or requiring a vulnerable adult to engage in activity or labor which is improper, illegal, or against the reasonable and rational wishes of the vulnerable adult. Exploitation does not include requiring a vulnerable adult to participate in an activity or labor which is a part of a written plan of care or which is prescribed or authorized by a licensed physician attending the patient; or (b) an improper, illegal, or unauthorized use of the funds, assets, property, power of attorney, guardianship, or conservatorship of a vulnerable adult by a person for the profit or advantage of that person or another person.

"Vulnerable adult" means a person 18 years of age or older who has a physical or mental condition which substantially impairs the person from adequately providing for his or her own care or protection. This includes a person who is impaired in the ability to adequately provide for the person's own care or protection because of the infirmities of aging including, but not limited to, organic brain damage, advanced age, and physical, mental, or emotional dysfunction. A resident of a facility is a vulnerable adult.

"Caregiver" means a person who provides care to a vulnerable adult, with or without compensation, on a temporary or permanent or full or part-time basis and includes, but is not limited to, a relative, household member, day care personnel, adult foster home sponsor, and personnel of a public or private institution or facility.

SOUTH DAKOTA: S.D. Codified Laws § 22-46-1 (2001)

"Abuse" means physical harm, bodily injury, or attempt to cause physical harm or injury, or the infliction of fear of imminent physical harm or bodily injury on a disabled adult.

"Neglect" means harm to a disabled adult's health or welfare, without reasonable medical justification, caused by the conduct of a person responsible for the adult's health or welfare, within the means available for the disabled adult, including the failure to provide adequate food, clothing, shelter, or medical care. If a disabled adult is under treatment solely by spiritual means, the court may, upon good cause shown, order that medical treatment be provided for that disabled adult.

"Exploitation" means the wrongful taking or exercising of control over property of a disabled adult with intent to defraud him of it.

"Disabled adult" means a person eighteen years of age or older who suffers from a condition of mental retardation, infirmities of aging as manifested by organic brain damage, advanced age, or other physical dysfunctioning to the extent that the person is unable to protect himself or provide for his own care.

TENNESSEE: Tenn. Code Ann. § 71-6-102 (2001)

"**Abuse or neglect**" means the infliction of physical pain, injury, or mental anguish, or the deprivation of services by a caretaker which are necessary to maintain the health and welfare of an adult or a situation in which an adult is unable to provide or obtain the services which are necessary to maintain that person's health or welfare. Nothing in this part shall be construed to mean a person is abused or neglected or in need of protective services for the sole reason that the person relies on or is being furnished treatment by spiritual means through prayer alone in accordance with a recognized religious method of healing in lieu of medical treatment; further, nothing in this part shall be construed to require or authorize the provision of medical care to any terminally ill person if such person has executed an unrevoked living will in accordance with the provisions of the Tennessee Right to Natural Death Law, compiled in title 32, chapter 11, and if the provisions of such medical care would conflict with the terms of such living will.

"**Exploitation**" means the improper use by a caretaker of funds which have been paid by a governmental agency to an adult or to the caretaker for the use or care of the adult.

"**Adult**" means a person 18 years of age or older who because of mental or physical dysfunctioning or advanced age is unable to manage such person's own resources, carry out the activities of daily living, or protect such person from neglect, hazardous or abusive situations without assistance from others and who has no available, willing, and responsibly able person for assistance and who may be in need of protective services.

"**Advanced age**" means 60 years of age or older.

"**Caretaker**" means an individual or institution who has the responsibility for the care of the adult as a result of family relationship, or who has assumed the responsibility for the care of the adult person voluntarily, or by contract, or agreement.

TEXAS: Tex. Hum.Res. Code § 48.002 (2000)

"**Abuse**" means: (A) the negligent or willful infliction of injury, unreasonable confinement, intimidation, or cruel punishment with resulting physical or emotional harm or pain to an elderly or disabled person by the person's caretaker, family member, or other individual who has an ongoing relationship with the person; or (B) sexual abuse of an elderly or disabled person, including any involuntary or nonconsensual sexual conduct that would constitute an offense under Section 21.08, Penal Code (indecent exposure) or Chapter 22, Penal Code (assaultive offenses), committed by the person's caretaker, family member, or other individual who has an ongoing relationship with the person.

"**Neglect**" means the failure to provide for one's self the goods or services, including medical services, which are necessary to avoid physical or emotional harm or pain or the failure of a caretaker to provide such goods or services.

"**Exploitation**" means the illegal or improper act or process of a caretaker, family member, or other individual who has an ongoing relationship with the elderly or disabled person using the resources of an elderly or disabled person for monetary or personal benefit, profit, or gain without the informed consent of the elderly or disabled person.

"**Elderly person**" means a person 65 years of age or older.

"**Disabled person**" means a person with a mental, physical, or developmental disability that substantially impairs the person's ability to provide adequately for the person's care or protection and who is: (A) 18 years of age or older; or (B) under 18 years of age and who has had the disabilities of minority removed.

UTAH: Utah Code Ann. §§ 62A-3-301, 76-5-111 (2001)

"**Abuse**" under § 62A-3-301 means: (a) attempting to cause, or intentionally or knowingly causing physical harm or intentionally placing another in fear of imminent physical harm; (b) physical injury caused by criminally negligent acts or omissions; (c) unlawful detention or unreasonable confinement; (d) gross lewdness; or (e) deprivation of life-sustaining treatment, except: (i) as provided in Title 75, Chapter 2, Part 11, Personal Choice and Living Will Act; or (ii) when informed consent, as defined in Section 76-5-111, has been obtained.

"**Elder abuse**" under § 62A-3-301 means abuse, neglect, or exploitation of an elder adult. "Emotional or psychological abuse" means deliberate conduct that is directed at a disabled or elder adult through verbal or nonverbal means, and that causes the disabled or elder adult to suffer emotional distress or to fear bodily injury, harm, or restraint.

"**Abuse**" under § 76-5-111 means: (i) attempting to cause, or causing physical harm; (ii) placing another in fear of imminent physical harm; (iii) physical injury caused by acts or omissions; (iv) unlawful detention or unreasonable confinement; (v) gross lewdness; or (vi) deprivation of life-sustaining treatment, except: (A) as provided in Title 75, Chapter 2, Part 11, Personal Choice and Living Will Act; or (B) when informed consent has been obtained.

"**Neglect**" under § 62A-3-301 means: (a) the failure of a caretaker to provide habilitation, care, nutrition, clothing, shelter, supervision, or medical care; (b) a pattern of conduct by a caretaker, without the disabled or elder adult's informed consent, resulting in deprivation of food, water, medication, medical services, shelter, cooling, heating, or other services necessary to maintain minimum physical or mental health; or (c) the failure or inability of a disabled adult to provide those services for himself.

"**Exploitation**" under § 62A-3-301 means exploitation of a disabled or elder adult as that offense is described in Subsection 76-5-111(4).

"**Elder adult**" under § 62A-3-301 means a person 65 years of age or older.

"**Caretaker**" under § 62A-3-301 means any person, corporation, or public institution that has assumed by relationship, contract, or court order the responsibility to provide food, shelter, clothing, medical, and other necessities to a disabled or elder adult.

VERMONT: 33 V.S.A. § 6902 (2001)

"**Abuse**" means: (A) Any treatment of an elderly or disabled adult which places life, health, or welfare in jeopardy or which is likely to result in impairment of health; (B) Any conduct committed with an intent or reckless disregard that such conduct is likely to cause unnecessary harm, unnecessary pain or unnecessary suffering to an elderly or disabled adult; (C) Unnecessary confinement or unnecessary restraint of an elderly or disabled adult; (D) Any sexual activity with an elderly or disabled adult by a caregiver, either, while providing a service for which he or she receives financial compensation, or at a caregiving facility or program; (E) Any pattern of malicious behavior which results in impaired emotional well-being of an elderly or disabled adult.

"Neglect" means the lack of subsistence, medical or other care necessary for well-being.

"Exploitation" means: (A) Willfully using, withholding, or disposing of funds or property of an elderly or disabled adult without legal authority for the wrongful profit or advantage of another; (B) Acquiring possession or control of or an interest in funds or property of an elderly or disabled adult through the use of undue influence, harassment, duress, or fraud; (C) The act of forcing or compelling an elderly or disabled adult against his or her will to perform services for the profit or advantage of another; (D) Any sexual activity with an elderly or disabled adult when the elderly or disabled adult does not consent or when the actor knows or should know that the elderly or disabled adult is incapable of resisting or declining consent to the sexual activity due to age or disability or due to fear of retribution or hardship.

"Elderly adult" means an individual who is 60 years of age or older.

"Caregiver" means a person, agency, facility, or other organization with responsibility for providing subsistence or medical or other care to an elderly or disabled adult, who has assumed the responsibility voluntarily, by contract or by an order of the court; or a person providing care including but not limited to medical care, custodial care, personal care, mental health services, rehabilitative services, or any other kind of care provided which is required because of another's age or disability.

VIRGINIA: Va. Code Ann. §§ 18.2-369, 63.1-55.2 (2001)

"Abuse" under § 63.1-55.2 means the willful infliction of physical pain, injury, or mental anguish or unreasonable confinement.

"Abuse" under §18.2-369 means (i) knowing and willful conduct that causes physical injury or pain or (ii) knowing and willful use of physical restraint, including confinement, as punishment, for convenience or as a substitute for treatment, except where such conduct or physical restraint, including confinement, is a part of care or treatment and is in furtherance of the health and safety of the incapacitated person.

"**Neglect**" under § 63.1-55.2 means that an adult is living under such circumstance that he is not able to provide for himself or is not being provided such services as are necessary to maintain his physical and mental health and that the failure to receive such necessary services impairs or threatens to impair his well-being. "Neglect" under §18.2-369 means the knowing and willful failure by a responsible person to provide treatment, care, goods or services which results in injury to the health or endangers the safety of an incapacitated adult.

"**Exploitation**" under § 63.1-55.2 means the illegal use of an incapacitated adult or his resources for another's profit or advantage.

"**Incapacitated person**" under § 63.1-55.2 and § 18.2-369 means any adult (18 or older) who is impaired by reason of mental illness, mental retardation, physical illness or disability, advanced age or other causes to the extent that the adult lacks sufficient understanding or capacity to make, communicate or carry out responsible decisions concerning his or her well-being.

"**Responsible person**" under § 18.2-369 means a person who has responsibility for the care, custody or control of an incapacitated person by operation of law or who has assumed such responsibility voluntarily, by contract or in fact.

WASHINGTON: Rev. Code Wash. (ARCW) §§ 70.124.020, 74.34.020 (2001)

"**Abuse**" under § 74.34.020 means the willful action or inaction that inflicts injury, unreasonable confinement, intimidation, or punishment on a vulnerable adult. In instances of abuse of a vulnerable adult who is unable to express or demonstrate physical harm, pain, or mental anguish, the abuse is presumed to cause physical harm, pain, or mental anguish. Abuse includes sexual abuse, mental abuse, physical abuse, and exploitation of a vulnerable adult, which have the following meanings: (a) "Sexual abuse" means any form of nonconsensual sexual contact, including but not limited to unwanted or inappropriate touching, rape, sodomy, sexual coercion, sexually explicit photographing, and sexual harassment. Sexual abuse includes any sexual contact between a staff person, who is not also a resident or client, of a facility or a staff person of a program authorized under chapter 71A.12 RCW, and a vulnerable adult living in that facility or receiving service from a program authorized under chapter 71A.12 RCW, whether or not it is consensual. (b) "Physical abuse" means the willful action of inflicting bodily injury or physical mistreatment. Physical abuse includes, but is not limited to, striking with or without an object, slapping, pinching, choking, kicking, shoving, prodding, or the use of chemical restraints or physical restraints unless the restraints are consistent with licensing requirements, and includes restraints that are otherwise being used inappropriately. (c) "Mental abuse" means any willful action or inaction of mental or verbal abuse. Mental abuse includes, but is not limited to, coercion, harassment, inappropriately isolating a vulnerable adult from family, friends, or regular activity, and verbal assault that includes ridiculing, intimidating, yelling, or swearing. "Exploitation" means an act of forcing, compelling, or exerting undue influence over a vulnerable adult causing the vulnerable adult to act in a way that is inconsistent with relevant past behavior, or causing the vulnerable adult to perform services for the benefit of another.

INSTITUTIONAL ABUSE/ NEGLECT: "Abuse or neglect" or "patient abuse or neglect" under § 70.124.020 means the nonaccidental physical injury or condition, sexual abuse, or negligent treatment of a state hospital patient under circumstances which indicate that the patient's health, welfare, or safety is harmed thereby.

"Neglect" under § 74.34.020 means (a) a pattern of conduct or inaction by a person or entity with a duty of care to provide the goods and services that maintain physical or mental health of a vulnerable adult, or that avoids or prevents physical or mental harm or pain to a vulnerable adult; or (b) an act or omission that demonstrates a serious disregard of consequences of such a magnitude as to constitute a clear and present danger to the vulnerable adult's health, welfare, or safety.

"Exploitation" under § 74.34.020 means an act of forcing, compelling, or exerting undue influence over a vulnerable adult causing the vulnerable adult to act in a way that is inconsistent with relevant past behavior, or causing the vulnerable adult to perform services for the benefit of another. "Financial exploitation" means the illegal or improper use of the property, income, resources, or trust funds of the vulnerable adult by any person for any person's profit or advantage.

"Vulnerable adult" under § 74.34.020 includes a person: (a) 60 years of age or older who has the functional, mental, or physical inability to care for himself or herself; or (b) Found incapacitated under chapter 11.88 RCW; or (c) Who has a developmental disability as defined under RCW 71A.10.020; or (d) Admitted to any facility; or (e) Receiving services from home health, hospice, or home care agencies licensed or required to be licensed under chapter 70.127 RCW; or (f) Receiving services from an individual provider.

WEST VIRGINIA: W.Va. Code §§ 9-6-1, 61-2-29 (2001)

"Abuse" under § 9-6-1 means the infliction or threat to inflict physical pain or injury on or the imprisonment of any incapacitated adult or facility resident.

"Abuse" under § 61-2-29 means infliction or threat to inflict physical pain or injury on an incapacitated adult.

"Neglect" under § 9-6-1 means: (A) The failure to provide the necessities of life to an incapacitated adult or facility resident with intent to coerce or physically harm the incapacitated adult or resident; and (B) the unlawful expenditure or willful dissipation of the funds or other assets owned or paid to or for the benefit of an incapacitated adult or resident. "Neglect" under § 61-2-29 means (i) the failure to provide the necessities of life to an incapacitated adult or (ii) the unlawful expenditure or willful dissipation of the funds or other assets owned or paid to or for the benefit of an incapacitated adult.

"Incapacitated adult" under § 9-6-1 and § 61-2-29 means any person who by reason of physical, mental, or other infirmity is unable to independently carry on the daily activities of life necessary to sustaining life and reasonable health.

"Caregiver" under § 61-2-29 means an adult who has or shares actual physical possession or care of an incapacitated adult on a full-time or temporary basis, regardless of whether such person has been designated as a guardian of such adult by any contract, agreement, or legal proceeding. Caregiver includes health care providers, family members, and any person who otherwise voluntarily accepts a supervisory role towards an incapacitated adult.

WISCONSIN: Wis. Stat. §§ 46.90, 55.01, 940.285, 940.295 (2000)

"Abuse" under § 46.90 means the willful infliction on an elder person of physical pain or injury or unreasonable confinement.

"**Abuse**" under § 55.01 means any of the following: (a) An act, omission, or course of conduct by another that is inflicted intentionally or recklessly and that does at least one of the following: 1. Results in bodily harm or great bodily harm to a vulnerable adult. 2. Intimidates, humiliates, threatens, frightens, or otherwise harasses a vulnerable adult. (b) The forcible administration of medication to a vulnerable adult, with the knowledge that no lawful authority exists for the forcible administration. (c) An act that constitutes first degree, second degree, third degree, or fourth degree sexual assault as specified under § 940.225.

"**Maltreatment**" under § 940.285 includes any of the following conduct: 1. Conduct that causes or could reasonably be expected to cause bodily harm or great bodily harm. 2. Restraint, isolation, or confinement that causes or could reasonably be expected to cause bodily harm or great bodily harm or mental or emotional damage, including harm to the vulnerable adults psychological or intellectual functioning that is exhibited by severe anxiety, depression, withdrawal, regression, or outward aggressive behavior or a combination of these behaviors. This subdivision does not apply to restraint, isolation, or confinement by order of a court or other lawful authority. 3. Deprivation of a basic need for food, shelter, clothing or personal or health care, including deprivation resulting from the failure to provide or arrange for a basic need by a person who has assumed responsibility for meeting the need voluntarily or by contract, agreement, or court order.

"**Neglect**" under § 55.01 means an act, omission, or course of conduct that, because of the failure to provide adequate food, shelter, clothing, medical care or dental care, creates a significant danger to the physical or mental health of a vulnerable adult.

> INSTITUTIONAL NEGLECT: "**Neglect**" under § 940.295 means an act, omission, or course of conduct by another that, because of the failure to provide adequate food, shelter, clothing, medical care or dental care, creates a significant danger to the physical or mental health of a patient or resident.

"**Material abuse**" under § 46.90 means the misuse of an elder persons property or financial resources.

"**Misappropriation of property**" under § 55.01 means any of the following: (a) The intentional taking, carrying away, use, transfer, concealment, or retention of possession of the property of a vulnerable adult without the vulnerable adult's informed consent and with intent to deprive the vulnerable adult of possession of the property. (b) Obtaining the property of a vulnerable adult by intentionally deceiving the vulnerable adult with a representation that is known to be a false representation, is made with intent to defraud, and does defraud the vulnerable adult.

"Elder person" under § 46.90 means a person who is age 60 or older or who is subject to the infirmities of aging.

"Vulnerable adult" under § 940.285 means any person 18 years of age or older who either is a developmentally disabled person or has infirmities of aging, mental illness, or other like incapacities and who is: 1. Substantially mentally incapable of providing for his or her needs for food, shelter, clothing or personal or health care; or 2. Unable to report cruel maltreatment without assistance.

"Caretaker" under § 55.01 means the person, if any, who takes care of a vulnerable adult voluntarily or under a contract for care.

WYOMING: Wyo. Stat. § 35-20-102 (2001)

"Abuse" means the willful infliction, whether by another person or self-inflicted, of physical pain, injury, unreasonable confinement or deprivation, which conduct threatens the welfare and well being of a disabled adult.

> *Defined separately: Abandonment* means leaving a disabled adult without financial support or the means or ability to obtain food, clothing, shelter, or health care.

"Neglect" means the deprivation, including self-deprivation, of the minimum food, shelter, clothing, supervision, physical and mental health care, and other care necessary to maintain a disabled adult's life or health, or which may result in a life-threatening situation. The withholding of health care from a disabled adult is not neglect if: (A) Treatment is given in good faith by spiritual means alone, through prayer, by a duly accredited practitioner in accordance with the tenets and practices of a recognized church or religious denomination; or (B) The withholding of health care is in accordance with a declaration executed pursuant to W.S. 35-22-101 through 35-22-109.

"Exploitation" means taking advantage of a disabled adult or of his physical or financial resources for personal or pecuniary profit by the use of undue influence, harassment, duress, deception, false representation, or false pretenses.

"**Disabled adult**" means any person 18 years of age or older who is unable unassisted to properly manage and take care of himself or his property as a result of the infirmities of advanced age, physical or mental disability, or the use of alcohol or controlled substances.

"**Caretaker**" means any person or agency responsible for the day to day care of a disabled adult because of: (A) A family relationship; (B) Voluntary assumption of responsibility for day to day care; (C) Court ordered responsibility or placement; (D) Rendering services on adult workshop or adult residential programs; or (E) Rendering services in an institution or in community-based programs.

APPENDIX
C
Elder Abuse and Neglect: History and Concepts

Rosalie Wolf

Good afternoon and thank you for the opportunity to address you on this important topic. I am going to quickly cover definitions, history, theories, risk factors, consequences, assessment instruments, prevalence, and interventions, if we have enough time.

DEFINITIONS

Elder abuse has been used as an all-inclusive term that is often used to represent physical abuse. So that already indicates that there are differences in the way elder abuse is interpreted. It may involve relationships between spouses, adult children, other relatives, maybe friends, and anyone else in whom the older person has placed trust. Other behavior that is considered abusive may depend on its duration, its frequency, its intensity, its intentionality, and the consequences.

HISTORY

Although elder abuse first appeared on the national scene in the late 1970s, the formal efforts to help vulnerable elders began at least two decades before that time. Public welfare officials were faced with an increas-

---

NOTE: This is an edited transcript of the text of a presentation to the Panel on Elder Abuse and Neglect, May 24, 2001.

ing number of older persons who were unable to manage on their own and began to develop a new approach to providing services, which they called "protective services units." It was an approach that would provide not only social services, but also legal assistance, particularly guardianship.

As a result of this interest in the 1950s, Congress passed legislation, as part of the Social Security Act, providing funds to the states on a three-to-one matching basis for setting up these protective service units. Some states took advantage of these federal dollars. In addition, Congress provided funds for six demonstration projects (they might represent the very first research on adult protective services).

One of those demonstration projects supported a team at the Benjamin Rose Institute in Cleveland under Margaret Blenkner and her associates. She matched a group of elders receiving protective services with a group from the community who were receiving traditional services and found that, during the grant period, those who received protective services had a higher mortality rate and higher nursing home placement rate than those who received traditional services.

But the advocates for the system went right ahead with their work in the Congress and in 1974, despite some of the findings of that study and five other studies that showed these protective services units to be very costly and of questionable effect (U.S. Department of Health, Education, and Welfare, 1966), Congress amended the Social Security Act to mandate protective service units in all states for adults over the age of 18. The target populations were people with mental and physical impairments who were unable to manage on their own and who had been or were being exploited or neglected. There was a lot of criticism of these programs, partly because they were so costly and partly because they seemed to infringe on the rights of the elders.

Interest temporarily waned on adult protective services, but at about the same time (middle to late 1970s), renewed interest in elder abuse became apparent, in part due to congressional hearings (U.S. House of Representatives, 1978, 1979). At one of those hearings, a witness spoke about "granny battering." The topic began to interest some of the members of Congress, particularly the late Claude Pepper of Florida. He and his Special Subcommittee on Aging sponsored other investigations and hearings, and there were, I think, two research projects submitted to the Administration on Aging for a discretionary grant that were of questionable methodology, but they did, at least, confirm that cases existed.

This congressional interest in elder abuse served to revive interest in adult protective services. When members of Congress looked around to see what was happening to these abused and neglected adults, they saw the adult protective service units and concluded that it wasn't necessary to establish a new system. Instead, they decided to continue trying to raise awareness of the problem.

In 1981, Congress proposed legislation to establish a national center on elder abuse, but the bill never reached the floor of Congress. Finally, in 1989, Claude Pepper introduced that proposal as an amendment to the Older Americans Act. The national center was funded the following year and began the federal government's specific commitment to this area, albeit with very small amounts of money. But at least elder abuse had been recognized in federal legislation.

Initially the conceptualization of this issue was not of adults needing protection and safety. It became an aging issue, whereas initially the response involved public welfare and the social services and legal services. By gaining the interest of the aging network, a larger constituency of interested people became involved.

It is interesting that the emphasis was on elder abuse and abused elders in the context of caregiving. The portrait of the problem was that of an impaired victim, usually an elderly parent being cared for by an adult caregiver, who wasn't able to manage the caregiving because of stresses in life, job, family, and so forth.

This picture of elder abuse seemed to resonate with Congress. The media really helped to promote this issue. Together the media and Congress provided the real push for interest in this problem.

In the 1980s, Surgeon General Louis Sullivan held a workshop on family violence, declaring it to be a public health and criminal justice issue that included the problems of elder abuse and neglect. Elder abuse was included under the umbrella of family violence. That had a very positive effect, because it brought in the medical community, and the criminal justice community and broadened the range of constituency groups interested in the topic

This was a real positive step forward. Sometimes the social service people are concerned about the so-called criminalization of the issue, but in terms of the breadth and depth of interest, it was a very positive step.

THEORIES

A number of theories have been promoted or proposed to explain elder abuse (Phillips, 1986). I'm not going to review them in depth, but I want to focus specifically on the "situational theory" because it represented a particularly popular theory in relation to the image of the overburdened caregiver. It is true that some caregivers are overburdened, and it is true that some of them do abuse or neglect the person for whom they are caring. When you look at some of the cases and some of the studies, you see perpetrators who are caregivers and who show a history of emotional problems, so psychopathology seems to be another way of explaining what takes place.

Several additional theories have been used to explain elder abuse:

- the exchange theory, which describes how some of the dependencies that exist between a victim and a perpetrator relate to tactics and responses developed in family life, which continue into adulthood;
- social learning theory, which brings in the whole issue of how abuse was learned and that spouse abuse among the elderly does exist; and
- political economic theory, which focuses on the challenges faced by elders in a society that leaves people in poverty and takes away their importance in community life. Political economic theory addresses the marginalization of elders in society.

People in the field have come to realize that you can't really explain such a complicated construct as elder abuse with one theory, and that perhaps what is needed is something that looks at factors across several domains. Heist has examined this issue in relation to child abuse, but it has subsequently been presented in a broader context by the Committee on Interventions of Family Violence (National Research Council and Institute of Medicine, 1998) as an ecological model that incorporates and links individual-level psychopathology and interpersonal relationships in the context of the overall sociocultural environment. That could be exchange dependency in the caregiver, for example, in the context of the elder community. For instance, are there services to take care of caregivers with alcohol problems? And it highlights some of the societal issues, such as the loss of the importance of older persons in transmitting values and traditions and certain cultural issues.

RISK FACTORS

In the absence of an overarching theoretical framework, research has thus far focused on the characteristics of situations and victims and perpetrators that constitute risk factors for abuse. I will mention victim dependency, abuser dependence/deviance, social isolation, and living arrangements as examples.

There is no question that there are some people who are impaired and neglected, but is impairment necessary? There is a model of family violence in which victims are generally seen as people unable to leave the situation. When you think of a younger victim of what I will refer to as intimate partner violence, this represents the classic "battered woman syndrome." When you look at those younger victims, you know that they find it very difficult to leave a situation. There is a concerted effort on the part of the perpetrator to isolate the victim. In child abuse, the child goes to school, but the family itself is isolated. This may be even more so for older persons who may be isolated because of physical impairments or loss of friends and family. Living arrangements are a major focus for examination. Generally, abuse or neglect takes place in the context of people living together, yet there is an obligation on the part of adult children, for example, to not neglect their elders. Theoretical frameworks are in need of great attention.

RISK ASSESSMENT

Moving into risk assessment instruments, since elder abuse first emerged as a problem, the focus has been on developing some instrument that determine whether a person is at risk. There are a number of groups working on this. Hwalek and Sengstock (1986) did some of the earliest work with funding from the Administration on Aging. They asked many people from various agencies what items in fact should be considered and came up with a list in the hundreds, if not thousands; they then conducted a multivariate analysis and came down to 15 and later to 10 statements from self-reports on elder abuse. Another study tested those original 15 statements by using the Australian longitudinal study on health, in which they had a sample of 12,000 women age 65 and older (Kurrle, 1993). They added two additional intimate family violence questions, coming up with a brief screening tool of six questions, which were reliable as a test for elder abuse. The idea is that a physician or any other screener could use these questions in the interview and could at least identify an at-risk elder.

A team from Montreal (Reis and Nahmiash, 1998) developed a completely different screening effort. They had nurses and social workers conduct a comprehensive interview of clients who had been seen by a social service agency and screened to determine who was abused. Their original research across demographics came out with three categories of risk factors relating to: (1) the abusive caregiver, (2) interpersonal characteristics (personal alcohol or substance abuse, characteristics of depression, personality disorder, mental outlook, behavioral problems), and (3) reluctance to discuss abusive behavior. The last is quite important, but it has not been followed up. The second category, interpersonal characteristics, includes poor relationships with the caregiver, marital or family conflict, lack of empathy for the elder, and financial dependence.

CONSEQUENCES

There has been very little work done on the consequences of elder abuse, in terms of both the effect on physical health and on mental health. We know from the family violence area that abuse has a substantial effect on the health of women, and that they make up a good proportion of emergency room admissions. But research on the effects of elder abuse has been inhibited because of the complexity of untangling the synergistic effects of aging, and disease in old age from the impact of abuse or neglect.

There is only one study on the consequences of abuse on physical health. Lachs and colleagues (1998) used an existing National Institute on Aging cohort study that looked at the status of the abused elders over a period of 13 years, examining statistics of physical health, mental health, social situations, even religious habits, and so forth. They merged that dataset with one from the adult protective services unit serving New Haven, Connecticut. That unit, which is in a mandatory reporting state, has been collecting data since 1978. There were 7 cases of abuse that had been investigated for corroboration, 57 cases of neglect, and 2,608 cases not reported but investigated by researchers. They looked at the rate of mortality and found there was no difference in the first few years, but by the 13th year there was a decided difference in outcomes: 40 percent of the non-reported elders were still alive, 13 percent of the "self-neglect" category were still alive, and 9 percent of the "reported abused" category were still alive.

What was interesting is how closely this followed the Blenkner results, from 30 years earlier. Both showed a higher rate of institutionalization and a higher rate of nursing home placement. It suggests to me that the intervention itself may be a factor. This would be an important area for research.

Let me go back to depression. Depression is the only aspect of psychological abuse that has been explored by researchers at all, and those studies are very small and the methodology is subject to question. But indeed, if you look at groups of elders who have been abused, neglected, and exploited, you find more depression in this group. Commentators have suggested that other causes of emotional distress are also provoked by the acts of elder abuse or exploitation—depression, fear, guilt, shame, stress, learned helplessness, and post-traumatic stress syndrome (see, for example, Goldstein, 1996).

PREVALENCE AND INCIDENCE

Five studies have been done on prevalence in five different countries, using three or four or five different methodologies, some better than others.

The first was the Pillemer and Finkelhor (1988) study of the metropolitan Boston area. A representative sample of elders was interviewed over the telephone, or if the older person was unable to respond on the telephone, they conducted face-to-face interviews. They found that 3.2 percent of that sample was abused or neglected. However, they did not include financial exploitation, which is a real shortcoming of that study. Another shortcoming was the very strict definition in terms of physical abuse and neglect. They used scales that had been used in the national family violence surveys to describe physical abuse, which may have been too limiting.

The Conflict Tactics Scale was also used on a national sample of Canadian elders (Podnieks, 1992). In that sample, Podnieks added financial exploitation and found several different results: 5 percent of the sample was financially abused, which was the largest category, followed by physical abuse and neglect. Podnieks concluded that 4 percent of the population had been abused, neglected, or financially exploited.

Researchers in the United Kingdom wanted to do a similar study but they couldn't get it through their human subjects review panel, so they added a few questions from the Boston study to another annual survey in the United Kingdom (Ogg and Bennett, 1992). They concluded that overall, 5 percent of the elders 65 and over had been abused or neglected or exploited (about 2 percent had been physically abused).

The next study was done in a small town in Finland (Kivela et al., 1992). It was a geriatric mental health study by geriatricians in a health center. They used a completely different methodology, with the subjects saying whether they were abused or neglected. They defined abuse simply as the infliction of unnecessary pain or injury. The researchers asked the subjects if they knew anybody who had been abused, if they had ever been abused, and then asked the same questions about the issues of exploitation, sexual abuse, and neglect. They found that 5.7 percent of that representative sample had been abused.

The latest study was reported in 1998 in Amsterdam (Comijs et al., 1998). The researchers added some questions about elder abuse and neglect from the Boston study to a health study being done in a representative sample of persons 69 and older. They came out with 5.6 percent prevalence.

An incidence study funded by the Administration for Children and Families and the Administration on Aging (National Center on Elder Abuse, 1998) attempted to answer some of these questions. Its methodology was questioned, but it was based on the iceberg theory and the assumption that what is reported to adult protective services is only part of what exists in the community.

Because of the shortage of time, I won't go into it in too great detail. The study showed that there were 70,942 new cases in 1996. But when these cases are added to the cases that came in from the sentinels (people, working in hospitals, senior centers, police departments, and banks), the total amounted to over 379,000 cases. Although the methodology has been questioned, there is much to examine in this study.

One criticism of the methodology stems from the fact that many older, vulnerable people do not have any contact with people outside their home or institution. The National Center on Elder Abuse has tried to find out how to reach these isolated elders. Currently some demonstration projects are trying to do that.

About 470,790 reports came to adult protective services units in the year 1999, with all states reporting (including Guam and the District of Columbia) except Mississippi. Of that number, 332,000 were investigated. That means the others did not meet minimal criteria for conducting an investigation. It is interesting that some states investigate every report, while some states do so in a triage arrangement. If it doesn't seem to be abuse, they pass it along or refer that case to whatever agency is appropriate. Of those that were investigated, 45 percent were validated.

Q & A SESSION

Richard Bonnie: In the beginning of your talk, you referred to different images of the problem, as you put it, which appealed to different constituencies. One was the adult in need of protection, then "elder" abuse and neglect and exploitation, which obviously borrowed from the child abuse tradition, and then the family violence orientation. You made the observation that, overall, you thought that this had a positive impact, at least from the standpoint of building constituencies. But I detected some reservations among some people, as to whether this interweaving of strands has been a good thing or not. Could you comment on that?

Rosalie Wolf: I think it comes mostly from the social service field. I'm not sure whether that is true today. It was true a few years ago, I believe.

Bonnie: One thing I am wondering about, in terms of the agenda for this panel, is that elder abuse is a very complicated construct. There are these three different strands that you have mentioned, and each one focuses on a different thing. For example, in the context of adult protective services, the "perpetrator," the third party, is not the centerpiece. It is the vulnerability of the individual. From the other two perspectives, at least, a third-party focus emerges.

I think this explains at least in part some of the confusion about definitions. For a sound research base to develop, isn't greater cohesion needed about the concept of elder abuse itself?

Wolf: I think that the whole criminal justice perspective has brought in an emphasis on the perpetrator—you're right, let me say, that the emphasis previously was totally on the victim. If you look at the laws of the states, I'm not sure the perpetrator is mentioned at all. Yet, as we know, it could be a mutual problem, but the perpetrator certainly bears the guilt in these situations.

I think when you bring in the criminal justice system, this was definitely a result of what had happened earlier with family violence. I think that as focus has been brought on the perpetrator, prosecution is now an intervention, where it never was before. In the social service field, they felt that prosecution was not anything that should be done, partly because older people don't want to prosecute, they don't want to bring charges against their children or their grandchildren. So it was more in keeping with the wishes of the victim, and prosecution was not a possibility. Then there were difficulties with perpetrators; it is hard to find them sometimes.

Constantine Lyketsos: Given that the dementia problem increases with age, if you look at reports of sentinel events or reports of events in much higher age groups in which dementia is more prevalent, do you see an increase of reports of abuse from communities as people get much older? Do you have any data on that?

Wolf: There are data in terms of reporting through adult protective services, which show that the highest number of reports of abuse within the age categories is among the 85 and over category. However, the prevalence study showed no difference in age. Since the author of that study is here, later on he can explain more about that.

Karl Pillemer: I think one of the reasons for some of the confusion is that there are two strands or traditions of research that have been used. One is the Murray Strauss school of family violence research, which is equally applicable to child abuse or wife abuse when you take a survey approach. The other has come out of the gerontological family caregiving tradition, which has looked at caregivers as samples—and hasn't used the general population. That typically doesn't include elderly spouse abuse, for example, which might occur among healthy elders.

That is where these lines become a lot less clear. So I think that is one reason for some of the confusion.

Wolf: I won't try to answer the first part, because it raises the whole issue of why do we segregate a whole service system, how do we approach the needs of elders. It is a separate service system. Why do we have the Administration on Aging, for instance?

Most states use the criterion of people age 18 and over who are vulnerable. So the vulnerability risk factor shows up very strongly in adult protective services. Some of the states don't use that criterion and instead serve all adults who are 60 or over; in those states, one doesn't see such a strong showing of vulnerability as a risk factor.

For instance, I think the statistics show that in states in which adult protective services serve younger and older persons with disabilities, about 40 percent of the reports that come in for people age 18 and over are collected from caregivers. In contrast, the state that I come from, Massachusetts, doesn't include vulnerability as a criterion. It has physical abuse and neglect without any necessary indicators. Illinois, which doesn't have vulnerability as a criterion, either, shows a much higher rate of financial abuse. The bottom line is that there are all sorts of issues that have to be taken into account.

REFERENCES

Comijs, H.C., A.M. Pot, H.H. Smit, and C. Jonker
    1998   Elder abuse in the community: Prevalence and consequences. *Journal of the American Geriatrics Society* 46:885-888.

Goldstein, M.
    1996   Elder mistreatment and PTSD. In *Aging and Post Traumatic Stress Disorder*, P.E. Ruskin and J.A. Talbots, eds. Washington, DC: American Psychiatric Association.

Hwalek, M.A., and M.C. Sengstock
    1986   Assessing the probability of abuse in the elderly: Toward development of a clinical screening instrument. *Journal of Applied Gerontology* 5(2):153-173.

Kivela, S.L., P. Kongas-Saviaro, E. Kesti, K. Pahkala, and M.L. Ijas
    1992   Abuse in old age: Epidemiological data from Finland. *Journal of Elder Abuse and Neglect* 4(3):1-18.

Kurrle, S.E.
    1993   Elder abuse: A hidden problem. *Modern Medicine of Australia* (September):58-71.

Lachs, M.S., et al.
    1998   The mortality of elder mistreatment. *Journal of the American Medical Association* 280:428-432.

National Center on Elder Abuse
    1998   *National Elder Abuse Incidence Study: Final Report.* Washington, DC: American Public Human Services Association in collaboration with Westat, Inc.

National Research Council and Institute of Medicine
    1998   *Violence in Families: Assessing Prevention and Treatment Programs.* Committee on the Assessment of Family Violence Interventions. R. Chalk, and P.A. King, eds. Washington DC: National Academy Press.

Ogg, J., and G.C.J. Bennett
    1992   Elder abuse in Britain. *British Medical Journal* 305:998-999.

Phillips, L.
    1986   Theoretical explanations of elder abuse: Competing hypotheses and unresolved issues. In *Elder Abuse: Conflict in the Family*, Rosalie Wolf and Karl Pillemer, eds. Dover, MA: Auburn House.

Pillemer K., and D. Finkelhor
    1988   The prevalence of elder abuse: A random sample survey. *Gerontologist* 28:51-57.

Podnieks, E.
    1992   National survey on abuse of the elderly in Canada. *Journal of Elder Abuse and Neglect* 41(1/2):5-58.

Reis, M., and D. Nahmiash
    1998   Validation of the Indicators of Abuse (IOA) Screen. *The Gerontologist*, 38(4): 471-480.

U.S. Department of Health, Education, and Welfare
    1966   Four Model Demonstration Projects: Services to Older Adults in the Public Wel-
            fare Program. State Letter No. 925. Washington, DC: U.S. Department of
            Health, Education, and Welfare.
U.S. House of Representatives, Select Committee on Aging
    1979   *Elder Abuse: The Hidden Problem.* Washington, DC: U.S. Government Printing
            Office.
U.S. House of Representatives, Subcommittee of Domestic and International Scientific Plan-
ning, Analysis, and Cooperation
    1978   *Hearings of the Committee on Science and Technology.* 14 February to 16
            February, 1978. Washington, DC: U.S. Government Printing Office.

Biographical Sketches

Richard J. Bonnie (*Chair*) is John S. Battle professor of law at the University of Virginia School of Law and director of the University's Institute of Law, Psychiatry, and Public Policy. He writes and teaches in the fields of criminal law and procedure, mental health law, bioethics, and public health law. He has been deeply interested in issues involving psychiatry and human rights. In 1991, he was elected to the Institute of Medicine (IOM) and he has been an active participant in the National Academies' work. He serves or has served on the IOM Board on Neuroscience and Behavioral Health, the IOM Committee to Assess the Science Base for Tobacco Harm Reduction, the National Research Council's Committee on Data and Research for Policy on Illegal Drugs, and the IOM Committee to Assess the System for Protection of Human Research Subjects. He chaired the IOM Committee on Injury Prevention and Control, the IOM Committee on Opportunities in Drug Abuse Research, and was vice-chair of the IOM Committee on Preventing Nicotine Dependence in Children and Youths. He is a fellow of the Virginia Law Foundation, a charter fellow of the College on the Problems of Drug Dependence, and is on the board of directors of the college. He received the American Psychiatric Association's Isaac Ray award in 1998 for contributions to forensic psychiatry and the psychiatric aspects of jurisprudence. He has a B.A. (1966) from Johns Hopkins University and a J.D. (1969) from the University of Virginia.

Terry Fulmer is co-director of the John A. Hartford Foundation Institute for Geriatric Nursing, Division of Nursing, at New York University. She is also professor of nursing at New York University's Division of Nursing and president of the Eastern Nursing Research Society. Her research focuses on acute care of the elderly, specifically on the subject of elder abuse and neglect. Her work on dyadic vulnerability/risk profiling for elder neglect is funded by the National Institute on Aging in partnership with the National Institute of Nursing Research. Her books include *Inadequate Care of the Elderly: Health Care Perspective on Abuse and Neglect* and *Critical Nursing Care of the Elderly.* Two of her books have received the American Journal of Nursing book of the year award. She is a fellow of the American Academy of Nursing, a fellow of the Gerontological Society of America and the New York Academy of Medicine, and distinguished practitioner of the National Academies of Practice. She completed a Brookdale fellowship and is a distinguished practitioner of the National Academies of Medicine. She was honored by the New York State Nurses Association with the distinguished nurse researcher award. She has chaired the clinical medicine section of the Gerontological Society of America and has been on the congress of nursing economics for the American Nurses Association. She has an undergraduate degree from Skidmore College and M.A. and Ph.D. degrees from Boston College.

Marisa A. Gerstein is a research assistant for the Committee on National Statistics and has worked on several of its panels, including the Panel to Review the 2000 Census, the Panel on Formula Allocations, and the Panel on Methods for Assessing Discrimination. She came to the Committee from Burch Munford Direct, a direct-mail company, and previously worked for the National Abortion and Reproductive Rights Action League. She has a B.A. in sociology from New College of Florida (1999).

Lora Flattum Hamp is a fellow of the Borchard Foundation Center on Law and Aging at the University of Georgia School of Law. Previously, she worked as an assistant director of an area agency on aging and served on the board of the Virginia Association on Aging. She has conducted research on state statutes governing elder abuse and studied factors contributing to the unmet legal needs of the elderly. She assisted in drafting the *National Handbook on Laws and Programs Affecting Senior Citizens* and was awarded the title of Virginia's Ambassador for the Aging by the Virginia Department for the Aging. Hamp has a B.S. in chemistry from the College of William and Mary, an M.S. in gerontology from the Medical College of Virginia, and a J.D. from the University of Virginia School of Law.

Richard A. Kulka is senior research vice president of statistics, health, and social policy at the Research Triangle Institute in Research Triangle Park, NC. Previously, he was senior vice president for survey research at the

National Opinion Research Center. He has been involved in the design, conduct, and analysis of numerous statistical surveys on health, mental health, and other social policy issues for over two decades, while also conducting a broad range of applied research on survey research methods in these areas. Kulka is a member of several professional associations, including the American Statistical Association, the American Association for Public Opinion Research, and the American Public Health Association. He has a Ph.D. in social psychology from the University of Michigan.

Eva Kutas is the director of the Office of Investigations and Training of the Oregon Department of Human Resources, which is the adult protective services agency that responds to all allegations of abuse and neglect of people with mental illness or developmental disabilities in Oregon. The office also provides training about abuse and neglect to providers and clients, mandatory abuse reporters, and the public. She has criminal and civil law experience and worked at the Oregon Advocacy Center (Oregon's protection and advocacy agency for people with disabilities) for 10 years as an advocate. She has conducted approximately 600 investigations over 15 years, specializing in complex cases and unusual or questionable deaths. She has also lectured extensively on the subject of interviewing people with disabilities who are victims of abuse or neglect. She is the current president of the National Association of Adult Protective Services Administrators, an organization that strives to improve the quality and availability of services to vulnerable adults who are abused, neglected, and exploited, to promote advocacy, training, and research in the field and to educate the public and government leaders on behalf of this population. She received her B.A. and M.S. from the University of Oregon, and her J.D. from Northwestern School of Law of Lewis and Clark College.

Edward O. Laumann is the George Herbert Mead distinguished service professor in the Department of Sociology and the College at the University of Chicago, chairman of the Department of Sociology, and director of the Ogburn Stouffer Center for Population and Social Organization. Previously he was editor of the *American Journal of Sociology*, dean of the Social Sciences Division, and provost (chief academic officer) at the university. Before coming to Chicago, he taught at the University of Michigan. Laumann's research interests include social stratification, the sociology of the professions, occupations, and formal organizations, social network analysis, the analysis of elite groups and national policy making, and the sociology of human sexuality. Among his published books are three volumes on human sexuality: *The Social Organization of Sexuality*, *Sex in America*, and *Sex, Love and Health in America*. He is vice president of the board of trustees of the National Opinion Research Center, a fellow of the

American Association for the Advancement of Science, a fellow of the Society for the Scientific Study of Sexuality, an associate director of the Center for Clinical Medical Ethics at the Pritzker School of Medicine, a member of the board of directors of the Metropolitan Chicago Information Center, current chair of the section on economic and political sciences of the American Association for the Advancement of Science, a former member of the University of Chicago board of governors for the Argonne National Laboratory, and a former member of the board of trustees of the University of Chicago Hospitals. He has a B.A. from Oberlin College (1960) and M.A. (1962) and Ph.D. (1964) degrees from Harvard University.

Tanya M. Lee is a project assistant for the Committee on National Statistics. Before joining the staff in September 2001, she worked for the Institute of Medicine's Committee on Strategies for Small Number Participants Clinical Research Trails and the Committee on Creating a Vision for Space Medicine during Travel Beyond Earth Orbit. She has been with the National Academy of Sciences since April 2000. She attended the University of Maryland, Eastern Shore, and Prince Georges Community College, pursuing a degree in sociology.

Constantine G. Lyketsos is a board-certified geriatric psychiatrist who directs the Johns Hopkins Neuropsychiatry Service and the Comprehensive Alzheimer Program. He is an active clinician with an expertise in dementia and Alzheimer's disease. With Peter Rabins and Cindy Steele he authored *Practical Dementia Care* and has contributed numerous publications to the international scientific literature on dementia, geriatrics, depression, neuropsychiatry, Alzheimer's disease, and HIV/AIDS. His ongoing research focuses on the impact and treatment of psychiatric disturbances in Alzheimer's disease, its diagnosis and prevention, the epidemiology of cognitive decline and dementia, and on the care of persons with dementia. He has special expertise in the design and conduct of clinical epidemiological and intervention studies. He was recently cited in Best Doctors in America. He has a B.A. from Northwestern University, an M.D. from Washington University in St. Louis, and an M.H.S. from Johns Hopkins School of Public Health with a focus on clinical epidemiology.

Gary B. Melton is professor of psychology and director of the Institute on Family and Neighborhood Life at Clemson University. A past president of the American Psychology-Law Society and the American Psychological Association (APA) Division of Child, Youth, and Family Services, he has received awards for distinguished scholarship in the public interest from APA itself (twice), two of its divisions, the American Psychological Foundation, Psi Chi, and Prevent Child Abuse America. He has written or edited numerous scholarly publications, and his work has been cited by U.S. courts at all levels. He has consulted, lectured, or conducted research in 24 countries and territories abroad, and he is nearing completion of two three-year terms as president of Childwatch International, a global network of child research centers. He received his B.A. from the University of Virginia, and his M.A. and a PhD in clinical-community psychology from Boston University.

Laura Mosqueda is director of geriatrics and associate clinical professor of family medicine at the Irvine College of Medicine, University of California, Irvine. She also is an associate clinical professor in family medicine at the college. She is the principal investigator of a 3-year project to create, implement, and evaluate an interdisciplinary elder abuse medical response team. This team works closely with adult protective services, law enforcement, and the district attorney's office in addressing the abuse and neglect of older adults and adults with disabilities. She also serves as the co-director of the Rehabilitation Research and Training Center on Aging with a Disability at Rancho Los Amigos National Rehabilitation Center. Previously she served as the co-chief of the Elder Abuse Domain of the California Medical Training Center, where she was responsible for creating and implementing courses designed to train physicians and health care professionals in the medical forensic aspects of elder abuse. She has an M.D. from the University of Southern California School of Medicine.

Gregory Paveza is currently professor in the School of Social Work and one of the founding faculty in the interdisciplinary Aging Studies Program at the University of South Florida. He has been a clinical social work practitioner, a social service agency administrator, and a health sciences researcher. His research deals with issues related to the social consequences of caregiving and Alzheimer's disease, including a specific interest in elder mistreatment in these families. He also has a general interest in elder mistreatment and its impact on the broader aging community. He is a member of the Institute of Medicine's Committee on the Training Needs of Health Professionals to Respond to Family Violence and a member of the Leadership Council of the Mental Health and Aging Network of the American Society on Aging. He has published extensively on issues related to geriatric assessment, the caregiving consequences of Alzheimer's disease, including the cost of providing community-based care, and elder mistreatment. He has a B.A. from Lewis College (1969), an M.S.W. from the University of Hawaii (1973), and a Ph.D. in public health sciences (psychiatric epidemiology, 1986) from the School of Public Health at the University of Illinois at Chicago.

Karl Pillemer is professor of human development and director of the Cornell Gerontology Research Institute at Cornell University. His interests center on human development over the life course, with a special emphasis on family and social relationships in middle age and beyond. His research, funded over the past 10 years by the National Institutes of Health, involves family members who provide care to Alzheimer's disease victims, examining the relationships among social network structure, social support, and psychological well-being. A second major interest is in intergenerational relations in later life, with a focus on determinants and consequences of the quality of adult child-parent relationships (including international comparative work on this topic). Over the past two decades, Pillemer has conducted a long-term program of research on conflict and abuse in families of the aged, including several related studies of the domestic abuse of elderly persons. These have included large-scale prevalence surveys in the United States and Canada, evaluations of abuse prevention and treatment programs, and longitudinal research that examines the health consequences of maltreatment. Pillemer has also conducted several studies of abuse in long-term care facilities. He has a Ph.D. in sociology from Brandeis University.

Earl S. Pollack is a member of the staff of the Committee on National Statistics and served as study director for this panel. Previously, he was chief of biometry at the National Cancer Institute and director of the Division of Biometry and Epidemiology at the National Institute of Mental Health. More recently, he was research professor at the Biostatistics Center, George Washington University, and served as statistician for the Center to Protect Workers Rights, the construction research arm of the AFL/CIO. His interests are in chronic disease epidemiology and the analysis of observational data from large health and medical databases. He is a fellow of the American Statistical Association, the American College of Epidemiology, and the American Public Health Association. He has B.S. and M.A. degrees in statistics from the University of Minnesota and an Sc.D. in biostatistics from Harvard University.

Lori A. Stiegel is associate staff director of the American Bar Association's Commission on Legal Problems of the Elderly in Washington, DC. She is currently directing three projects on elder abuse and older battered women with funding from the U.S. Department of Justice, as well as the commission's activities in its role as a partner in the National Center on Elder Abuse funded by the U.S. Administration on Aging. She serves on the board of directors of the National Committee for the Prevention of Elder Abuse and is the author of *Elder Abuse in the State Courts: Three Curricular Judges and Court Staff* and *Recommended Guidelines for State Courts*

Handling Cases Involving Elder Abuse. She has a B.A. from the University of Florida, and a J.D. from George Washington University National Law Center.

Robert B. Wallace is professor of epidemiology and internal medicine at the University of Iowa's College of Public Health and Medicine and interim director of the university's Center on Aging. He has been a member of the U.S. Preventive Services Task Force and is now a senior adviser to it, and was also a member of the National Advisory Council on Aging of the National Institutes of Health. He is currently chair of the Board on Health Promotion and Disease Prevention of the Institute of Medicine. He served on the executive committee of the Association of Teachers of Preventive Medicine and was chair of the epidemiology section of the American Public Health Association. He is the author or coauthor of numerous publications and book chapters and has been the editor of four books, including the current edition of *Public Health and Preventive Medicine.* His research interests concern the causes and prevention of disabling conditions of older persons. He has had substantial experience in the conduct of both observational cohort studies of older persons and clinical trials, including preventive interventions related to osteoporotic fracture and coronary disease prevention. He is the site principal investigator for the Women's Health Initiative (WHI), a national intervention trial exploring the prevention of breast and colon cancer and coronary disease. He has been a collaborator in several international studies of the prevention of chronic illness in older persons. He has a B.S.M in medicine (1964) and an M.D. (1967) from Northwestern University and an M.Sc. in epidemiology from the State University of New York, Buffalo (1972).

OTHER CONTRIBUTORS

Ronald Acierno is assistant professor of psychiatry at the National Crime Victims Research and Treatment Center of the Medical University of South Carolina. He specializes in the assessment and treatment of psychopathology in older adults who have been victims of assault, abuse, neglect, and exploitation. He has a B.A. (with distinction) in psychology from the University of Virginia (1989) and M.S. and Ph.D. degrees in clinical psychology from Nova-Southeastern University (1996).

Marie-Therese Connolly, a senior trial counsel in the Civil Division of the U.S. Department of Justice, coordinates its Nursing Home Initiative and elder justice activities. In that capacity, she coordinates the department's internal efforts and works with federal, state, and local entities (and in particular with the U.S. Department of Health and Human Services), academics, advocates, providers, and others on nursing home and elder-related issues and cases. She has a B.A. from Stanford University, and her J.D. from Northeastern University School of Law.

Rebecca Susan Dresser is Daniel Noyes Kirby professor of law at the Washington University School of Law. She has written extensively on legal and ethical issues in the progression of dementia, the end of life, and informed consent, among other areas. She has a B.A. in psychology and sociology (1973) and an M.S. in education (1975) from Indiana University, Bloomington, and a J.D. from Harvard Law School (1979).

Carmel Bitondo Dyer is associate professor of medicine at Baylor College of Medicine as well as co-director and founder of the Texas Elder Abuse and Mistreatment Institute established in 1997. Her clinical interests include care of the elderly poor, elder mistreatment, dementia, delirium, depression, and geriatric assessment. She is board certified in internal medicine and geriatrics and has been the director of the geriatrics program at the Harris County Hospital District since completing her postgraduate training in 1993. She has an M.D. from Baylor College of Medicine (1988).

Thomas L. Hafemeister is the director of legal studies at the Institute of Law, Psychiatry, and Public Policy of the University of Virginia. He is also an instructor at the University of Virginia Law School and an associate professor of medical education in the Department of Psychiatric Medicine at the University of Virginia Medical School. He has conducted research on a wide range of topics, including end-of-life decision making, guardianship and conservatorship proceedings, public health law and the public health system, and tort law in the health care system. He has a J.D. from the University of Nebraska Law School (1982) and a Ph.D. in social psychology (1988) from the University of Nebraska as part of a joint J.D./Ph.D. degree program.

Catherine Hawes is professor in the Department of Health Policy and Management, School of Rural Public Health, at the Texas A&M University's Health Science Center. She is also director of the Southwest Rural Health Research Center, one of six federally funded rural health research centers nationwide. She has been active in research, teaching, and policy making in long-term care for more than 25 years. She has a B.A. from Principia College and a Ph.D. from the University of Texas at Austin.

Patricia J. McFeeley is assistant chief medical investigator for the state of New Mexico. She is certified in anatomic and forensic pathology by the American Board of Pathology. She has an undergraduate degree from Ohio

Wesleyan University and an M.D. from the University of New Mexico School of Medicine.

Rosalie S. Wolf was executive director of the Institute on Aging at UMass Memorial Health Care, the clinical partner of the University of Massachusetts Medical School, and assistant professor of family medicine and community health. She passed away in fall 2001. A major portion of her time in the past two decades was devoted to the study of elder abuse in domestic settings. With Karl A. Pillemer, she co-edited *Elder Abuse: Conflict in the Family* and co-authored *Helping Elderly Victims: The Reality of Elder Abuse*. She had a B.S. from the University of Wisconsin and a Ph.D. in social welfare policy with a concentration in aging from the Florence Heller Graduate School at Brandeis University.

David Wolfe is professor of psychology and psychiatry at the University of Western Ontario and director of the Center for Research on Violence Against Women and Children. He has broad research and clinical interests in abnormal child psychology, with a special focus on child abuse, domestic violence, and developmental psychopathology. He has a B.A. in psychology from University of Rochester (1973) and an M.A. in psychology (1978) and a Ph.D. in clinical psychology (1980) from the University of South Florida.

Part II
Background Papers

10
Elder Mistreatment: Epidemiological Assessment Methodology

Ron Acierno, Ph.D. *

Epidemiological data on elder mistreatment can be obtained through (1) agency record review, (2) sentinel reports (trained observers in agencies that serve older adults but do not document abuse in official adult protective service [APS] records), (3) translation of criminal justice statistics using age and perpetrator data fields, (4) caretaker/family member interviews (in person or via telephone), and (5) interviews of elderly respondents themselves (in person or via telephone). Each of these assessment formats has been used with older adults, either in isolation or in combination with other methods to generate population estimates of physical, sexual, or emotional abuse, neglect, and financial exploitation. These mistreatment categories are typically divided according to perpetrator identity as either familial/spousal abuse or caretaker abuse. A final category of stranger abuse (i.e., stranger assault: physical, sexual, or emotional) may arguably be included under the heading elder mistreatment (with the caveat that risk factors will probably be different) because (a) psychological and health effects are similar to those caused by abuse by family members; (b) a significant proportion of elder mistreatment, particularly in the area of financial exploitation, is perpetrated by strangers; and (c) failure to assess similarly assaultive behaviors by strangers ignores potential mediating factors that might interact with familial abuse to predict medical health and mental health outcome.

---

*Ron Acierno, Ph.D., is an assistant professor of psychiatry at the National Crime Victims Research and Treatment Center of the Medical University of South Carolina.

Another assessment issue of considerable importance that has not received sufficient attention, at least insofar as elder abuse is concerned, is the categorization of elder mistreatment along lines of cognitive impairment. Although the same behavior of physical abuse might be manifest against two individuals, one demented and the other nondemented, by the same class of perpetrator, the optimal method of assessing these two events may vary widely. Research to date has not thoroughly considered cognitive status as *the* major parameter determining relevance of assessment methodology. Rather, as mentioned above, assessment of elder mistreatment has been divided into abuse versus assault studies according to perpetrator identity. This is problematic in that researchers attempting to document the extent and rate of elder abuse (irrespective of cognitive status) have adopted methodologies that are better suited for one class or the other of older adults. That is, methods 1, agency record review, and 2, sentinel reports, may be effective in assessing abuse against cognitively impaired elders, whereas they will not be very effective in assessing abuse against nonimpaired elders, who may actually avoid these individuals and agencies. Similarly, method 5, anonymous older adult assessment, is probably preferred when cognitive status is intact but is precluded in instances of dementia. Method 4, caretaker assessment, walks the line between these two, in that its effectiveness is not determined by an elder's cognitive status and may therefore be an appropriate stopgap or supplemental technique (see Pillemer and Finkelhor, 1988). However, this method is less statistically sensitive than respondent interviews (i.e., when cognitive status is intact) and probably should not be relied on exclusively.

A distinction based on the mistreated elder's cognitive status is *conceptually*, as well as methodologically, important in that the social context of abuse or assault of nondemented older adults by family members appears to more closely resemble domestic violence, whereas the social context of abuse of cognitively impaired older adults appears to be more akin to child abuse. This is particularly the case when one considers the nature of the relationship between violence perpetrators and recipients (Finkelhor and Pillemer, 1988; Utech and Garrett, 1992; Whittaker, 1996). Thus, violence between two individuals of equal or near-equal societal status, and of equal or near-equal cognitive development, describes both domestic violence and abuse of noncognitively impaired elders (Finkelhor and Pillemer, 1988). By contrast, violence between individuals of varied social status and dependency resulting from differences in cognitive functioning or independence (due to either dementia or lack of development) describes both child abuse and abuse of cognitively impaired elders.[1]

---

[1]Additional justification for this conceptual distinction is provided by empirical, sociopolitical, and legal sources. For example, epidemiological data demonstrate that most

This conceptual distinction becomes even more important when considering that risk factors for violence against older adults probably vary as a function of cognitive status. Hence primary prevention strategies for abuse of cognitively impaired elders will differ from those for abuse of unimpaired elders, just as strategies to prevent child abuse differ from those used to prevent domestic violence.

Thus, cognitive status of the respondent is *pragmatically* important in that it will determine the risk factors and intervention strategies most useful and important for a particular class of individuals. Cognitive status of the respondent is *methodologically* and *conceptually* important in that it will largely determine which assessment strategies from the domestic violence field and from the child abuse field, both of which are more developed than those of the elder mistreatment field, may be applied to older adults. The appropriateness of this application will vary in terms of the cognitive status of the respondent in that an assessment strategy that does not rely on victim report (which will be significantly affected by cognitive status) is indicated in cases of abuse of young children and cognitively impaired older adults. The National Elder Abuse Incidence Study methodology, for example, is appropriate in these instances. By contrast, methods involving some degree of self-report will be indicated in instances where cognitive impairment is not severe. These methods are described at length below.

---

elder abuse is in fact spouse abuse, leading Pillemer and Finkelhor (1988) to state: "In the past, elder abuse was described primarily in analogy with child abuse. The present study suggests that elder abuse has much more in common with spouse abuse than child abuse" (p. 55). Utech and Garrett (1992) go even further, writing, " . . . such parallels with child abuse have had an unfortunate impact on the study of elder abuse, including a tunnel vision effect, which precludes a comprehensive analysis of the problem" (p. 419). Considering sociopolitical factors, investigators have warned against the dangers of infantilizing the older adult victim, as illustrated by Finkelhor and Pillemer (1988): "much elder abuse does not conform to the child abuse model, and elder abuse victims are not necessarily in a structural relationship to their abusers parallel to that of children. . . . We argue that it may be useful to start examining elder abuse for more parallels with the spouse abuse situation: legally independent adults, living together out of choice for a variety of emotional and material reasons" (see also Whittaker, 1996). Finally, legal support for the conceptualization of mistreatment of non-cognitively impaired elders as spouse abuse, rather than child abuse, is provided by the fact that a debate is currently underway regarding mandatory reporting of mistreatment of unimpaired elders (the same debate is underway across the nation with respect to domestic violence), whereas no such debate exists with respect to mandatory reporting mistreatment of cognitively impaired elders (see Daniels, Baumhover, and Clark-Daniels, 1989; Gordon and Tomita, 1990; Macolini, 1995).

ISSUES RELEVANT TO ASSESSMENT OF VIOLENCE
AGAINST OLDER ADULTS

There are two major points to consider when interviewing older adults, relative to younger adults. First, older adults are frequently more reluctant to disclose psychological and interpersonal problems of the past or present. Second, their verbal reports are more affected by physical factors (e.g., fatigue, hearing difficulty) (Ouslander, 1984; Patterson and Dupree, 1994). With respect to the first point, older adults may actually be less likely to disclose abuse than are their abusers (see Homer and Gilleard, 1990, Pillemer and Finkelhor, 1988). Older adults who have been abused or assaulted by family members may be unlikely to report these events for a variety of reasons. Among hypothesized explanations that require further study is the supposition that older adults feel responsible, at least in part, for their children's abusive behavior because they "taught them to be that way." That is, they blame their own parenting style for their adult child's behavior. Another hypothesized explanation is that older adults may also feel extremely embarrassed that their offspring or spouses are abusing them and that they are powerless to stop the abuse. They may be very motivated to hide this powerlessness, both out of pride, and in order to deny any physical or cognitive declines associated with aging. Older and younger adults also report that simply being stigmatized or labeled as a victim is aversive, particularly in instances of sexual assault (Kilpatrick et al., 1992). As with younger victims of domestic violence, abused older adults may fear retribution or more intense assaultiveness from the perpetrator or other abusive parties. Financially or physically dependent older adults also face the very real fear that if the perpetrator is arrested or removed from the household following disclosure, they may be institutionalized or lose other freedoms. Indeed, adults of all ages who have never made or experienced a report of abuse probably do not have information about resources or outcomes of reporting abuse and hence may deny any query, considering truthful responses as potentially damaging but not potentially helpful. Finally, older adult victims may care deeply for or love the perpetrator and may try to avoid hurting or embarrassing the perpetrator in any way through disclosure to epidemiological researchers or authorities.

Physical health barriers to reporting victimization events include deficits in cognitive functioning, hearing loss, increased susceptibility to fatigue, inability to remain sitting for extended durations (e.g., due to arthritis), and effects of medication on concentration and memory. Other factors to consider when assessing older adults include ageism, interview stress, increased somatic presentations that may mirror psychopathological symptoms, increased time needed to build trust and rapport, and increased medication use. Ageism refers to "a personal revulsion to, and distaste for, growing old, and a fear of powerlessness, uselessness, and death" (Patterson and Dupree, 1994:374). Not only must assessors be trained to avoid ageist thinking or actions, but the assessment instrument itself must not be ageist in tone or content. Focusing on specific behaviors and events during assessment (e.g., using very clear, specific descriptions of behavioral events, rather than culturally or generationally defined phrases) appears to be an objective means by which to limit ageism, and, as illustrated below, is an important methodological strategy to increase sensitivity and accuracy of victimization assessment (Patterson and Dupree, 1994).

In addition, it is important to conduct some assessment of cognitive functioning in order to determine the best form of violence assessment, and whether or not assessment of the older adult is even appropriate. Greater susceptibility to fatigue and concentration problems related to disclosure of highly personal content make it advantageous to limit stress during interviews (Gurland et al., 1978). This is particularly the case when interview disclosures potentially affect the interviewee's life, or at least such potential impact is perceived (e.g., disclosing abuse, which then might be reported, leading to social service intervention).

ASSESSMENT OF ELDER MISTREATMENT: EXISTING METHODS AND MEASURES

The following review summarizes specific measures of elder mistreatment and their advantages and disadvantages. Measures are categorized in terms of the five forms of elder mistreatment assessment methodology outlined above. In general, factors such as feasibility, sensitivity, reliability, validity, and cost guide overall conclusions and recommendations for each strategy and measure.

Agency Record Review

Agency records provide a readily available source of information regarding investigated and substantiated cases of elder abuse, neglect, and exploitation. These data are not collected for the purpose of epidemiological or preventive research, however, and the specific information is not always exactly what a particular researcher desires. Moreover, the criteria by which cases are designated substantiated or not and the definitions for particular forms of elder mistreatment vary widely across social service agency, county, and state.

The National Center on Elder Abuse (Tatara, 1997) collects and compiles into reports nationwide data from those social service agencies charged with protecting the health and welfare of older adults. Thus, these reports describe actual investigated and indicated cases of abuse and neglect in which family members were interviewed, households were visited, and inspections were conducted. Although the rate of reported cases has been increasing each year, the sensitivity of this method is extremely low because most cases of elder mistreatment are not reported to any social service authorities (Pillemer and Finkelhor [1988] found only 7 percent of cases reported to authorities), and those incidents that are reported must be judged as valid to be considered substantiated. Again, the criteria by which a report is considered founded vary widely by center, as do the definitions of abuse. Ultimately, it is the judgment of individual caseworkers that determines whether or not a mistreatment event has occurred.

A notable strength of agency record review studies such as that conducted by the National Center on Elder Abuse is the highly detailed nature of the data regarding the abuse event. Specifically, the context of elder mistreatment, the perpetrator characteristics, demographic variables, and social structures are usually specified and documented somewhere in agency records. Moreover, there is a relatively strong level of confidence that indicated cases did, in fact, occur. Relative to epidemiological surveys that are conducted solely for data collection and analysis (as opposed to service delivery), information from agency records exists independent of research protocols and is therefore relatively inexpensive to transfer to the research realm.

By contrast, several significant weaknesses characterize agency record-based investigations. This method requires collecting data from a wide variety of agencies that may use dissimilar definitions of mistreatment. Even more problematic is that individual agencies vary widely in the resources directed to investigation of cases, training of caseworkers, and follow-up and substantiation of cases. Thus, even when standard definitions and criteria are used, the means by which agencies determine whether an event meets these criteria will differ. As such, sensitivity and reliability of findings will suffer. The utility of this approach for epidemiological researchers is further affected by the quality of agency record maintenance, accessibility to records, accessibility of the agency personnel, and overall quality of record keeping by an agency.

Overall, the agency record review methodology is indicated when the population of older adults suffers from cognitive impairment and cannot otherwise be interviewed. However, this method is less sensitive than in other methods applicable to cognitively impaired populations and should probably be used only to guide initial efforts insofar as gross approximations of elder mistreatment are needed.

Sentinel Reports

The National Elder Abuse Incidence Study (NEAIS) sponsored by the Administration for Children and Families and the Administration on Aging expanded its data sources from APS reports to include trained sentinel reports of substantiated or presumed substantiated cases. The NEAIS-targeted people living in their own homes, age 60 and above. This was an incidence study (new cases during a set time frame), not a prevalence study. Importantly, this study did not interview older adults themselves. Sentinels were professionals who served older adults and were randomly selected from more than 200 agencies. Sentinels were trained to complete data entry forms identical to those used by APS workers for elder abuse. The logic of the sentinel approach is based on the supposition that sentinels enhance sensitivity by detecting those older adult victims of abuse who are nonreporters or are not involved with APS but who nonetheless interact in some way with community-based service agencies. NEAIS data were gathered on domestic (i.e., noninstitutionalized) elder abuse and neglect cases from a nationally representative sample of 20 counties in 15 states. Reports from APS agencies were considered only when substantiated and reports from sentinels were presumed to be substantiated.

The methodology of combining agency record reviews with sentinel reports to detect mistreatment has previously demonstrated success in three studies of child abuse. Moreover, the method is cost-effective, and identified cases are very likely true positives. Multiple data sources are consulted, and these typically have a very thorough familiarity with cases. Finally, multiple forms of mistreatment are identifiable.

Weaknesses of this method include the fact that no direct assessment is made of the population in question. Thus, it is very likely that mistreatment rates derived from this study greatly underestimate the true scope of the problem of elder victimization because a great majority of cases go both unreported and undetected by existing formal and informal monitoring agents. Although this approach has been used three times with child abuse, there are several problems with this method when applied to elder abuse. First, and perhaps most relevant, is the fact that child abuse reporting statutes and subsequent education of an extremely wide range of service providers (e.g., schoolteachers, doctors, nurses, counselors, day-care workers, etc.) regarding these statutes is formally established and mature. That is, awareness of the problem of child abuse is far greater among the general and professional public, and thus sentinels in the child arena will be more familiar with the problem and its symptoms. Moreover, child abuse mandatory reporting and provisions for anonymous voluntary reporting have been in place nationwide and have been accompanied by national education campaigns. As such, it is likely that child protective services receive a significantly larger proportion of existing cases than APS. Indeed, *mandatory* reporting of elder abuse is not consistent across the nation and is still actively debated. National education campaigns for the general public and for health and social service providers on child abuse also increase the likelihood that noncompelled reporters will approach sentinels for child abuse, relative to elder abuse. Thus, sentinels for child abuse have access to greater conduits of information than their older adult counterparts.

Overall, the unresolved issue of mandatory reporting of elder abuse, the relative infancy of elder abuse public education, and the limited conduits of information on elder abuse cases flowing to potential sentinels may severely limit the application of this form of child abuse assessment to elder mistreatment in that the method may lack sensitivity. This lack of sensitivity will be particularly problematic for the population of non-cognitively impaired, relatively independent mistreated older adults who wish to avoid formal service agency involvement in their abuse situations.

Criminal Justice System Statistics Translation

There are several sources of victim statistics describing rates of violent crime in this country (e.g., National Crime Victimization Survey [NCVS], Federal Bureau of Investigation [FBI] Uniform Crime Reports [UCR], FBI National Incident Based Reporting System [NIBRS]). Official police or government estimates of assaultive violence are typically lower than those obtained by social scientists conducting epidemiological research. These differences are largely attributable to methodological variance across surveys (e.g., use of gateway versus behaviorally specific preliminary screening questions, or aggregation of official police reports versus population surveys, see discussion of this below). This variance is informative: failure to use direct, behavioral questions leads to failed case identification.

The FBI's UCR is a frequently cited index of violent crime that has been reported to police. The UCR is a case-based report, in which the worst FBI index crime (murder, rape, robbery, aggravated assault, burglary, larceny, motor vehicle theft, arson) reported by an individual is the only one that is recorded for that individual. However, since many crimes are not reported to police, and because many individuals are multiply victimized, UCR results are somewhat misleading.

The Bureau of Justice Statistics overcomes this weakness in its annual NCVS of approximately 80,000 to 100,000 adults aged 12 years and older from approximately 45,000 households. Randomly contacted U.S. citizens are asked about both reported and unreported victimization experiences. In 1992, older adults (age 65 years and older) comprised 14 percent of survey respondents (Bachman, 1992). According to the NCVS, adults over age 50 were the least likely to be physically or sexually assaulted, with an annual violent crime rate of 12.5 per 1,000. However, once assaulted, older adults were more than twice as likely to be seriously injured and require hospitalization following crime. Fully half of older injured victims, compared to about 25 percent of younger injured victims, required hospitalization. Moreover, elderly victims were more likely than younger victims to be assaulted or robbed by a stranger and were more likely to be victimized in or around their home. Half of elderly victims, compared to 26 percent of those under 65, experienced violence in or around their homes and were more likely than younger adults to face offenders armed with a gun (Bachman, 1992). Elderly men were at greater risk of violent crime than elderly women. Low income, minority racial status, and geography also contributed to increased risk of assault (Bachman, 1992). For example, African American older adults were victimized at twice the rate of Caucasian elderly, and older adults living in urban settings were three times as likely to experience crime.

McCabe and Gregory (1998) used the FBI's NIBRS to assess crime against the elderly. This system differs from the UCR in that each incident, not only the worst incident, of crime is recorded. Moreover, like the NCVS, the NIBRS includes information on the perpetrator's relationship to the victim, permitting assessment of abuse versus assault rates. The NIBRS also includes demographic and gender information, providing some ability to conduct risk-factor research. Finally, the NIBRS differs from the UCR in that additional, nonindex crimes are also covered. Unfortunately, only crime reported to police is included in these records.

An advantage of using criminal justice system (CJS) statistics is its nationwide data collection frame. That is, many CJS studies are actual population derivations, not sample estimates. In addition, information on reported (to police) crime includes data regarding gender, race, and perpetrator status. Moreover, older adults are more likely to report some forms of crime to police than younger adults, increasing the relative validity of published rates of *reported* crime. However, crimes of abuse and neglect are less likely to be reported, mitigating this advantage somewhat.

In contrast to these strengths, CJS data generally have very poor sensitivity (excepting the NCVS). Furthermore, CJS data collection requires criminal justice system interaction for case identification (excepting NCVS), an activity that may be specifically avoided by older adults. Another weakness is that UCR and NIBRS data are entirely record-based and are removed from direct reports of victims. As a result, they are affected by subjective interpretations by police officers of (1) whether an event actually occurred and (2) classification of the event by police departments across the country. Overall, these forms of assessment methodology represent preliminary, as opposed to comprehensive, epidemiological data regarding elder mistreatment.

Caretaker/Family Member Assessment

Caretakers do, in fact, report their abusive behaviors. Coyne et al. (1993) reported that 12 percent of caregivers calling a dementia care hot line indicated that they had abused the individual under their care. Homer and Gilleard (1990) studied respite care patients and caregivers in England and found that 45 percent of caregivers admitted either verbal (41 percent) or physical (14 percent) abuse. Interestingly, frequency of patient reports of abuse was less than that of caregivers. Similarly, Pillemer and Suitor (1992) interviewed family members of dementia patients and found that 6 percent reported violence. Pillemer and Finkelhor (1988) interviewed proxies when older adults were unable to participate as respondents and found higher rates of abuse than in victim reports (although this group of proxies arguably represented elders at increased risk, and higher levels should be expected). These studies, and studies cited below, demonstrate that caregiver assessment may be an acceptable, albeit unidimensional, method of detecting elder abuse in the subset of abusers willing to disclose these behaviors. Sensitivity can be expected to be increased if provisions for anonymity are enhanced.

When using caregivers as the data source, researchers have either assessed abusive behaviors directly through interviews or screens, or assessed risk factors associated with perpetrating elder mistreatment. Risk factors include alcoholism, social isolation, psychopathology, low socioeconomic status, overdependence on the older adult, and inexperience or reluctance to provide care (Reis and Nahmiash, 1998). In addition, caregiver risk-factor assessment can be augmented by studying care-receiver risk factors, such as being older, female, isolated, aggressive, or provocative.

Reis and Nahmiash (1998) developed the 29-item (from an original 48 items) Indicators of Abuse (IOA) screen based on previous risk factor research (Kosberg, 1988) with both caregivers and receivers. Although this is a screen, it requires prior in-depth knowledge of caregiver and care-receiver characteristics obtained through interview. The items were selected based on their discriminant ability to detect elder mistreatment derived as part of the major health and social services assessment offered in a North American city. Using the 29 items of the IOA that discriminated abuse from nonabuse, sensitivity was about 85 percent and specificity was 99 percent. Approximately 70 cases were reexamined by a panel to assure criterion accuracy. Using these criterion references, 28 of the original 29 items (caregiver age was dropped) achieved a sensitivity of 78.4 percent and a specificity of 100 percent. Factor analyses failed to identify separate thematic problem areas. Notably, items such as needing help with activities of daily life or cognitive or physical impairment did not contribute to discriminant ability. The overall findings indicate that caregiver rather than care receiver risk factors were most important in predicting abuse and neglect. Using a cutoff of 16, about 22 percent of cases were missed (compared to 36 percent of cases missed by the Hwalek-Sengstock Elder Abuse Screening Test, see below, which is completed by seniors, not interviewers). A notable strength of this tool is that it assesses multiple forms of abuse and assesses both caregiver and care-receiver. Weaknesses include a high false negative rate, limited applicability of the scale to assess domestic violence in elder marital relationships (the Conflict Tactics Scale is useful for this, see below), and the requirement of in depth knowledge of both caregiver and care receiver.

While risk factor assessment is most certainly a clinically valid tool for social service workers, its usefulness in epidemiological studies, particularly in initial investigations, is limited. This is because epidemiological studies are often conducted with the aim, at least in part, of identifying risk factors. Thus, using risk factors to select perpetrators in order to identify additional risk factors is a tautological methodology, and should be avoided in epidemiological efforts.

The Caregiver Abuse Screen (CAS) (Reis and Nahmiash, 1995) is completed by caregivers, not interviewers, as was the case with the IOA. The CAS is very short, only eight items, which somewhat superficially assess forms of abuse and neglect. That is, direct questions regarding mistreatment behaviors are avoided. The authors state that wording is based on "control theory" in which a perpetrator's sense of external locus of control predicts abuse (Bendik, 1992). Conceptualization is also based on neutralization theory, in which abuse is seen as justified and rationalized by the abuser (Tomita, 1990). The CAS is specifically worded so as to be non-blaming. The instrument was validated on 44 abusive caregivers and 45 nonabusive caregivers (the abusive caregivers and 45 controls were receiving services from a social services center). Designation as an abuser was made on the basis of a thorough interview. Results indicated that overall scores of abusers were significantly higher on the CAS (mean = 3.2) than nonabusers (mean = 1.9). CAS scores were positively correlated (0.41) with IOA scores. Unfortunately, no discriminant analyses were conducted, and classification accuracy and optimal cutoff scores for detecting abuse and neglect were not available (rather, only the mean scores of each group were reported as significantly different; note, however, that scores differed by only about one point). Weakness of this measure in terms of its applicability to epidemiological efforts mirrors those of the IOA. Specifically, it is clinically relevant but lacks detailed descriptions of mistreatment events, as well as comprehensive psychometric validation.

The health, attitudes toward aging, living arrangements, and finances (HALF) is presented by Ferguson and Beck (1983) with no psychometric data. This is a clinician-based tool to identify elders at risk in a health service setting. Questions are answered by the interviewer following a meeting with both the caretaker and older adult. Items are categorized in terms of the scale's name on a three-point Likert scale from "almost always" to "never." The instrument is based on previous risk factor research and probably covers relevant areas of assessment for elder mistreatment. However, items in each section often bear no resemblance to the section heading (e.g., under "health" and regarding "caregiver" comes the item "limited capacity to express own needs," or "poor self-image"). Neither factor analysis nor discriminant analysis were conducted to validate constructs measured by item groups or to identify sensitivity or specificity. Many items (e.g., "negative attitudes toward aging") are extremely vague and open to cultural speculation or subjectivity. Other items are clearly physician-relevant (e.g., "shows evidence of dehydration or malnutrition"). Although the screen generally addresses areas of mistreatment, including physical abuse, neglect, and exploitation, no area is specifically assessed. Moreover, the screen is clinically oriented and requires interviews of both caregivers and care receivers. The lack of psychometric validation combined with the vagueness of questions and the need for medical expertise renders this screen of little use in epidemiological efforts. However, its use in medical settings is probably justified.

Fulmer and Cahill (1984) developed the Elder Assessment Protocol, a tool for critical care nurses. The measure is relatively unstructured and intended for use in clinical settings. A checklist of physical symptoms that could be the result of abuse forms the core of the mistreatment assessment protocol. However, these symptoms could have other origins. For example, physical abuse is measured by the item, "physical abuse: present or absent, suspect high risk." In effect, this protocol is a reminder checklist for clinicians but does not directly apply victimization assessment techniques (discussed below) to enhance sensitivity. No psychometric data are provided.

Fulmer also developed the Elder Assessment Instrument (EAI) a 35-item screen that includes subjective and objective items regarding mistreatment (Fulmer and O'Malley, 1987; Fulmer and Cahill, 1984). This screen is designed to identify individuals at high risk of mistreatment who should be referred for further assessment. There is no scoring system, and the tool is designed for clinical rather than epidemiological use.

Overall, several indices and interviews exist and have been used successfully with caregivers to measure elder mistreatment. Caregivers can be asked directly about their abusive or neglectful behaviors, or they can be assessed in terms of risk factors. However, risk factor assessment is more appropriate in clinical than in epidemiological settings. Caregiver assessment can be used in cases where older adults suffer from cognitive deficits and to augment direct assessment of care receivers. Caretaker assessment appears to be the most sensitive method of detecting elder mistreatment in instances where older adults live with family members and suffer from significant cognitive impairment. Indeed, when older adults cannot serve as reliable historians or reporters of mistreatment, family caretaker assessment maybe the only available alternative. However, when cognitively impaired older adults reside in care facilities, the usefulness of caretaker assessment is less well established. This is because there are multiple caretaking staff for any single individual, the turnover rate of these staff is extremely high, precluding accurate long-term (i.e., multiyear retrospective) assessment, and the consequence of disclosure of abusive behavior is more immediately apparent (e.g., immediate suspension or termination).

Assessment of Older Adults

Epidemiological investigations with young adults and adolescents support direct interviewing of potential victim populations to determine the extent and character of mistreatment. It is logical to conclude that, for cognitively unimpaired older adults, direct assessment will also be useful. The following measures have been used with older adults. An additional interview methodology is proposed later.

The Hwalek-Sengstock Elder Abuse Screening Test (HSEAST) is a paper-and-pencil index of elder mistreatment with some psychometric evaluation. Neale et al. (1991) validated the 15-item screen and found that 9 of these items identified abused or exploited individuals. Items are scored yes or no, and a score of 3.5 or higher is indicative of abuse. Three domains of elder abuse are assessed: overt symptoms, victim risk characteristics, and victim symptom characteristics (the authors categorize these as violation of personal rights or direct abuse, characteristics of vulnerability, and potentially abusive situation). The test has some psychometric support of its construct, concurrent, and discriminant validity. The authors compared responses from 170 older adults who were agency referred with founded abuse cases with agency-referred nonfounded cases ($n = 47$) and a non-APS agency comparison group of elderly women ($n = 47$). Significantly higher scores were noted for the abused group, and item-level analysis indicated that nine items provided the basis for this difference. Discriminant function analyses of the nine relevant items revealed correct classification 74 percent of the time, with false negatives (35.7 percent) more likely than false positives (9.3 percent).

Advantages of the HSEAST include its preliminary psychometric validation, along with the fact that it is based on factor analysis of a large item pool. The test is able to assess risk factors along victim and situation lines and can facilitate direction or allocation of additional resources or assessment measures when risk is present. Although it assesses aspects of physical abuse, exploitation, and neglect, no specific assessment of any type of mistreatment is made. One replication study of 100 elders in public housing (Moody et al., 2000) was recently completed to measure discriminant ability of the test again. Factor analysis indicated some differences in loadings from the original study; however, discriminant analyses indicated that the test again classified correctly about 70 percent of respondents as abused or not abused. False positives (17 percent) were more likely in this study than false negatives (12 percent).

The HSEAST suffers from some specific deficits. Several items are extremely vague and lack behavioral specificity when describing events. That is, actual events cannot be determined from this screen, as they can from the Conflict Tactics Scale. However, this screen is designed to be followed by a more in-depth interview when indicated by higher scores. Some items are not directly related to abuse (e.g., a response of "someone else" to the question, "who makes decisions about your life?" or the question, "Do you feel that nobody wants you around?"). Some questions measure potentially abusive situations instead of actual events (e.g., "Can you take your own medication and get around by yourself?" "Are you helping to support someone?"). As a screen, the typical preference is that false-positive rates exceed false-negative rates, and the opposite was observed here. Moreover, there is limited replication of discriminant ability at this point. Overall, this tool may be useful more clinically than epidemiologically.

According to the NEAIS, two-thirds of elder mistreatment cases involved spouses or children. Similarly, Pillemer and Finkelhor (1988) found that 65 percent of elder abuse cases involved spouses as perpetrators. For this reason, and for the conceptual similarities between domestic violence and mistreatment of non-cognitively impaired elders, inclusion of domestic violence assessment methods when measuring elder mistreatment is justified.

The Conflict Tactics Scale (CTS) (Straus, 1979) and the Revised Conflict Tactics Scale (CTS2) are well known, studied, and used indexes of relationship violence. The CTS2 (Straus et al., 1996), originally developed by Straus (1979), is a widely used (over 70,000 empirical studies have used it) and thoroughly evaluated (approximately 400 papers) measure of interpersonal violence for married or cohabiting partners; it has been modified for use with caregivers to the elderly (Pillemer and Finkelhor, 1988). Note that it is not a measure of attitudes toward violence, but rather a measure of conflict-resolution events that involve violence. The scale also measures psychological abusiveness and the use of negotiation and reasoning by either party to reduce conflict. Although the CTS has undergone numerous revisions in the past 15 years, its basic structure has remained the same. The most recent version contains several scales: reasoning/negotiation (6 items), psychological aggression (8 items), physical assault (12 items), sexual coercion (7 items), and consequence (physical injury) (6 items). The 39 items are rated on an 8-point frequency scale (never, once, twice, 3 to 5 times, 6 to 10 times, 11 to 20 times, and more than 20 times, not in the past year but it did happen before). Interpersonal problem-resolution behaviors range from benign (e.g., "When you had a dispute has spouse discussed the issue calmly?") to dangerous (e.g., "Has your spouse threatened you with a knife or gun?"). Each question is asked in terms of both respondent's and partner's behavior. Reliability ranges from 0.79 to 0.95, and initial evidence of construct validity has been obtained (reliability and validity of the scale are well established, and early factor analysis revealed constructs representing (1) verbal reasoning, (2) psychological abuse/aggression, (3) physical aggression, and (4) life-threatening violence. The CTS allows different types (physical and sexual) and intensities of violence to be documented and collects data on specific behavioral aspects of violent events. It can be used in both clinical and epidemiological settings. Weaknesses of the CTS include a potential overfocus on physical and sexual violence incident identification in that the CTS does not assess financial exploitation or neglect.

Using a modified version of the CTS (in addition to other queries) Pillemer and Finkelhor (1988) directly studied over 2,000 randomly selected older adults in the Boston metropolitan area. A two-stage interview was used in which a 30-minute screening interview (conducted either via telephone or in person) was followed by a more thorough interview to assess the context and specific aspects of abuse. The decision to use telephone or in person interviews was made on the basis of respondent availability, ability, and preference to use the telephone (telephone was the default method). An oversample of older adults living with others (a major abuse risk factor) was studied to increase likelihood of interviewing abuse victims. Proxy interviews were also conducted in instances where older adults were incapable of being interviewed. Modified CTS questions were used to assess physical abuse. Modified Older Americans Resources and Services questions were used to assess neglect. Precise wording of assessment questions was not provided in the report.

The strengths of this modified elder mistreatment assessment methodology included combining the CTS with a prescreen to limit assessment time. In addition, multiple assessment formats were used, including telephone, in-person, and proxy interviews. Weaknesses were few. Most notably, event-based interviews cannot study neglect and abuse of demented individuals, and of course caregivers or proxies must be assessed in these instances, but this weakness is not inherent in this assessment method, per se.

Several other measures have been used to study elder abuse, ranging from simple questions regarding mistreatment behaviors to clinical interview protocols. Some of these measures provide little or no psychometric validation or actual specification of items. Others measure constructs related to elder mistreatment, but not mistreatment per se. They are mentioned here in the interest of achieving comprehensiveness.

The modified Elder Abuse Attitudes and Behavior Intention Scale-revised (Childs et al., 2000) assesses attitudes toward abuse, intentions to abuse, and actual behaviors of abuse in caregivers. Although this scale measures both attitudes and intentions (e.g., potential risk factors) as well as behaviors, it is not specifically designed to measure prevalence or incidence of abuse. Childs and colleagues report some indication that perpetrators tend to "fake good."

Coyne and colleagues (1993) sent anonymous questionnaires to 1,000 caregivers who called a dementia hot line. Three hundred forty-two completed and returned questionnaires, which contained 30 items assessing caregiver characteristics, demented senior characteristics, and specific abusive behaviors. Functioning was also assessed. The manner and type of abusive behaviors for which data were collected were not specified further than "punching, shoving, biting, kicking, and striking." This measure was inexpensive, and confidence in reports of abuse is high. However, confidence in nonreports is low. Moreover, no psychometric data were available on reliability or validity. No assessment of financial exploitation, neglect, or psychological abuse was indicated in the article, and a low response rate to the mailed questionnaire mitigated results.

Cooney and Mortimer (1995) also sent anonymous postal questionnaires to 200 British caretakers who participated with a dementia support organization. Questions followed the format of Pillemer and Finkelhor (1988), thus apparently some form of the CTS was used for physical abuse, although the report gave no specifics. Physical abuse, verbal abuse, threats and verbal aggression, and neglect were measured. Data were collected on caregivers (substance use, psychiatric history, length of care) and victims (physical dependency, behavioral disturbance). The response rate was 33.5 percent. Strengths included assessment of multiple forms of abuse and seemingly high sensitivity, with 55 percent of respondents reporting some abuse. However, low response rate to survey must be considered.

Finally, Sengstock and Hwalek (1986) reviewed items (not the measures as complete indices) from seven assessment indices from the early 1980s. Most of the items on these scales assessed risk rather than incidents of elder mistreatment (57.6 percent of all items). Sixteen percent measured neglect and 14.3 percent measured physical abuse. Sexual abuse, emotional abuse, and exploitation were largely omitted. The measures from which items were collected consisted of two social service intake-screening sheets (South Carolina, Ohio), an index from a conference paper presentation

(Hooyman, 1982; Tomita, 1982), an unpublished index from the University of Massachusetts Medical Center, and three published manuscripts (Block and Sinnott, 1979; Johnson, 1981). The review authors described these measures as largely driven by caseworker familiarity with the older adult's case and indicated that "such depth of information may require many months to develop." Moreover, these measures were described as depending "a great deal upon the judgment of the service provider" and may be overly subjective, producing results of questionable validity.

A final group of purely clinical assessment protocols includes the Screening Protocol for Identification of Abuse and Neglect of the Elderly (Johnson, 1981), the Elder Abuse Detection Indicators (Bloom et al., 1989), Tomita's (1982) Detection and Treatment of Elderly Abuse and Neglect: Protocol for Health Care Professionals, and the Community Based Education Model for Identification and Prevention of Elder Abuse (Weiner, 1991). Although clinically useful, these tools have little or no psychometric validation, generally use little behavioral description (see "Issues Pertaining to Assessment of Victimization," below) when posing queries about mistreatment, and are inappropriate for epidemiological efforts. They may also lack sensitivity in clinical realms due to the method and context within which questions are vaguely asked. Examples come from Johnson (1981): "8. Can patient relate instances of: being shaken, shoved?" and from Tomita (1982): "Ask patient if he/she experiences: (a) being shoved, shaken, or hit." These questions, while seemingly relevant, lack specificity and do not employ contextually orienting preface statements or behaviorally specific descriptions about queried events. Research with younger adults indicates that these two characteristics are essential for violence assessment, and further definition and discussion of these aspects is provided in the following section. As such, these protocols represent guidelines, rather than specific assessment manuals or strategies.

ISSUES PERTAINING TO ASSESSMENT OF VICTIMIZATION: WHAT WE'VE LEARNED FROM RESEARCH ON VIOLENCE AGAINST CHILDREN AND YOUNG ADULTS

The following discussion involves techniques used with cognitively intact adolescents and young adults to determine violence prevalence and characteristics. These methods are not appropriate for use with cognitively impaired or demented older adults. For these individuals, the NEAIS methodology in which APS reports and sentinel reports are used to estimate the rate of abuse, combined with caretaker interviews, are indicated to assess the multiple forms of elder mistreatment (see below).

The research on violence against young adults and children, particularly that research involving direct assessment of victims (as opposed to agency/sentinel report sources of data) is more advanced than that on older adults. From this research it is evident that prevalence estimates for criminal victimization, including sexual assault, physical assault, and domestic violence may vary widely according to parameters of assessment methodology, including assessment context, assessment structure, assessor characteristics, and trauma definition (Breslau et al., 1991; Hanson et al., 1995; Kilpatrick et al., 1989; Koss et al., 1993; Resnick et al., 1993, 1996). For example, in interview studies, contextual cues may prime participants to respond in a particular manner. That is, assessment by medical doctors conducted in a primary care facility may be less likely to detect victimization than assessment by criminal justice system epidemiologists conducting crime surveys because respondents in the former situation are primed to answer questions about their health, whereas respondents in the latter situation are expecting to answer questions about victimization. Moreover, definitions of assault vary among respondents (Koss et al., 1993). For example, asking, "Have you ever been raped?" may mean different things to different people (e.g., "It's not rape if my husband does it."). Such culturally, generationally, or ethnically charged questions, if not restructured, will produce inaccurate estimates of violence prevalence.

In addition to definitional and contextual problems, violent crime, particularly that type of crime associated with interpersonal, psychological, or cultural stigma (e.g., elder abuse), is not readily reported by all victims, particularly older adults. Indeed, victims of assault do not openly identify themselves as such. For example, only 2 percent of sexually abused young adult women discuss their victimization history with their doctor (Spring and Friedrich, 1992). Therefore, victim self-identification to strangers conducting epidemiological surveys cannot be taken for granted. In fact, in order to report to an investigator that a particular type of mistreatment or crime has occurred, a victim must (1) recall the assault, (2) label the assault as such, (3) be queried by an investigator who is using a matching label/definition, (4) be willing and psychologically able to disclose the assault, and (5) not feel that safety is jeopardized (e.g., when the perpetrator lives with the respondent and might be listening to the interview). While straightforward, these factors must not be overlooked. For example, many respondents do not label aggravated assault as such when the perpetrator is a relative or spouse, or when there was only limited force or *threat* of force used, or when the psychological effects of such a label are too distressing. Furthermore, many victims are very reluctant to disclose their victimization experiences. Reasons for willful nondisclosure include: (1) fear of retribution by an assailant, particularly if the assailant is known or proximate to victim; (2) fear of stigma attached to being a victim of a particular type of crime (e.g., rape, domestic violence); (3) fear of being blamed; (4) history of negative outcomes following previous disclosure (e.g., placement in a nursing home, court involvement leading to acquittal); (5) lack of encouragement to discuss victimization; and (6) fear of psychological consequences of disclosure (e.g., depression, anxiety on revisiting the event) (Kilpatrick, 1983; Koss et al., 1993; Resnick et al., 1996). It should be obvious that investigators conducting prevalence studies must not *assume* that all victimization events will be specifically and easily reported. Unfortunately, this stipulation has not always been met (e.g., FBI Uniform Crime Reports, 1991; Bachman, 1992; Helzer et al., 1987).

Given that the above factors will combine to reduce the likelihood that a crime event will be reported, what procedural modifications have been used with young adults and children to maximize sensitivity? Two components appear crucial: (1) contextually orienting, empathetic preface statements and (2) extremely specific behavioral descriptions of index events that elicit closed-ended responses. Because traumatic events such as violent crime are associated with extremely aversive emotional and cognitive states, it is important, both to respondent welfare and to experimental integrity, to preface criminal victimization queries in such a way as to convey acceptance, empathy, normalization, and encouragement. Obviously, victims will disclose extremely personal and frequently humiliating information only when they feel that such disclosure is worthwhile and relevant. Of equal import, preface statements must also provide contextual orientation so that the likelihood of reporting that information sought by the investigator is maximized. For example, if questions regarding elder abuse follow a crime survey in which *reported* crimes are investigated, and no preface statement is used to specifically direct respondents to disclose *all* assaults, including those not reported to authorities, then respondents might be biased toward disclosing only those events that have been reported to police (Koss et al., 1993). Similarly, if questions regarding assault follow a psychopathology survey, then respondents might be biased toward disclosing only those assaults that are of a relatively bizarre nature (Koss et al., 1993). Epidemiological researchers studying violence against younger adults and children are typically interested in *all* experienced events. Thus, it must be made clear to the respondent that the individual collecting these data is interested in *any* assault perpetrated by *any* individual, at *any* time in their lives (e.g., assaults by family members years ago, as opposed to just assaults by strangers in the recent past). The National Women's Study (Kilpatrick et al., 1992) and the National Survey of Adolescents (Kilpatrick et al., 2000), both population-based violence assessment projects, employed contextually orienting preface statements similar to the one below. Note that after normalizing the experience somewhat, respondents are oriented to disclose all assaults (reported to authorities or not), by all perpetrators (including family members), occurring at any time (even distant past events).

Another type of stressful event that many people have experienced is unwanted sexual advances. These experiences are not always reported to the police or other authorities or even discussed with family or friends. The person making the advances isn't always a stranger, but can be a friend, boyfriend, or even a family member. Such experiences can occur anytime in a person's life—even as a child. Regardless of how long ago it happened or who made the advances.

In successful studies of violence against younger populations, contextually orienting preface statements are followed by detailed, behaviorally specific, closed-ended descriptions of trauma events under investigation. Early CJS surveys of violence employed gateway screening questions characterized by very limited behavioral specificity (e.g., "Have you ever been physically abused?"). If respondents endorsed the gateway question, further questions about assault followed. Gateway questions shorten the overall interview process for those respondents not endorsing the gateway item. Unfortunately, gateway questions without preface statements lack specificity and do not adequately orient respondents to the type of responses the assessor is seeking (i.e., they fail to state that one is interested in all abuse/assaults, not just those reported to police or perpetrated by strangers). Most problematic, however, is that gateway questions are extremely subject to an individual's interpretation of queries (i.e., definitional variance) (Koss et al., 1993), and a respondent's own victimization history will affect his or her personal definitions of elder abuse (Childs et al., 2000). Behaviorally specific, closed-ended (i.e., yes/no) questions are an alternative to gateway questions. Behaviorally specific descriptions of assault events minimize variance associated with cultural differences, personal differences in intellect, psychological stability, general willingness to disclose, or understanding of criminal justice terminology (e.g., rape, aggravated assault). These questions should be designed with great detail and require only yes or no answers in response to whether or not a specifically described event was experienced. In addition to removing definitional and cultural variance associated with gateway questions, closed-ended yes or no questions simplify the role of the respondent and minimize the risk that anyone will overhear disclosure of highly personal events, particularly during telephone interviews, where at least the queries are unintelligible to others not on the phone. The following are examples of behaviorally specific questions from the National Womens Study. These questions follow directly after the preface statement outlined above and leave very little room for interpretation or error in assessment of a particular type of victimization, in this instance, rape.

1. *Has a man or boy ever made you have sex by using force or threatening to harm you or someone close to you? Just so there is no mistake, by sex we mean putting a penis in your vagina. 2. Has anyone, male or female, ever made you have oral sex by using force or threat of harm? Just so there is no mistake, by oral sex we mean that a man or a boy put his penis in your mouth or someone, male or female, penetrated your vagina or anus with their mouth or tongue. 3. Has anyone ever made you have anal sex by using force or threat of harm? Just so there is no mistake, by anal sex we mean that a man or boy put his penis in your anus. 4. Has anyone, male or female, ever put fingers or objects in your vagina or anus against your will by using force or threats?* (Kilpatrick et al., 1992)

Note that each of the above questions is entirely event-based. That is, priority is given to establishing that mistreatment has or has not occurred. Follow-up questions are asked only in instances where affirmative responses to violence type queries have been given. Thus, secondary questions about the event context and perpetrator status are skipped out when the respondent says "no" to a query. Importantly, computerized protocols can be programmed with complex skip-out patterns resulting in dramatically shortened interview times for those respondents who do not endorse victimization events. For those who indicate that a specific form of violence has occurred, additional questions regarding relationship to the perpetrator, whether or not the event was one in a series, the first and most recent times the event occurred, etc., can be asked. Combining highly specific behavior-based questions with computer-assisted skip out patterns achieves the same brevity of interviews found in gateway surveys, without a loss in sensitivity. Most importantly, this method allows assessment of both abuse by family or caretakers *and* assault by strangers.

TELEPHONE VERSUS IN-PERSON INTERVIEW SURVEY METHODOLOGY

The previous discussion involved methodology used with younger adults in at least three prior population-based studies. This survey technique can be conducted in person or via telephone using random digit dialing methodology, in which stratified samples are derived and randomly called. Several advantages exist for each format. In-person interviews permit visual contact between interviewers and respondents. In-person interviewers can also modulate their volume to a relatively greater extent than telephone interviewers. In addition, conducting in-person interviews allows surveyors to select an appropriate assessment location (i.e., a quiet, undisturbed room, as opposed to wherever the respondent happens to have his or her phone). In-person interviews may also facilitate expressions of empathy, honesty, and respect, which then might encourage more complete self-disclosure (Goodstein, 1980). Finally, in-person interviews can be conducted in households that do not have telephones. (However, the advantage of in-person interviews over telephone interviews insofar as telephone availability is concerned may be illusory. For example, according to the 1990 census, only 5 percent of U. S. households did not have telephones.)

By contrast, data indicate that telephone-based interviewing is an efficient method for collecting information from large representative samples of respondents at a relatively low cost with insignificant response bias in detection of critical variables of interest when compared to in-person interview approaches (Weeks et al., 1983; Bradburn, 1984). These issues have been examined specifically in terms of detection of rates of victimization using in-person versus telephone interview methods (Catlin and Murray, 1979). Based on objective police report data, no differences in rates of detection of victimization were observed, supporting both the reliability and validity of the telephone method. One study (Paulsen et al., 1988) compared telephone and in-person assessment of DSM-III Axis I disorders, including anxiety disorders, affective disorders, alcoholism, and no mental disorder using a structured diagnostic interview. Kappa ranging from 0.69 to 0.84 was obtained, even with a delay between in-person and telephone methods of 12 to 19 months.

There are several additional advantages to telephone assessment of victimization and psychopathology, particularly when considering interviewing older adult respondents. Many older adults indicate that they are hesitant to allow a stranger into their home for a variety of reasons (e.g., safety, feeling compelled to clean the house for the interviewer). The telephone format may also be perceived as relatively more anonymous and less intimidating than in-person disclosures of personal victimization, particularly when perpetrators are family members. Indeed, this anonymity may facilitate disclosure of embarrassing or potentially problematic material. Moreover, this anonymity may reduce the risk of negative outcomes on disclosure of abuse events. That is, if an interview is conducted in person, the interviewer is present in the house and clearly noticed by the abuser. The abuser may even overhear the interview questions and be aware of the older adult's responses. This is not a problem during telephone-based interviews.

Telephone-based interviewing also has the advantage of improving access to participants from across the socioeconomic status range. Thus, the very rich, rich, middle class, lower class, and poor are equally approachable, if they have a telephone. It is unlikely that the upper and lower ends of the socioeconomic spectrum would be available for in-person interviews. Another important concern and advantage of telephone assessment is interviewer safety. In order to achieve national representativeness, all geographic and economic areas must be surveyed and interviewers must enter high-crime areas where they will be at increased risk for victimization. Telephone-based assessment overcomes the risk of victimization that interviewers would certainly face. Another advantage of telephone interviews, particularly those that employ computer-assisted telephone interview technology, is greater and more easily verified standardization (e.g., supervisor spot checks via remote computers). That is, interviewers following a computer generated script with computer-prompted skip-outs who are randomly monitored by supervisors are far less likely to suffer from interviewer drift than interviewers who are not so prompted or supervised. Thus, the integrity of the interview and subsequent collected data are more thoroughly preserved by the telephone interviewing methodology. Moreover, telephone interviews are far less expensive than in-person interviews and generally require significantly less time to complete. Finally, logistic factors such as scheduling, dealing with mandatory reporting issues, overcoming participant hesitation at having strangers in the house, and so on, are relatively less problematic for telephone-based interviews.

COLLECTING SUPPLEMENTAL DATA IN
ADDITION TO THE VIOLENT EVENT

In addition to verifying that a particular form of assault has occurred, social and health science researchers are typically interested in determining health outcomes of such events. In order to derive conceptual models that outline assault-to-pathology pathways, multiple aspects of trauma and traumatic response must be considered. Unfortunately, most studies of assault-related pathology have been somewhat limited in their assessment of variables that play potentially important roles in emotional and physical functioning. Specifically, assault events are routinely examined in isolation, with little consideration given to the differential effects of multiple versus single assault, early-childhood versus later-life assault, assault by stranger versus acquaintance assault, and so on. This point is particularly relevant when considering that approximately 50 percent of physically and sexually assaulted individuals have prior victimization histories (e.g., Kilpatrick et al., 1992). Kilpatrick et al. (2000) suggest that new studies be designed in accord with the following: (1) Temporal boundaries of prevalence rates should be widened to include all adult, or even all lifetime, events. Failure to attend to crime occurring across the life span (e.g., the NCVS) produces artificially bounded prevalence rates. Such methodology might oversimplify causal models involving events that contribute to mental and medical pathology. (2) Multiple or complex victimization histories for each respondent should be collected and considered in causal models of psychopathology, as opposed to focusing on one type of crime, occurring at one point in time, committed by one type of assailant (e.g., the FBI's UCR, in which only the most serious victimization is included in prevalence rates; assessment of abuse by family members or caretakers, but not by strangers). (3) Studied samples should be representative of the population of interest. (4) Both quantitative aspects (e.g., level of physical injury experienced, number of perpetrators, presence of weapon during assault) and qualitative aspects (e.g., perceptions of life threat during assault, fear of crime) of victimization history should be obtained and studied. (5) Other contextual factors that influence postviolence outcome, including familial and personal history of psychopathology, social and vocational adjustment, and level of social support, should be assessed.

CONCLUSIONS AND SUGGESTIONS FOR FUTURE RESEARCH

There are two very distinct groups of elderly victims: those without significant cognitive impairment living independently, with a relative or caretaker, or in a care setting, and those with cognitive impairment, typically in the last two settings. These two classes of victims very likely require different assessment methodologies for two major reasons. First and most obvious, the nature of cognitive impairment limits one's ability to participate in survey research. Second, the type of elder mistreatment very likely varies with the level of cognitive impairment. Moreover, the location of the elder also determines, in some part, the type of mistreatment to which she or he will be exposed (e.g., familial abuse is less likely in institutionalized elders). Existing methods to identify elder abuse fall into five groups: (1) agency record review, (2) sentinel reports, (3) criminal justice statistics, (4) caretaker/family member interview, and (5) interviews of elderly respondents themselves (in person or via telephone).

In the past, research made a distinction when studying victimization of older adults in that assessment efforts were confined to investigating either elder abuse/neglect by family members (including caregivers) or nonfamilial criminal violence, but not both. This distinction may be artificial for three reasons. First, the physical and emotional effects of such events, particularly elder abuse and nonfamilial physical and sexual assault, are often very similar, or at least share a number of similarities (Acierno et al., 1997). Second, both forms of violence appear to have several risk factors in common (e.g., poverty, limited resources, previous victimization), indicating that victims of one type of assault may be more likely to experience the other type of assault than nonvictims. Third, both forms of victimization are amenable to assessment through similar methodological strategies. Studies that endeavor to delineate risk factors for abuse or violence toward older adults should, therefore, simultaneously assess both forms of victimization when possible. Similarly, studies conducted to outline effects of these events on the elderly, and studies conducted to inform preventive interventions for both violence and effects of violence should use a methodology that assesses both forms of victimization. One such method is event-based interviewing such as that used in the National Women's Study and National Survey of Adolescents, in which all forms of elder mistreatment are first identified, followed by perpetrator specification. As such, both assault by strangers and abuse by caretakers/relatives are measured in the same population with the same instrument.

Feasibility, Sensitivity, and Cost:
Older Adults Without Cognitive Impairment

For the group of elderly victims with no cognitive impairment, the most feasible methodology to produce population prevalence estimates for physical, sexual, and emotional forms of violence, as well as for financial exploitation, is direct respondent survey via telephone, similar to that used by Pillemer and Finkelhor (1988). However, a major departure from previous efforts would be to widen the net of assessed violence against older adults to include all violent events using behaviorally specific close-ended questions, with a determination of perpetrator status following determination of event occurrence. This methodology has been used with adolescents and young adults effectively to measure both domestic violence and stranger assault, and could be applied to older adults as well. Thus, combining the methodology of Pillemer and Finkelhor with the content structure of Kilpatrick et al. (National Women's Study) yields "comprehensive violence against the elderly" assessment data. In the past, telephone survey random digit dialing (RDD) procedures were precluded when the target population was significantly represented by individuals in institutions that used internal telephone switchboards for residents' telephones. However, newer and upgraded assisted care institutions and facilities for those who are physically, as opposed to cognitively, disabled often have direct lines to residents' rooms and apartments. As such, this group is also potentially reachable by RDD techniques. This methodology also has the significant advantage of assessing a variety of categories of elder mistreatment simultaneously, compared to record review or FBI UCRs, in which types of mistreatment are largely limited to specific crime types that may or may not be in line with elder abuse definitions (e.g., verbal assault and emotional abuse). Finally, comparisons of criminal justice system/victimization studies using incident-based methodology (FBI UCR) to RDD methodology indicate tremendously improved sensitivity for the latter. Although in-person interviewing is also extremely sensitive, telephone methodology is far more cost-effective.

Feasibility, Sensitivity, and Cost:
Older Adults with Significant Cognitive Impairment

For the group of older adults suffering from dementia, survey interview methodology, whether in person or over the telephone, is probably not feasible or sensitive. For this group, a combination of agency record review and sentinel reporting, such as that employed in the NEAIS, would be indicated. However, until elder abuse statutes that compel reporting are unified and implemented across states, and until service-providing professionals are educated about this compulsion to report instances of elder abuse and neglect—that is, until elder abuse is treated similarly to child abuse for cognitively disabled elders—estimates derived by agency records and sentinel systems will lack sensitivity. To improve sensitivity, these methods might be augmented by caretaker interviews. Note that studies with victims of domestic violence have asked potential perpetrators of assault about their sexually and physically abusive behaviors. Interestingly, these respondents reported significant levels of abuse. Precedent also exists in the elder abuse literature for such methodology. For example, Pillemer and Finkelhor (1988), who interviewed proxies when the older adults designated respondent was incapable of providing self report, found even higher rates of elder abuse (of course, the conclusion that use of proxy report is more sensitive is premature because the group of disabled older adults has been identified as at greater risk of abuse, and hence higher numbers were expected). Thus, interviewing potential perpetrators may provide good information, particularly if used in conjunction with other methodologies. Random sample in person epidemiological interviews are very likely the most sensitive at detecting cases of elder abuse by virtue of their ability to allow interviewers to "lay eyes on" the respondent and his or her environment. However, in-person interviewing is the least feasible and most costly of all methodologies. Tables 10-1 and 10-2 outline the author's impressions of the aforementioned assessment methodologies, and those covered above, in terms of feasibility, sensitivity, and cost.

SUMMARY

Abuse assessment of older adults with significant dementia or other cognitive impairment is most appropriately accomplished by agency record review and sentinel reports, as in the NEAIS. However, these endeavors could be significantly enhanced by including caretaker interviews. For those older adults who are not cognitively impaired, direct interview appears most appropriate. Assessment of this group might also be enhanced

TABLE 10-1 Assessment of Seniors with No Significant Cognitive Impairment

	Feasibility	Sensitivity	Cost
Record review	+	_	+
Sentinel reports	?	_	?
Criminal justice statistic translation	+	_	+
RDD telephone survey: victims	+	+	+
RDD telephone survey: family/caretakers	+	?	+
In-person interview: victims	_	+	_
In-person interview: family/caretakers	_	?	_

TABLE 10-2 Assessment of Seniors with Significant Cognitive Impairment

	Feasibility	Sensitivity	Cost
Record review	+	?	+
Sentinel reports	?	?	?
Criminal justice statistic translation	+	_	+
RDD telephone survey: victims	_	_	+
RDD telephone survey: family/caretakers	+	?	+
In-person interview: victims	_	_	_
In-person interview: family/caretakers	_	?	_

by caretaker interview; however, care must be taken to protect respondents in such studies from perpetrator violence triggered by assessment (e.g., if the perpetrator is aware that the older adult has participated in a survey of violence and has incriminated the perpetrator, albeit anonymously, the perpetrator may be angered). Research with young adults and children demonstrates specific techniques to enhance sensitivity of assessment protocols, and these methodologies should be incorporated into assessment studies of elder mistreatment.

REFERENCES

Acierno, R., H. Resnick, and D. Kilpatrick
   1997   Health impact of interpersonal violence. Section I: Prevalence rates, case identifi-
           cation, and risk factors for sexual assault, physical assault, and domestic violence
           in men and women. *Behavioral Medicine* 23:53–64.
Anetzberger, G.J., B.R. Palmigano, M. Sanders, D. Bass, C. Dayton, S. Eckert, and M.R.
Schimer
   2000   A model intervention for elder abuse and dementia. *The Gerontologist* 40:492–
           497.
Bachman, R.
   1992   *Bureau of Justice Statistics Special Report: Elderly Victims.* NCJ-138330. Wash-
           ington, DC: U.S. Government Printing Office.
Baron, S., and A. Welty
   1996   Elder abuse. *Journal of Gerontological Social Work* 25:336–457.
Bendik, M.F.
   1992   Reaching the breaking point: Dangers of mistreatment in elder caregiving situa-
           tions. *Journal of Elder Abuse and Neglect* 4(3):39–59.
Block, J.D., and M.R. Sinnott
   1979   *The Battered Elder Syndrome: An Exploratory Study.* College Park, MD: Uni-
           versity of Maryland Center on Aging (Abuse Report Form).
Bloom, J., P. Ansell, M. and M. Bloom
   1989   Detecting elder abuse: A guide for physicians. *Geriatrics* 44:40–44.
Bradburn, N.M.
   1984   *Discussion: Telephone Survey Methodology.* Proceedings of the 4th Conference
           on Health Survey Research Methods, Washington, DC. DHHS Publication No.
           (PHS) 84-3346. Washington, DC: U.S. Government Printing Office.
Breslau, N., G.C. Davis, P. Andreski, and E. Petersen
   1991   Traumatic events and posttraumatic stress disorder in an urban population of
           young adults. *Archives of General Psychiatry* 48:216–222.
Catlin, G., and S. Murray
   1979   *Report on Canadian Victimization Survey Methodology Pretests.* Ottawa, ON:
           Statistics Canada.
Childs, H.W., B. Hayslip, Jr., L.M. Radika, and J.A. Reinberg
   2000   Young and middle-aged adults' perceptions of elder abuse. *The Gerontologist*
           40:75–85.
Comijs, H.C., B.W.J.H. Pennix, K.P.M. Knipsheer, and W. Tilburg
   1999   Psychological distress in victims of elder mistreatment: The effects of social
           support and coping. *Journal of Gerontology* 54B:P240–P245.
Comijs, H.C., A.M. Pot, J.H. Smit, L.M. Bouter, and C. Jonker
   1998   Elder abuse in the community: Prevalence and consequences. *Journal of Ameri-
           can Geriatrics Society* 46:885–888.
Cooney, C., and A. Mortimer
   1995   Elder abuse and dementia: A pilot study. *International Journal of Social Psychia-
           try* 41:276–283.
Coyne, A.C., W.E. Reichman, and L.J. Berbig
   1993   The relationship between dementia and elder abuse. *American Journal of Psy-
           chiatry* 150:643–646.
Daniels, R., L. Baumhover, and C. Clark-Daniels
   1989   Physicians' mandatory reporting of elder abuse. *The Gerontologist* 29:321–327.

Federal Bureau of Investigation
    1991   *Uniform Crime Reports for the United States: 1990*. Washington, DC: United States Government Printing Office.

Ferguson, D., and C. Beck
    1983   H.A.L.F.—A tool to assess elder abuse within the family. *American Journal of Nursing* 4:301–304.

Finkelhor, D., and K. Pillemer
    1988   Elder abuse: Its relationship to other forms of domestic violence. In *Family Abuse and Its Consequences: New Directions in Research*, G. Hotaling and D. Finkelhor, eds. Thousand Oaks, CA: Sage Publications.

Floyd, J.
    1984   Collecting data on abuse of the elderly. *Journal of Gerontological Nursing* 10:11–15.

Fulmer, T.T., and V.M. Cahill
    1984   Assessing elder abuse: A study. *Journal of Gerontological Nursing* 10:16–20.

Fulmer, T., and T. O'Malley
    1987   *Inadequate Care of the Elderly*. New York: Springer.

Goodstien, R.K.
    1980   The diagnosis and treatment of elderly patients: Some practical guidelines. *Hospital and Community Psychiatry* 31:19–24.

Gordon, R., and S. Tomita
    1990   The reporting of elder abuse and neglect: Mandatory or voluntary. *Canada's Mental Health* 38:1–6.

Gurland, B., J. Kuriansky, L. Sharpe, R. Simon, P. Stiller, and P. Birkett
    1978   The comprehensive assessment and referral evaluation (CARE)-rationale, development and reliability. *International Journal of Aging and Human Development* 8:9–42.

Hanson, R.F., D.G. Kilpatrick, S.A. Falsetti, and H.S. Resnick
    1995   Violent crime and mental health. In *Traumatic Stress: From Theory to Practice*, J.R. Freedy, and S.E. Hobfoll, eds. New York: Plenum Press.

Helzer, J.E., L.N. Robins, and L. McEvoy
    1987   Post-traumatic stress disorder in the general population. *New England Journal of Medicine* 317.1630–1634.

Homer, A.C., and C. Gilleard
    1990   Abuse of elderly people by their carers. *British Medical Journal* 301:1359–1362.

Hooyman, T.
    1982   *Intervention in Cases of Elderly Abuse within Medical Settings*. Paper presented to the Western Gerontological Society, San Diego, CA.

Hwalek, M.A., and M.C. Sengstock
    1986   Assessing the probabilty of abuse of the elderly: Toward development of a clinical screening instrument. *Journal of Applied Gerontology* 5:153–173.

Hwalek, M.A., A.V. Neale, C.S. Goodrich, and K. Quinn
    1996   The association of elder abuse and substance abuse in the Illinois elder abuse system. *The Gerontologist* 36:694–700.

Jang, M., H.S. You, K. Malley-Morrison, and R. Mills
    1999   Recollections of parental acceptance and control and perceptions of elder abuse: Korean and American college students. *Gerontology and Geriatrics Education* 19:67–80.

Johnson, D.
    1981   Abuse of the elderly. *Nurse Practitioner* 6(1):29–34.

Jones, G.M.
    1987   Elderly people and domestic crime. *British Journal of Criminology* 27:191–201.
Kallman, H.
    1987   Detecting abuse in the elderly. *Medical Aspects of Human Sexuality* 21:89–99.
Kilpatrick, D.G., R. Acierno, H. Resnick, B. Saunders, and C. Best
    2000   Risk factors for adolescent substance abuse: Data from a national sample. *Journal of Consulting and Clinical Psychology* 68:19–30.
Kilpatrick, D.G.
    1983   Special feature: Assessment and treatment of rape victims. *The Clinical Psychologist* 36(4).
Kilpatrick, D.G., C.S. Edmunds, and A.K. Seymour
    1992   *Rape in America: A Report to the Nation.* Arlington, VA: National Victims Center and Medical University of South Carolina.
Kilpatrick, D.G., B.E. Saunders, A. Amick-McMullan, C.L. Best, L.J. Veronen, and H.S. Resnick
    1989   Victim and crime factors associated with the development of crime-related post-traumatic stress disorder. *Behavior Therapy* 20:199–214.
Kosberg, J.I.
    1988   Preventing elder abuse: Identification of high risk factors prior to placement decisions. *The Gerontologist* 28:43–50.
Koss, M.P., L.A. Goodman, A. Browne, and L.F. Fitzgerald, et al.
    1993   *No Safe Haven: Violence Against Women at Home, at Work, and in the Community.* Final report of the American Psychological Association Women's Programs Office Task Force on Violence Against Women.
Lachs, M.S., and K. Pillemer
    1995   Abuse and neglect of elderly persons. *The New England Journal of Medicine* 332:437–443.
Lachs, MS., C.S. Williams, S. O'Brien, K.A. Pillemer, and M.E. Charlson
    1998   The mortality of elder mistreatment. *The Journal of the American Medical Association* 280:428–432.
Macolini, R.
    1995   Elder abuse policy: Considerations in research and legislation. *Behavioral Sciences and the Law* 13:349–363.
McCabe, K.A., and S.S. Gregory
    1998   Elderly victimization: An examination beyond the FBI's index crimes. *Research on Aging* 20:363–372.
Moody, L.E., A. Voss, and C.A. Lengacher
    2000   Assessing abuse among the elderly living in public housing. *Journal of Nursing Measurement* 8:61–70.
Neale, A.V., M.A. Hwalek, R.O. Scott, and C. Stahl
    1991   Validation of the Hwalek-Sengstock elder abuse screening test. *The Journal of Applied Gerontology* 10:406–418.
Ouslander, J.G.
    1984   Psychiatric manifestations of physical illness in the elderly. *Psychiatric Medicine* 1:63–388.
Patterson, R.L., and L.W. Dupree
    1994   Older adults. In *Diagnostic Interviewing*, M. Hersen, and S. M. Turner, eds. New York: Prentice Hall.
Paulsen, A.S., R.R. Crowe, R. Noyes, and B. Pfohl
    1988   Reliability of the telephone interview in diagnosing anxiety disorders. *Archives of General Psychiatry* 45:62–63.

Penhale, B.
1993   The abuse of elderly people: Considerations for practice. *British Association of Social Workers* 23:95–112.

Phillips, L.R., and V.F. Rempusheski
1984   A decision-making model for diagnosing and intervening in elder abuse and neglect. *Nursing Research* 34:134–139.

Pillemer, K., and R. Bachman-Prehn
1991   Helping and hurting. *Research on Aging* 13:74–95.

Pillemer, K., and D. Finkelhor
1988   The prevalence of elder abuse: A random sample survey. *The Gerontologist* 28:51–57.

1989   Causes of elder abuse: Caregiver stress versus problem relatives. *American Journal of Orthopsychiatry* 59:179–187.

Pillemer, K., and J.J. Suitor
1992   Violence and violent feelings: What causes them among family caregivers? *Journal of Gerontology* 47:S165–S172.

Pittaway, E.D., A. Westhues, and T. Peressini
1995   Risk factors for abuse and neglect among older adults. *Canadian Journal on Aging* 14:21–44.

Reay, A.M.C., and K.D. Browne
2001   Risk factors characteristics in carers who physically abuse or neglect their elderly dependents. *Aging and Mental Health* 5:56–62.

Reis, M., and D. Nahmiash
1995   Validation of the caregiver abuse screen (CASE). *Canadian Journal on Aging* 14:45–60.

1998   Validation of the indicators of abuse (IOA) screen. *The Gerontologist* 38:471–480.

Resnick, H.S., D.G. Kilpatrick, B.S. Dansky, B.E. Saunders, and C.L. Best
1993   Prevalence of civilian trauma and PTSD in a representative national sample of women. *Journal of Consulting and Clinical Psychology* 61:984–991.

Resnick, H.S., S.A. Falsetti, D.G. Kilpatrick, and J.R. Freedy
1996   Assessment of rape and other civilian trauma-related PTSD: Emphasis on assessment of potentially traumatic events. In *Theory and Assessment of Stressful Life Events*, T.W. Miller, ed. Madison, CT: International Universities Press.

Rudolph, M.N., and D.H. Hughes
2001   Emergency assessments of domestic violence, sexual dangerousness, and elder and child abuse. *Psychiatric Services* 52:281–282.

Saveman, B.-I., A. Norberg, and I.R. Hallberg
1992   The problems of dealing with abuse and neglect of the elderly: Interviews with district nurses. *Quantitative Health Research* 2:302–317.

Schiamberg, L.B., and D. Gans
2000   Elder abuse by adult children: An applied ecological framework for understanding contextual risk factors and the intergenerational character of quality of life. *International Journal of Aging and Human Development* 50:329–359.

Sengstock, M.C., and M. Hwalek
1986   Domestic abuse of the elderly: Which cases involve the police. *Journal of Interpersonal Violence* 1:335–349.

1987   A review and analysis of measures for the identification of elder abuse. *Journal of Gerontological Social Work* 10:21–37.

Shiferaw, B., M.B. Mittelmark, J.L. Wofford, R.T. Anderson, P. Walls, and B. Rohrer
1994   The investigation and outcome of reported cases of elder abuse: The Forsyth county aging study. *The Gerontologist* 34:123–126.

Spring, F.E., and W.N. Friedrich
  1992   Health risk behaviors and medical sequelae of childhood sexual abuse. *Mayo Clinic Procedures* 67:527–532.
Stokes, S.S., and S.E. Gordon
  1988   Development of an instrument to measure stress in the older adult. *Nursing Research* 37:16–19.
Straus, M.A.
  1979   Measuring intrafamily conflict and violence: The Conflict Tactics (CT) Scales. *Journal of Marriage and the Family* 41:75–88.
Straus, M.A., S.L. Hamby, S. Boney-McCoy, and D.B. Sugarman
  1996   The revised conflict tactics scales (CTS2). *Journal of Family Issues* 17:283–316.
Tatara, T.
  1997   *The National Elder Abuse Incidence Study: Executive Summary.* New York: Human Services Press.
Tomita, S.K.
  1982   Detection and treatment of elderly abuse and neglect: A protocol for health care professionals. *Physical and Occupational Therapy in Geriatrics* 2:37–51.
Tomita, S.K.
  1990   The denial of elder mistreatment by victims and abusers: The application of neutralization theory. *Violence & Victims* 5:171–184.
Utech, M., and R. Garrett
  1992   Elder and child abuse: Conceptual and perceptual parallels. *Journal of Interpersonal Violence* 7:418–428.
Vida, S.
  1994   An update on elder abuse and neglect. *Canadian Journal of Psychiatry* 39:S34–S40.
Weeks, M.F., R.A. Kulka, J.T. Lessler, and R.W. Whitmore
  1983   Personal versus telephone surveys for collecting household health data at the local level. *American Journal of Public Health* 73:1389–1394.
Weiner, A.
  1991   A community-based education model for identification and prevention of elder abuse. *Journal of Gerontological Social Work* 16:107–119.
Wetle, T.
  1986   An elder abuse assessment team in an acute hospital setting. *The Gerontologist* 26:115–118.
Whittaker, T.
  1996   Violence, gender and elder abuse. In *Violence and Gender Relations: Theories and Interventions*, B. Fawcett and B. Featherston, eds. Thousand Oaks, CA: Sage Publications.
Wolf, R.S.
  1988   Elder abuse: Ten years later. *Journal of American Geriatrics Society* 36:758–762.
  1992   Victimization of the elderly: Elder abuse and neglect. *Reviews in Clinical Gerontology* 2:269–276.
  1997   Elder abuse and neglect: An update. *Reviews in Clinical Gerontology* 7:177–182.
Wolf, R.S., and K. Pillemer
  1994   What's new in elder abuse programming? Four bright ideas. *The Gerontologist* 34:126–129.
  2000   Elder abuse and case outcome. *The Journal of Applied Gerontology* 19:203–220.

APPENDIX
ASSESSMENT TOOLS

From Hwalek and Sengstock (1986).

Elder Abuse Screening Test

1.** Do you have anyone who spends time with you, taking you shopping or to the doctor?[3]

2.*** Are you helping to support someone?

3.** Are you sad or lonely?

4.* Who makes decisions about your life—like how you should live or where you should live?

5.*** Do you feel uncomfortable with anyone in your family?

6.** Can you take your own medication and get around by yourself?

7.*** Do you feel that nobody wants you around?

8.*** Does anyone in your family drink a lot?

9.* Does someone in your family make you stay in bed or tell you you're sick when you're not?

10.* Has anyone forced you to do things you didn't want to do?

11.* Has anyone taken things that belonged to you without your OK?

12.*** Do you trust most of the people in your family?

13.*** Does anyone tell you that you give them too much trouble?

14.*** Do you have enough privacy at home?

15.* Has anyone close to you tried to hurt you or harm you recently?

---

[3]A response of "no" to items 1, 6, 12, and 14; a response of "someone else" to item 4; and a response of "yes" to all others was scored in the "abused" direction.

Identified factors: *violation of personal rights or direct abuse, **characteristics of vulnerability, and ***potentially abusive situation

From Fulmer and Cahill (1984).

Elder Assessment Tool

1. Date_____
2. Person completing form_____
3. Patient age_____
4. Patient sex   Male____   Female____
5. PAYMENT STATUS   __Medicare   __Private Pay   __Other
6. RESIDENCE   __Home   __Nursing Home __Other
7. ACCOMPANIED BY   __Family   __Friend   __Alone
8. MENTAL STATUS   __Alert   __Confused __Unresponsive
9. REASON FOR VISIT   __Orthopedic   __Changed Mental Status
__Other

GENERAL ASSESSMENT
10. Hygiene   ____yes   ____no
11. Nutrition ____good   ____fair   ____poor
12. Clothing ____good   ____fair   ____poor

USUAL LIFESTYLE
13. Maintenance of hygiene   ____self   ____assist
14. Continent of bowel/bladder   ____self   ____assist
15. Feedings   ____self   ____assist
16. Ambulatory   ____self   ____assist

17. ____Housebound   ____Outings
18. ____Sedentary   ____Active
19. Personal contact with   ____family   ____friends
    ____nursing home personnel
20. Happy with living situation   ____yes   ____no
21. Who manages finances   ____self   ____family   ____other?
22. Does financial arrangement work well ____yes   ____no?
23. If care provider is present, is the observed relationship
    ____good   ____poor   ____indifferent   ____doesn't apply
24. History of recent life crisis   ____yes   ____no   ____unsure

25. PHYSICAL ASSESSMENT (evidence of)
    __bruising   __lacerations   __abrasions
    __diarrhea   __urine burns   __decubiti
    __dehydration   __malnutrition   __alcohol abuse

MEDICATIONS

26. Any duplication of similar medications? (i.e., multiple laxatives, seda-tives, etc.)   ___yes   ___no

27. Any unusual doses of medications?   ___yes   ___no

28. If yes to #26, please comment_____

29. Who gives medications?   ___self   ___family   ___nursing home

30. If patient or family gives medications, do they have an adequate under-standing of medications?

                       ___yes   ___no

ASSESSMENT

31. Physical Abuse   ___present   ___absent   ___suspect/high risk

32. Psychological Abuse   ___present   ___absent   ___suspect/high risk

33. Material Abuse   ___present   ___absent   ___suspect/high risk

34. Outcome   ___Referral to Elder Abuse team

    ___Referral to Clinical Advisor

35. Summary Statement   ___Too busy to fill out

    ___No abuse/neglect suspected

From Reis and Nahmiash (1998).

INDICATORS OF ABUSE

Indicators of abuse are listed below, numbered in order of importance.[4] After two- to three-hour home assessment (or other intensive assessment) please rate each of the following items on a scale of 0 to 4. Do not omit any items. Rate according to your current opinion.

Scale: Estimated extent of problem: 0 = nonexistent
                                           00 = not applicable
                                           000 = don't know
                                           1 = slight
                                           2 = moderate
                                           3 = probably/moderately severe
                                           4 = yes/severe

Caregiver Age ____years
Caregiver and Care Receiver Kinship   ___spouse
                                               ___nonspouse

Caregiver   Care Receiver

__ 1. Has behavior problems   __ 4. Has been abused in the past
__ 2. Is financially dependent   __ 5. Has marital/family conflict
__ 3. Has mental/emotional   __ 8. Lacks understanding of
       difficulties   medical condition
__ 6. Has alcohol/substance   __ 11. Is socially isolated
       problem   __ 15. Lacks social support
__ 7. Has unrealistic expectations __ 16. Has behavior problems
__ 9. Lacks understanding of   __ 18. Is financially dependent
       medical condition   __19. Has unrealistic expectations
__ 10. Caregiver reluctancy   __ 20. Has alcohol/medication
__ 12. Has marital/family conflict   problem
__ 13. Has poor current   __ 21. Has poor current
       relationship   relationship
__ 14. Caregiver inexperience   __ 22. Has suspicious falls/injuries
__ 17. Is a blamer   __ 23. Has mental/emotional
__ 24. Had poor past relationship   difficulties
                                    __ 25. Is a blamer
                                    __ 26. Is emotionally dependent
                                    __ 27. No regular doctor

---

[4]The majority of the most important indicators are the caregiver ones.

From Reis and Namiash (1995).

Caregiver Abuse Screen

Please answer the following as a helper or caregiver	YES	NO
1. Do you sometimes have trouble making (___) control his/her temper or aggression?	___	___
2. Do you often feel you are being forced to act out of character or do things you feel bad about?	___	___
3. Do you find it difficult to manage (___'s) behavior?	___	___
4. Do you sometimes feel that you are forced to be rough with (___)?	___	___
5. Do you sometimes feel you can't do what is really necessary or what should be done for (___)?	___	___
6. Do you often feel you have to reject or ignore (___)?	___	___
7. Do you often feel so tired and exhausted that you cannot meet (___'s) needs?	___	___
8. Do you often feel you have to yell at (___)?	___	___

From Ferguson and Beck (1983).

HALF Assessment

HEALTH	Almost Always	Some of the Time	Never
1. Aged Adult Risk Dynamics			
1.1 Poor health	_____	_____	_____
1.2 Overly dependent on adult child	_____	_____	_____
1.3 Was extremely dependent on spouse who is now deceased	_____	_____	_____
1.4 Persists in advising, admonishing and directing the adult child on whom he/she is dependent	_____	_____	_____
2. Aged Adult Abuse Dynamics			
2.1 Has an unexplained or repeated injury	_____	_____	_____
2.2 Shows evidence of dehydration and/or malnutrition without obvious cause	_____	_____	_____
2.3 Has been given inappropriate food, drink, and/or drugs	_____	_____	_____
2.4 Shows evidence of overall poor care	_____	_____	_____
2.5 Is notably passive and withdrawn	_____	_____	_____
2.6 Has muscle contractures due to being restricted	_____	_____	_____
3. Adult Child/Caregiver Risk Dynamics			
3.1 Was abused or battered as a child	_____	_____	_____
3.2 Poor self-image	_____	_____	_____
3.3 Limited capacity to express own needs	_____	_____	_____

HEALTH	Almost Always	Some of the Time	Never
3.4 Alcohol or drug abuser	_____	_____	_____
3.5 Psychologically unprepared to meet dependency needs of parent	_____	_____	_____
3.6 Denies parent's illness	_____	_____	_____

4. Adult Child/Caregiver Abuse Dynamics

	Almost Always	Some of the Time	Never
4.1 Shows evidence of loss of control, or fear of losing control	_____	_____	_____
4.2 Presents contradictory history	_____	_____	_____
4.3 Projects cause of injury onto third party	_____	_____	_____
4.4 Has delayed unduly in bringing the aged person in for care, shows detachment	_____	_____	_____
4.5 Overreacts or underreacts to the seriousness of the situation	_____	_____	_____
4.6 Complains continuously about irrelevant problems unrelated to injury	_____	_____	_____
4.7 Refuses consent for further diagnostic studies	_____	_____	_____

5. Attitudes Toward Aging

	Almost Always	Some of the Time	Never
5.1 Aged adult views self negatively due to aging process	_____	_____	_____
5.2 Adult child views aged adult negatively due to aging process	_____	_____	_____
5.3 Negative attitude toward aging	_____	_____	_____
5.4 Adult child has unrealistic expectations of self or the aged adult	_____	_____	_____

6. Living Arrangements

	Almost Always	Some of the Time	Never
6.1 Aged insists on maintaining old patterns of independent functioning that interfere with the child's needs or endanger aged adult	_____	_____	_____

HEALTH	Almost Always	Some of the Time	Never
6.2 Intrusive, allows adult child no privacy	_____	_____	_____
6.3 Adult child is socially isolated	_____	_____	_____
6.4 Has no one to provide relief when uptight with the aged person	_____	_____	_____
6.5 Aged adult is socially isolated	_____	_____	_____
6.6 Has no one to provide relief when uptight with adult child	_____	_____	_____

7. Finances

	Almost Always	Some of the Time	Never
7.1 Aged adult uses gift money to control others, particularly adult children	_____	_____	_____
7.2 Refuses to apply for financial aid	_____	_____	_____
7.3 Savings have been exhausted	_____	_____	_____
7.4 Adult child financially unprepared to meet dependency needs of aged adult	_____	_____	_____

M.T.C.S.

PLEASE COMPLETE IF YOU HAVE HAD A ROMANTIC PART-NER IN THE PAST YEAR. No matter how well a couple gets along, there are times when they disagree on major decisions, get annoyed about something the other person does, or just have spats or fights because they are in a bad mood or tired or for some other reason. They also use many different ways of trying to settle their differences. The following is a list of some things that you and your partner or spouse might have done when you had a dispute.

For each item on the list, please check the box that indicates how often each has occurred *in the past year*.

		Never	Once	Twice	3–5 Times	6–10 Times	11–20 Times	More Than 20 Times
1.	A. Have you discussed the issue calmly	o	o	o	o	o	o	o
	B. Has your spouse discussed the issue calmly	o	o	o	o	o	o	o
2.	A. Have you gotten information to back up your side of things	o	o	o	o	o	o	o
	B. Has your spouse/partner gotten information	o	o	o	o	o	o	o
4.	A. Have you tried to bring in someone to help settle things	o	o	o	o	o	o	o
	B. Has your spouse/partner	o	o	o	o	o	o	o
5.	A. Have you insulted or sworn at your spouse/partner	o	o	o	o	o	o	o
	B. Has your spouse/partner	o	o	o	o	o	o	o
6.	A. Have you sulked and/or refused to talk about it	o	o	o	o	o	o	o
	B. Has your spouse/partner	o	o	o	o	o	o	o
7.	A. Have you stomped out of the room, house, or yard	o	o	o	o	o	o	o
	B. Has your spouse/partner	o	o	o	o	o	o	o
8.	A. Have you cried	o	o	o	o	o	o	o
	B. Has your spouse/partner cried	o	o	o	o	o	o	o
9.	A. Have you done or said something to spite your spouse/partner	o	o	o	o	o	o	o
	B. Has your spouse/partner	o	o	o	o	o	o	o
13.	A. Have you threatened to hit or throw something at your spouse/partner	o	o	o	o	o	o	o
	B. Has your spouse/partner	o	o	o	o	o	o	o

	Never	Once	Twice	3–5 Times	6–10 Times	11–20 Times	More Than 20 Times
14. A. Have you thrown, smashed, hit, kicked something	o	o	o	o	o	o	o
B. Has your spouse/partner	o	o	o	o	o	o	o
15. A. Have you hit or tried to hit your spouse with something	o	o	o	o	o	o	o
B. Has your spouse/partner	o	o	o	o	o	o	o
16. A. Have you thrown something at your spouse/partner	o	o	o	o	o	o	o
B. Has your spouse/partner	o	o	o	o	o	o	o
17. A. Have you pushed, grabbed, or shoved your spouse/partner	o	o	o	o	o	o	o
B. Has your spouse/partner	o	o	o	o	o	o	o
18. A. Have you slapped your spouse/partner	o	o	o	o	o	o	o
B. Has your spouse/partner	o	o	o	o	o	o	o
19. A. Have you kicked, bit, or hit your spouse/partner with a fist	o	o	o	o	o	o	o
B. Has your spouse/partner	o	o	o	o	o	o	o
22. A. Have you beat up your spouse/partner	o	o	o	o	o	o	o
B. Has your spouse/partner	o	o	o	o	o	o	o
23. A. Have you threatened spouse/partner with a knife or gun	o	o	o	o	o	o	o
B. Has your spouse/partner	o	o	o	o	o	o	o
24. A. Have you used a knife or gun on your spouse/partner	o	o	o	o	o	o	o
B. Has your spouse/partner	o	o	o	o	o	o	o

11

Ethical and Policy Issues in Research on Elder Abuse and Neglect

*Rebecca Dresser**

R esearch on elder abuse and neglect poses a multitude of challenges. Besides presenting methodological and practical difficulties, studying maltreatment of older people raises formidable ethical and policy problems. Two general features of the research account for these problems. First, the study population includes older persons with various mental, physical, and social vulnerabilities. Second, the research involves collecting information that could have negative legal, financial, and social consequences for the older persons and caregivers being studied.

The ethical and policy analysis is further complicated by an absence of regulatory guidance and ethical consensus regarding the appropriate procedures to govern research involving persons who lack the ability to decide about research participation. A similar lack of guidance exists regarding the conduct of research in nursing homes and other residential facilities. Finally, current policy and ethics fail to resolve many questions about the appropriate approach to research seeking legally and socially sensitive information.

In this paper, I address ethical and policy issues raised by research on elder abuse and neglect. I use as a framework for ethical analysis the Belmont Report, a document that identifies ethical principles and guidelines

*Rebecca Dresser, J.D., M.S., is the Daniel Noyes Kirby Professor of Law, Washington University School of Law, and Professor of Ethics in Medicine, Washington Univesity School of Medicine.

for research involving human participants[1] (National Commission for the Protection of Human Subjects of Biomedical and Behavioral Research, 1979). I use as a framework for policy analysis the Federal Policy for the Protection of Human Subjects (U.S. Department of Health and Human Services, 1991), also known as the Common Rule. My analysis reviews general issues relevant to research on elder abuse and neglect. Because states vary in their approaches to regulating disclosures of private information, professional reporting duties, nursing home operations, and other relevant topics, issues raised by individual research projects must be separately evaluated by local institutional review boards (IRBs) and attorneys.

The Belmont Report describes the characteristic features of research involving human participants and articulates three ethical principles that apply to such research. These principles are (1) respect for persons, (2) beneficence, and (3) justice. The principle of respect for persons underlies the requirement for informed consent to study participation. The principle of beneficence underlies the requirement to evaluate and balance risks and expected benefits in human studies. The principle of justice addresses fairness in selection of research participants. Provisions in the Common Rule incorporate these Belmont Report principles and requirements.

Institutional review boards rely heavily on the Belmont Report and Common Rule when they evaluate research proposals. Thus, studies on elder abuse and neglect must take into account the concepts and considerations in these documents. Although the Department of Health and Human Services has adopted additional regulations to cover certain populations deemed especially vulnerable in research, it has no special regulations governing research involving older persons, persons with impaired decision making capacity, or residents of nursing homes and other institutions. Various individuals and groups have, however, made recommendations addressing ethical issues with particular relevance to these populations.

In addition, the Common Rule contains a few provisions that specifically bear on vulnerable populations in research. The Rule directs IRBs to "be particularly cognizant of the special problems of research involving vulnerable populations" and to ensure that "[w]hen some or all of the subjects are likely to be vulnerable to coercion or undue influence, . . . additional safeguards have been included in the study to protect the rights and welfare of these subjects" (1991:28,016). The Common Rule advises IRBs that regularly review research involving a vulnerable subject population to consider including "one or more individuals who are knowledgeable about and experienced in working with these subjects" (1991:28,015).

---

[1]In this paper, I use both the newer term "research participant" and the traditional term "research subject" to refer to persons from whom research data are collected.

In considering the issues raised by research involving elder abuse and neglect, one should keep in mind certain characteristics of U.S. policy governing research involving human subjects. Ethical principles and federal regulations establish a general framework for analyzing research proposals. In the current system, local IRBs, as well as funding agencies, interpret and apply the general principles and regulations to specific studies. The oversight system is based on the judgment that studies are sufficiently different and complex that it would be difficult (and probably futile) to set rules for every possible situation. Moreover, the current system reflects the government's desire to avoid a centralized approach in which federal officials are responsible for reviewing study proposals. Instead, the system is designed to allow staff at the local institution and people from the local community to decide how the general principles should apply to individual studies. One inevitable consequence of this system is variation in IRB decisions addressing matters not definitively resolved by the federal regulations.

WHICH PROJECTS ARE GOVERNED BY RESEARCH ETHICS PRINCIPLES AND FEDERAL POLICY?

An initial task is to determine which projects qualify as research and which research projects are covered by the Common Rule. Not all information gathering and interventions related to elder abuse and neglect involve research. Moreover, some research is exempt from federal oversight. The Belmont Report and the Common Rule address, but do not fully resolve, these classification issues.

Distinguishing Research from Other Information Gathering Activities

Underlying the research oversight system is the judgment that research presents particular ethical concerns. Past incidents illustrate that the rights and interests of participants may be compromised in research. As a result, individuals are owed certain special protections in research that may not be required in other data-collection contexts. The Common Rule and its underlying principles are intended to cover the process of producing generalizable knowledge, an activity that society labels desirable but not so important that people should be compelled to participate (Pritchard, 2000). A project's classification as research determines the nature of ethical and policy scrutiny it receives.

Data collection can occur in numerous contexts, including patient care, social services, public health, and program evaluation contexts. These activities fall under the general heading of practice and are not covered by the research oversight system. At the same time, these activities may be combined with research. When they are, they should undergo the same ethical and policy assessment as other research projects.

The Belmont Report relies primarily on the different goals of research and practice to distinguish the two activities. Medical and behavioral clinicians gather information or perform interventions to advance the interests of individual patients or clients. Researchers, on the other hand, collect data and perform interventions "to test an hypothesis, permit conclusions to be drawn, and thereby to develop or contribute to generalizable knowledge" (National Commission for the Protection of Human Subjects of Biomedical and Behavioral Research, 1979:3). Like the Belmont Report, the Common Rule's definition of research looks primarily to the intended aim of the activity. According to the Common Rule, "[r]esearch means a systematic investigation, including research development, testing, and evaluation, designed to develop or contribute to generalized knowledge" (U.S. Department of Health and Human Services, 1991:28,013).

The National Bioethics Advisory Commission (NBAC) recently called attention to flaws in the Common Rule definition. The NBAC observed that the definition omits the additional important point that research is done primarily to benefit society, while practice activities primarily aim to benefit patients, clients, or specific populations. In this respect, the NBAC noted, the Common Rule definition fails to recognize the possible conflict of interest that "always exists between investigators' desires to pursue knowledge and their obligation to protect the rights and welfare of research participants" (2001:35). Moreover, the NBAC noted that the Common Rule definition provides little assistance to those seeking to distinguish research from activities such as public health and quality improvement projects.

As a result of these regulatory shortcomings, it can be difficult to determine when various data-gathering activities should be considered research. Three authors addressing this problem suggested that as a general rule, "[r]esearch projects are done to change the way the [health or social services] community thinks about a specific issue," while "[n]onresearch investigations are done to give a specific group the information they need to make a specific decision" (Amdur et al., 2000).

Consistent with this approach, the Centers for Disease Control and Prevention Guidelines for Defining Public Health Research and Public Health Non-Research (1999) provide as follows:

> The major difference between research and nonresearch lies in the primary intent of the activity. The primary intent of research is to generate or contribute to generalizable knowledge. The primary intent of nonresearch in public health is to prevent or control disease or injury and improve health, or to improve a public health program or service. Knowledge may be gained in any public health endeavor designed to prevent disease or

injury or improve a program or service. In some cases, that knowledge may be generalizable, but the primary intention of the endeavor is to benefit clients participating in a public health program or a population by controlling a health problem in the population from which the information is gathered (1999).

Similarly, a health care organization's quality improvement efforts typically combine review of patient care data with a commitment to take corrective action if the findings warrant. When this commitment is absent, the organization's information gathering is conducted primarily to benefit others and ought to receive the ethical scrutiny appropriate to a research project (Bellin and Dubler, 2001).

When public-health, quality-improvement, and other data-gathering projects have both research and practice objectives, they should be classified as research. Although individual participants or populations may directly benefit from their involvement in such projects, they also are subjected to such measures as structured interviews, intrusions on privacy, and potentially distressing questions to advance the aim of collecting generalizable data. When the aim of collecting generalizable data exposes individuals to risks or burdens not present in standard practice, an activity should be evaluated in the research oversight system (Cassarett et al., 2000). Because participants in such activities fail to receive services tailored to their individual needs and interests, and because the dominant goal is to produce knowledge for the benefit of others, these activities present risks and inconveniences to participants that are not typically present in the practice setting.

Determining Which Research Projects Are Subject to Federal Oversight

Determining whether a project involves research is just the first step in evaluating the project's ethical and policy status. Not all activities that qualify as research are regulated by the federal government. The Common Rule explicitly applies only to research performed or funded by federal agencies that have adopted the Rule (U.S. Department of Health and Human Services, 1991:28,012). One of the Rule's provisions seeks to extend this coverage, however, by requiring all institutions receiving federal research support to "protect the rights and welfare of human subjects of research conducted at or sponsored by the institution, regardless of whether the research is subject to federal regulation" (U.S. Department of Health and Human Services, 1991:28,014). In addition, some research conducted in the private sector is subject to explicit federal oversight. In separate regulations, the U.S. Food and Drug Administration (1999) requires manufacturers seeking agency approval for their products to conform their studies to provisions similar to those in the Common Rule. Certain states also have laws regulating the conduct of human studies (Glantz, 1992).

The Common Rule itself excludes certain research activities from its coverage. The Rule applies only to "research involving human subjects" (U.S. Department of Health and Human Services, 1991:28,012). According to the Rule, "human subject" is "a living individual about whom an investigator . . . conducting research obtains (1) data through intervention or interaction with the individual, or (2) identifiable private information" (U.S. Department of Health and Human Services, 1991:28,013). According to the Rule, information is private if it concerns "behavior that occurs in a context in which an individual can reasonably expect that no observation or recording is taking place" (U.S. Department of Health and Human Services, 1991:28,013). The Rule also classifies as private personal information that is collected for a particular purpose and that the individual reasonably believes will not be publicly disclosed, such as a medical record. When access to medical records or other private information would enable an investigator to readily determine the identity of a person, obtaining such information qualifies as research involving human subjects.

The Common Rule's definition of research involving human subjects incorporates certain ethical judgments. First, if data are publicly available, researchers may use them without securing the permission of the individuals being studied (U.S. Department of Health and Human Services, 1991:28,012). For example, elder abuse and neglect research that involves the examination of public records, such as court or police records, is exempt from the Common Rule provisions. Second, if the information is not publicly available, researchers may gain access without a person's permission as long as that person cannot be individually identified (U.S. Department of Health and Human Services, 1991:28,012).[2] For example, elder abuse and neglect studies involving the examination of medical records lacking individual identifiers would be exempt from the Common Rule's coverage. Another provision of the Common Rule exempts from its coverage surveys and interviews in which no identifying information is recorded (U.S. Department of Health and Human Services, 1991:28,012).

In adopting these provisions, federal officials determined that a person's privacy interests do not extend to certain kinds of information (King, 1995). The Common Rule makes investigators and IRBs responsible for deciding whether people have reasonable expectations that personal information is

---

[2]Also exempt is research "in established or commonly accepted educational settings involving normal educational practices," research evaluating or examining public benefit or service programs, and research on food quality (1991:28,012).

private and when access to private information would enable investigators to identify individuals.

RESPECT FOR PERSONS IN RESEARCH ON ELDER ABUSE AND NEGLECT

The Belmont Report's principle of respect for persons expresses the moral judgment that no one should be used in research purely as a means to benefit others. In essence, the principle gives protection of individual rights and welfare priority over any medical or social benefits research might generate.

The Belmont Report describes two elements of the principle of respect for persons. The first element is that individuals capable of autonomous decision making should be permitted to make their own choices about whether to participate in research. To enable individuals to make autonomous choices, investigators must disclose important facts about a study, ensure that prospective participants understand that information, and ensure that decisions to enroll are not a response to undue pressures or incentives.

The second element of the principle is that individuals with impaired decision making capacities should be protected from harm in the research process. This dimension of the principle is reflected in legal requirements preventing investigators from enrolling decisionally incapable individuals in research without the informed consent of a family member or other appropriate person. Adequate protection may also require investigators to exclude decisionally incapable individuals from certain risky or burdensome studies that are permissible when conducted with capable, consenting individuals.

Standards and Procedures for Evaluating Decisional Capacity

Central to applying the principle of respect for persons is the determination of whether a prospective research participant can make autonomous decisions about study participation. Because capacity determinations have significant moral implications, evaluators must strive to avoid erroneous classifications. Treating a decisionally capable person as incapable leads to a demeaning and unjustified deprivation of that person's right to decide whether research participation would be consistent with his or her particular values and preferences. Treating a decisionally incapable person as capable exposes that person to exploitation to advance the interests of those who benefit from the research enterprise.

In research on elder abuse and neglect, both types of errors can have serious consequences. Delegating research decision-making authority to another individual can be especially problematic in this context, in light of the difficulties that may arise in selecting an appropriate research representative. Moreover, research on abuse and neglect can expose vulnerable individuals to physical, psychological, social, and other risks that ought not be assumed by someone who is unable to comprehend them or is acting in response to perceived pressure from others.

Although no single definition is enshrined in research ethics and policy, agreement exists on the basic features of decisional capacity. According to Paul Appelbaum and Thomas Grisso (1988), four abilities are relevant to decision-making capacity: (1) ability to communicate a choice, (2) ability to understand relevant information, (3) ability to appreciate how this information applies to one's current and future situation, and (4) ability to give comprehensible reasons for a decision. Similarly, a Hastings Center group considering capacity to decide about life-sustaining treatment declared that a "patient has the capacity to make the treatment decision when he or she can understand the relevant information, reflect on it in accordance with his or her values, and communicate with caregivers" (1987:23).

The presence or absence of a dementia diagnosis fails to indicate whether someone has the necessary abilities to make choices about study participation. Similarly, although they may furnish preliminary guidance, simple mental status assessments are insufficient to determine whether someone is able to make autonomous research decisions. Instead, investigators should evaluate decisional capacity in the context of the specific study being proposed.

In the research setting, decision-making capacity should be assessed through a discussion of the facts relevant to the particular choice facing a prospective participant. At minimum, a prospective participant should demonstrate the ability to "understand the purpose, procedures, risks, benefits, and alternatives to participation in the study (including nonparticipation), express a choice about participation; and understand that refusal to participate involves no penalty or loss of benefits to which the person should otherwise be entitled" (Advisory Work Group on Human Subject Research, 1998:23). In this respect, assessing a person's decision-making capacity goes hand in hand with assessing that person's understanding of the important study information:

> The concepts of capacity and adequate information are intertwined. To be informed, a subject must be cognitively capable of understanding the relevant facts about the decision at hand. To determine whether a subject has the requisite cognitive capacity, the examiner must disclose these facts and then ascertain the subject's level of comprehension (Dresser, 1996:68).

As the NBAC pointed out, "our society has not decided what degree of impairment counts as a lack of decision making capacity" (1998:10). Many groups support a sliding-scale approach to evaluating a person's capacity to decide about research. According to this approach, capacity standards may be lower in research presenting comparatively low risk, while a higher level of decisional ability should be required for research that presents comparatively high risks, particularly when the research fails to offer participants the prospect of direct benefit (NBAC, 1998:24).

The assessment process itself can be conducted using a variety of methods. The simplest method is to ask prospective participants to describe briefly and in their own words the basic study information noted above (Wendler and Prasad, 2001). Richard Bonnie has suggested as options "specially tailored follow-up questions to assess subject understanding, videotaping or audiotaping of consent interviews, second opinions, use of consent specialists, or concurrent consent by a family member" (1997:110). The device of concurrent consent is often adopted in dementia research when prospective participants have uncertain or fluctuating decisional capacity (High et al., 1994). This will not always be an option in studies on elder abuse and neglect, but it could be feasible in some such studies. Another suggestion is to adopt a two-part consent process, in which relevant study information is presented and the prospective participant is then asked questions about the study. If the individual exhibits a lack of adequate comprehension, the information is presented again, and the individual is reexamined (Ratzan, 1985). Such a process can detect individuals with problematic memory or other incapacitating cognitive deficits.

The capacity examination should enable researchers to ascertain when someone lacks the requisite abilities to make an autonomous choice about study participation. For people who appear to have adequate decision-making capacity, the next step is to ensure that they *actually* understand the significant information relevant to becoming a study participant.

Informed Choices About Research

People deciding to enter a study should understand certain facts. The Belmont Report lists the following general items essential for investigators to describe: "the research procedure[s], their purposes, risks, and anticipated benefits, alternative procedures (where therapy is involved), and a statement offering the subject the opportunity to ask questions and to withdraw at any time from the research" (National Commission for the Protection of Human Subjects of Biomedical and Behavioral Research, 1979:5). The Report describes the following risks, each of which is specifically relevant to elder abuse and neglect research: "psychological harm, physical harm, legal harm, social harm, and economic harm" (National Commission for the Protection of Human Subjects of Biomedical and Behavioral Research, 1979:7).

The Common Rule includes a more detailed list of the information that prospective participants should understand. Two items are particularly relevant to research on elder abuse and neglect. First, researchers must describe "the extent, if any, to which confidentiality of records identifying the subject will be maintained" (U.S. Department of Health and Human Services, 1991:28,016). Second, if the research presents more than minimal risk, prospective subjects must be told whether compensation or treatment, or both, will be available if injury occurs (U.S. Department of Health and Human Services, 1991:28,016).

Helping prospective participants to achieve adequate understanding is no small task. Surveys and interviews indicate that an appreciable number of people fail to understand important information about the studies in which they participate. A major problem is that participants often mistakenly think that studies are done primarily for their individual benefit, rather than to advance knowledge (Kass and Sugarman, 1996). The challenges may be especially great in research on elder abuse and neglect, given the educational levels and health problems of many prospective participants. Researchers could also encounter difficulties in ensuring that participants understand when elder abuse and neglect studies offer them no direct personal benefit.

Besides the methods described previously in the discussion of capacity assessment, investigators may enhance participants' comprehension by using graphics, videotapes, and other creative approaches to information disclosure (Sachs and Cassel, 1990). The NBAC suggested additional measures to enhance prospective participants' understanding. These include the use of translators when investigators and participants speak different languages, seeking advice from representatives of study populations regarding the appropriate content and presentation of information to prospective participants, and focusing less on the consent form and more on ensuring an effective disclosure and decision-making process (2001:88, 100).

Voluntary Choices About Research

According to the Belmont Report, decisions to enroll in research are voluntary if they occur in the absence of coercion or undue influence. Coercion exists "when an overt threat of harm is intentionally presented by one person to another in order to obtain compliance." Undue influence exists when there is "an offer of an excessive, unwarranted, inappropriate, or improper reward or other overture in order to obtain compliance" (National Commission for the Protection of Human Subjects of Biomedical and Behavioral Research, 1979:6).

A variety of factors may compromise the voluntariness of decisions to participate in elder abuse and neglect research. Older people who depend on health and social services professionals for assistance may agree to participate out of a desire to preserve good relationships. Older people may fear they will lose needed services if they refuse to participate. Residents of nursing homes may be especially vulnerable to these pressures. Offers of monetary or other incentives for study participation may also be unduly tempting to economically disadvantaged people.

The NBAC suggested ways to address some of these problems. This group's suggestions were to discuss possible research participation out of the presence of those to whom the prospective participant usually defers and to design studies so that staff in residential facilities are unaware which individuals are participating (2001:89). Others suggest that research discussions with nursing home residents be conducted in private and that the residents' own physician and nurses not be involved in conducting the research (Sachs et al., 1993). If a physician is conducting research, the Helsinki Declaration urges particular caution and advises that in such a case, "the informed consent should be obtained by a well-informed physician who is not engaged in the investigation and who is completely independent of this relationship" (World Medical Association, 2000:3044).

Procedures for Assessing the Quality of Research Decisions

Investigators must adopt procedures for determining whether research choices are sufficiently capable, informed, and voluntary. At minimum, investigators should develop an assessment plan and the IRB should review that plan. Some individuals and advisory groups believe the assessment should be performed by a qualified professional not otherwise involved in the research. This proposal responds to the concern that researchers eager to enlist participants may be insufficiently demanding about the level of capacity, understanding, and voluntariness necessary to consent.

Some groups say that IRBs should be authorized to decide when independent evaluations are needed in specific studies. The NBAC declared that when research proposals present greater than minimal risk, IRBs ordinarily "should require that an independent, qualified professional assess the potential subject's capacity to consent" (1998:58). In such cases, the proposal "should describe who will conduct the assessment and the nature of the assessment" (1998:58).

Although the use of independent evaluators will add to the costs of a study, supporters contend that the costs are justified by the need to protect individual rights and welfare. This is particularly true, they say, when individuals are asked to join studies that will expose them to significant risk (Dresser, 2001a).

Decisionally Incapable Persons

The screening process may identify individuals lacking decisional capacity. According to the principle of respect for persons, individuals incapable of autonomous choice should be protected from harm in the research process. Conferring such protection may require excluding them from research altogether, or excluding them from studies that present relatively high risk, approaches that are discussed below. If decisionally incapable individuals are considered for research participation, special protective measures are warranted. The most common protective safeguards are (1) to designate as a research decision maker someone "likely to understand the incompetent subject's situation and to act in that person's best interest" (National Commission for the Protection of Human Subjects of Biomedical and Behavioral Research, 1979), and (2) to require the decisionally incapable person's assent or lack of objection to study participation.

Selection of a Research Representative

The Common Rule allows a decisionally incapable person's "legally authorized representative" to consent to that individual's research participation, as long as the representative's consent is adequately informed and voluntary. The Rule fails to specify who may assume the position of representative; instead, it refers generally to "an individual or judicial or other body authorized under applicable law to consent on behalf of a prospective subject to the subject's participation in the procedure[s] involved in the research" (U.S. Department of Health and Human Services, 1991:28,013).

State laws provide for the appointment of legal guardians to make personal and financial decisions for individuals a court has declared legally incompetent. Some states also have laws explicitly authorizing courts, guardians, or family members to act as research decision makers, but many states lack clear rules in this area (Hoffman and Schwartz, 1998). In states without clear rules, possible decision makers include a court-appointed guardian, an individual the currently incapable person previously chose as a research or health care decision maker (also known as a research or health care proxy decision maker), or a relative or close friend of the decisionally incapable person (also known as a surrogate decision maker).[3]

In practice, people from all three of these groups make research choices

---

[3]Although research advance directives and proxies are sometimes discussed as possible mechanisms for authorizing research involving decisionally incapable individuals, it seems highly unlikely that competent persons will complete directives that authorize participation in research on elder abuse and neglect.

for decisionally incapable individuals. Indeed, relatives acting as informal surrogates are probably the most common research decision makers for older people unable to make their own choices. Limiting research decision making to court-appointed guardians is generally seen as burdensome, expensive, and unnecessary to supply adequate protection. Because guardianship proceedings typically fail to examine a prospective guardian's qualifications to act as a research decision maker, such proceedings are an ineffective research safeguard. Moreover, court-appointed guardians may be strangers lacking knowledge of an incapable person's current situation and former values and preferences.

At the same time, the practice of relying on informal surrogates for research decision making raises its own concerns. The primary worry is that such surrogates may have personal interests that conflict with those of the prospective research subject (Dresser, 1996). Conflicts of interest are an obvious possibility in research on elder abuse and neglect, particularly when an abusive or neglectful relative acts as the surrogate decision maker for an older incapable participant.

Investigators should make every effort to select research representatives genuinely concerned with the decisionally incapable individual's welfare. One way to do this is to conduct screening and education of potential representatives, with the aim of detecting inappropriate decision makers and increasing the odds that those chosen will adequately protect research participants' interests. Another is to ensure that the incapable person's research representative will not be the person asked to supply information relevant to abuse and neglect.

The U.S. Department of Health and Human Services regulations on research involving children suggest a third possible response to the conflict of interest problem. The regulations provide as follows:

> if the IRB determines that a research protocol is designed for conditions or for a subject population for which parental or guardian permission is not a reasonable requirement to protect the subjects (for example, neglected or abused children), it may waive the [usual parental] consent requirements . . . provided an appropriate mechanism for protecting the children who will participate as subjects in the research is substituted, and . . . that the waiver is not inconsistent with federal, state, or local law (1999, §46.408(c)).

The regulations also state that the "choice of an appropriate mechanism would depend upon the nature and purpose of the activities described in the protocol, the risk and anticipated benefit to the research subjects, and their age, maturity, status, and condition" (1999, §46.408(c)).

In discussing this research situation, the National Commission for the

Protection of Human Subjects of Biomedical and Behavioral Research suggested the following option:

> to appoint a social worker, pediatric nurse, or physician to act as surrogate parent when the research is designed, for example, to study neglected or battered children. Such surrogate parents would be expected to participate not only in the process of soliciting the children's cooperation but also in the conduct of the research, in order to provide reassurance for the subject and to intervene or support their desire to withdraw if participation becomes too stressful (National Commission for the Protection of Human Subjects of Biomedical and Behavioral Research, 1975:19).

An analogous approach might be adopted in studies of elder abuse and neglect involving decisionally incapable adults. Major considerations would be whether it would be justifiable or practical to withhold information about the appointment of such a designated surrogate from a close family member suspected of abuse. As two authors addressing the child abuse research regulation noted, "removing the parent's decision-making authority will not assuage a child's concerns about the consequences of disclosure, or prevent a parent from vigorously asking a child about what was discussed in interviews . . ." (King and Churchill, 2000:722). Similar concerns could arise in research involving older adults with impaired decisional capacity. Other important considerations would be the study's potential risks and direct benefits, variables that are addressed in the section on beneficence in research on elder abuse and neglect.[4]

Assent and Absence of Objection

Decisionally incapable persons ought not be completely excluded from research decision making. According to the Belmont Report, the principle of respect for persons "requires giving [such persons] the opportunity to choose to the extent they are able, whether or not to participate in re-

---

[4]It appears that the regulatory provision has rarely, if ever, been applied. My review of the literature failed to yield any discussion of the use of a surrogate parent or other alternative to parental or guardian consent in child abuse and neglect research. Moreover, neither an inquiry to the Department of Health and Human Services Office of Human Research Protections nor a request to subscribers to the major IRB listserv produced any reports of studies in which these alternatives were adopted.

One individual did report that his IRB had appointed an independent advocate for child research participants in foster care and other out-of-home placements, based on another provision of the pediatric research regulations that deals with children who are wards of the state or other institutions. The appointments had to be approved by the child's legal guardian. He noted that they had encountered several problems in determining the appropriate role for the advocate, as well as how to cover the costs of this mechanism.

search" (National Commission for the Protection of Human Subjects of Biomedical and Behavioral Research, 1979:6). This requirement has two components. One is to supply information and help decisionally incapable persons understand as much as they can about the proposed study experience. The other is to respect their verbal or physical opposition to participation.

The assent requirement is met when a decisionally incapable person verbally agrees to cooperate with study procedures. The lack of objection requirement is met when a decisionally incapable person fails to indicate verbal or physical opposition to study participation. Assent or lack of objection alone is insufficient to authorize an incapable person's research participation; the informed and voluntary permission of the legally authorized representative is required as well. The presence of the decisionally incapable person's assent or lack of objection is an additional precondition to proceeding with research.

The demand for assent or lack of objection rests on the moral judgment that vulnerable incapable individuals ought not be forced to contribute to the generation of knowledge for the benefit of others. Instead, imposed interventions are warranted solely when they are absolutely necessary to protect the objecting individual's personal welfare.

These moral judgments account for the current view that assent or lack of objection are mandatory in nearly all studies seeking the involvement of decisionally incapable persons. The one possible exception arises when research offers participants a direct health or behavioral benefit unavailable outside the research context. The rationale is that in this situation, "the decision is more akin to a treatment decision, and thus incompetent refusals may be overridden in some cases" (Berg, 1996:24). Although some individuals and groups support such an exception, others question its justification. As one group noted, "it is difficult to equate an intervention which is investigative in nature—with an intervention 'which would be ordered in a purely therapeutic context'" (Keyserlingk et al., 1995:342). Compelling direct benefit would be necessary to justify including actively resisting incapable individuals in research on elder abuse and neglect.

Exceptions to the Requirement for Informed Consent to Research

The Belmont Report acknowledges that imposing the customary informed consent requirements could eliminate or seriously impede some research projects. The Report suggests that incomplete information disclosure could be acceptable under certain circumstances. This view is incorporated in a Common Rule provision permitting exceptions to the general requirements for informed consent. An investigator seeking IRB approval to omit or alter information that must ordinarily be disclosed, or to waive the informed consent requirement altogether, must establish that (1) participants will be exposed to no more than minimal risk, (2) waiving or altering informed consent "will not adversely affect the rights and welfare of the subjects," (3) the study would be impracticable if the information had to be disclosed, and (4) in appropriate cases, the withheld information will be disclosed at the end of the study (U.S. Department of Health and Human Services, 1991:28,016).

According to the Belmont Report, withholding information is never justified simply to make it easier to enroll participants. Instead, withholding should be permitted only if full disclosure would "destroy or invalidate the research" (National Commission for the Protection of Human Subjects of Biomedical and Behavioral Research, 1979:6). This suggests that IRBs should be rigorous in demanding investigators show that their studies would be impracticable if the usual informed consent requirements were applied.

An investigator proposing a study on elder abuse and neglect might seek to withhold information about the study, such as its purpose or risks, from prospective participants or research representatives. For example, an investigator might propose to omit from the consent discussion and form a statement that evidence of possible abuse or neglect will trigger a referral to the appropriate adult protective services agency. The investigator might argue that disclosure of this information would generate too many refusals to participate or distort the responses of those who agree to participate. Another example would be an investigator who sought to modify the study description so that prospective participants would be unaware that its focus was elder abuse or neglect.

Withholding study information from prospective participants compromises their right to make informed research decisions. Thus, it should be done only for compelling reasons. One relevant IRB consideration in the above examples would be the degree of risk that the proposed study would create for participants. If study procedures would expose participants to more than minimal risk, the IRB ought not approve the information withholding. (This topic is discussed in greater detail in the section on balancing harms and benefits in research, below.) The IRB would also need to evaluate the investigator's claim that full disclosure would make the research impracticable.

Surprisingly, data from a study of parents' and teenagers' preferences suggest that disclosure of reporting plans might actually be a positive factor in participant recruitment. O'Sullivan and Fisher found that parents and adolescents would be more willing to enroll in studies on abuse and related behaviors if the investigator planned to notify the parents or help the child obtain independent assistance for any problems discovered in the course of the study (O'Sullivan and Fisher, 1997). These data suggest that IRBs should require persuasive evidence that research will be unduly compromised before granting requests to withhold information from prospective participants in elder abuse and neglect studies.

Conclusion

Choices to participate in research on elder abuse and neglect should be capable, informed, and voluntary. When someone is unable to make valid decisions to participate, researchers should obtain the capable, informed, and voluntary permission of a relative or other individual concerned with protecting the incapable person's well-being. Researchers should also seek the willing cooperation of the decisionally incapable person. Departures from these rules require compelling justification, including a showing that research interventions will not expose participants to significant risk.

BENEFICENCE IN RESEARCH ON ELDER ABUSE AND NEGLECT

The Belmont Report describes two dimensions of the beneficence principle in research. One is to avoid harm to study participants, and the other is to maximize possible benefits and minimize possible harms. Risks to research participants cannot be completely avoided. Instead, those evaluating the ethics of proposed studies must "decide when it is justifiable to seek certain benefits despite the risks involved, and when the benefits should be forgone because of the risks" (National Commission for the Protection of Human Subjects of Biomedical and Behavioral Research, 1979:4)

Two Common Rule provisions incorporate the beneficence principle. The first provision directs researchers to minimize risks to participants through the use of procedures that are "consistent with sound research design," do not impose "unnecessary risks," and, when possible, are "already being performed on the subject for diagnostic or treatment purposes" (1991:28,015). The second provision requires researchers to justify any unavoidable risks by discussing the benefits a study is expected to produce. According to the Common Rule, risks must be "reasonable in relation to anticipated benefits, if any, to subjects, and the importance of the knowledge that may reasonably be expected to result" (U.S. Department of Health and Human Services, 1991:28,015).

To apply the beneficence principle in research, investigators and IRBs must first determine the risks and potential benefits presented by specific studies. The Belmont Report directs study reviewers to be systematic in evaluating potential harms and benefits:

> The method of ascertaining risks should be explicit, especially where there is no alternative to the use of such vague categories as small or slight risk. It should also be determined whether an investigator's estimates of the probability of harm or benefits are reasonable, as judged by known facts

or other available studies (National Commission for the Protection of Human Subjects of Biomedical and Behavioral Research, 1979:7).

The material below describes types of harms and benefits possible in elder abuse and neglect research.

Potential Benefits Offered by Research

Research benefits are available primarily to two groups. First, people enrolled in elder abuse and neglect studies might receive personal benefits due to their study participation. Second, as noted earlier, research is conducted primarily to generate knowledge that could contribute to improved medical and social interventions for others.

Benefits to research participants are generally classified as direct or indirect. Biomedical and behavioral studies may offer a variety of direct benefits to participants. As the National Commission for the Protection of Human Subjects of Biomedical and Behavioral Research noted, "[t]o be considered 'direct,' the possibility of benefit to the subject must be fairly immediate [and t]he expectation of success should be well-founded scientifically" (1978:13).

Examples of research offering potential direct benefit are studies designed to enhance current biomedical or behavioral therapies or to create new training or educational materials (National Commission for the Protection of Human Subjects of Biomedical and Behavioral Research, 1978:13). Direct benefits in research on elder abuse and neglect could be available in studies comparing different interventions to reduce the occurrence of elder abuse and neglect or studies to determine the best methods of assistance to provide once maltreatment has occurred.

To be considered direct, potential benefits should be provided by the intervention(s) under study. In contrast, indirect benefits may be received independently of the primary study interventions (King, 2000). Such benefits may include added contact with health or social services professionals, opportunities to engage in social activities outside of one's usual routine, and a sense of satisfaction in contributing to a valuable social endeavor. Indirect benefits can be difficult to predict due to variations in individual responses. For example, although some older people may value the above elements of the research experience, others may be distressed by having their routines disrupted or receiving additional attention from health or social services professionals. For this reason, although indirect benefits may "count" as possible benefits to study participants, they ought not be assigned the same significance as potential direct benefits when studies are discussed with prospective participants or reviewed by IRBs (Keyserlingk et al., 1995). The NBAC asserted that indirect benefits should be recognized, but "should not weigh in the judgment of IRBs regarding the balance of risks and potential benefits to the participants" (2001:74). A similar approach should be taken regarding benefits studies offer to participants' relatives or other caregivers.

It is generally agreed that items such as financial incentives and reimbursement for transportation and other costs associated with research participation should not be considered benefits to participants. If payments were allowed to count as benefits, then a high payment could offset serious and otherwise unacceptable risks to participants (NBAC, 2001:74).

The evaluation of a study's potential benefits should also consider its possible benefits to society. Evaluating possible societal benefits involves scrutinizing study design, personnel, and other factors affecting the quality of information collected. Because poorly designed or conducted studies will not yield valid and reliable data, they fail to offer benefits to others. Involving people in low-quality studies imposes burdens and risks on them without an adequate social justification. Thus, investigators must propose, and IRBs must demand, studies that meet the relevant scientific standards. When studies are not expected to undergo rigorous peer review as part of the funding process, investigators and IRBs have a responsibility to obtain such a review (Office of Protection from Research Risks, 1993:4–11).

Another dimension of research benefit to others concerns the importance of the research aim. This dimension of research value has received relatively little attention in research ethics analysis, but it deserves more serious consideration. In elder abuse and neglect studies, as in all human research, there must be a good reason for exposing research participants to inconveniences, burdens, and possible harms. Investigators should be able to show why the specific study problem is socially significant and how information gained from the study will help address the problem (NBAC, 2001:73). For example, studies proposing to test minor variations in existing health or social service interventions might hold little prospect of material benefit to others.[5]

Potential Harms in Research

As noted above, the Belmont Report lists the following as risks to research participants: "psychological harm, physical harm, legal harm, social harm, and economic harm" (National Commission for the Protection of Human Subjects of Biomedical and Behavioral Research, 1979:7). More recently, the NBAC elaborated on these concepts. Included as physical

---

[5]An analogy would be clinical trials on so-called "me-too" drugs (Angell, 2000).

harms are "injury, illness, pain, suffering, or discomfort." Types of psycho-logical harm are "negative perceptions of self, emotional suffering (e.g., anxiety or shame), or aberrations in thoughts or behavior." The Commis-sion defined social harms as "negative effects on one's interactions or rela-tionships with others." Participants experience economic harm when they incur expenses as a direct or indirect result of research participation. Legal harms arise when research participation exposes people to actions such as "arrest, conviction, incarceration, or lawsuits" (NBAC, 2001:71–72).

These categories of research risk could exist in studies of elder abuse and neglect. Older participants in such studies could suffer physical harm from family or professional caregivers due to the participant's negative statements about these individuals. Older participants could also experi-ence anxiety or other emotional distress at being asked about a difficult living situation. Relationships with relatives could be damaged as a result of information provided to researchers. Older participants could incur financial costs if the research triggers removal of an unpaid family caregiver or another change in living situation. Information disclosures to research-ers could also lead to guardianship or other legal actions, which could be perceived as detrimental by older participants.

Family and professional caregivers participating in elder abuse and neglect studies could face an array of research harms as well. Although they would be unlikely to experience physical harm as a result of research, shame and other psychological harm from being asked to discuss poten-tially problematic behavior could be a common risk in such studies. In addition, family relationships could suffer if research triggers questions about a caregiver's conduct or abilities. Family caregivers could be de-prived of financial benefits if research leads to removal of relatives from an older person's home. Professional caregivers could experience economic harm if their research participation leads to employment termination. Per-sons reported for abuse and neglect based on information elicited in re-search could also be subjected to legal harm.

Of course, older persons and their caregivers face risks of this sort in their customary interactions with health care and social services personnel. In evaluating potential research harms, the emphasis should be on any additional risks that will arise due to the data gathering associated with a research project. If research participation will entail interviews, examina-tions, or other interventions that participants would not encounter in their usual contacts with health care and social services personnel, the risks accompanying these interventions are properly classified as research risks that should be minimized, justified, and, in many cases, disclosed to poten-tial participants.

Minimizing Risk in Research

Minimizing physical and other research-related risks to participants in elder abuse and neglect studies can raise complex issues. The Common Rule directs researchers to minimize risks "by using procedures already being performed on the subjects for diagnostic or treatment purposes" (U.S. Department of Health and Human Services, 1991:28,015). Investigators may also reduce risks by ensuring that (1) the research team is properly qualified and trained, (2) a system is in place to address harm arising in the research process, (3) confidentiality measures are appropriate, (4) participants are adequately monitored during the study, and (5) individuals are excluded or withdrawn from studies presenting unacceptable risk (NBAC, 2001:73).

Two general features of elder abuse and neglect research pose risks to participants. First, investigators often seek information that could produce harmful consequences if it were released to protective services or other authorities. A variety of methods allow investigators to obtain needed data while minimizing this risk. Sometimes data can be obtained from public records or other public sources. Sometimes data can be collected through the use of interviews or other procedures conducted in routine health care and social services activities; in such cases, data collection will not expose individuals to reporting risks beyond those they would encounter in clinical and social services settings. Sometimes data can be recorded without identifying participants. Sometimes identifying information can be destroyed shortly after it is collected. Strict security measures can also be adopted, including identifying participants by code and severely restricting access to documents linking codes with individual participants (Office of Protection from Research Risks, 1993:3–33). The Common Rule permits IRBs to waive the usual requirement for a signed consent form if such forms would be the sole record tying an individual participant to research and a breach of confidentiality constitutes the principal study risk (U.S. Department of Health and Human Services, 1991:28,017).

When investigators studying elder abuse and neglect seek information about a participant's mental health, illegal conduct, drug or alcohol use, or other conduct with potential negative financial or employment consequences, they may obtain special confidentiality protections from federal officials. Federal law authorizes the Secretary of the Department of Health and Human Services to issue certificates of confidentiality to protect participants' privacy in both government and privately funded projects (Public Health Service Act §310(d), U.S. Code 42 §241(d), 1994). The certificates allow investigators to withhold "from all persons not connected with the conduct of such research the names or other identifying characteristics of such individuals." Investigators with certificates "may not be compelled in any federal, state or local civil, criminal, administrative, legislative, or other proceedings to identify" research participants (Public Health Service Act, 1994). Certificates are granted only when officials deem them necessary to achieve the project aims.

Certificates of confidentiality may prevent researchers from being forced by government authorities to disclose private information about participants suspected to be victims or perpetrators of elder abuse and neglect. Yet some investigators and commentators question whether certificates legally exempt researchers from reporting requirements, and no definitive court ruling exists to resolve this question (Amaya-Jackson et al., 2000). Some federal agencies reportedly refuse funding for studies in which investigators with confidentiality certificates plan to refrain from reporting child abuse and neglect (Runyan, 2000). Moreover, confidentiality certificates do not prohibit investigators from voluntarily disclosing information about suspected abuse and neglect. Thus, researchers must address the ethical issues that arise when withholding information could leave older persons in serious jeopardy.

This point is related to the second risk-producing feature of elder abuse and neglect research. Older persons who participate and those whose relatives or professional caregivers participate may face physical and other serious risks. To minimize such risks to older persons, researchers should take measures to address suspected abuse and neglect. But such measures may cause harm to relatives or professional caregivers. Moreover, such measures may be opposed by older participants who prefer their risky situations to the available alternatives. Finally, social services interventions may do more harm than good for an older individual.

As this discussion reveals, the ethical and policy directive to minimize risks can present difficult trade-offs in elder abuse and neglect research. Measures to minimize harm to older participants, such as reporting suspected abuse and neglect to authorities and the protective interventions that follow, can increase psychological, social, financial, and legal risks to relatives and caregivers. Similarly, measures to safeguard private information about families and caregivers can leave older persons vulnerable to harm. And measures to minimize certain kinds of harm to older persons may increase their exposure to other kinds of harm. The conflicts that may arise in attempts to protect older persons and caregivers from research harms are addressed in further detail in the section on confronting major ethical conflicts.

Balancing Potential Harms and Benefits in Research

After investigators have reduced study risks as much as possible, some risks will almost always remain. The IRB must then determine that these remaining risks are justified by the benefits the study is expected to yield.

As noted above, the Common Rule requires that a study's risks are "reasonable in relation to anticipated benefits." "Reasonable" is a term subject to varied interpretation. In directing IRBs to decide whether a proposed study presents a reasonable balance of risks and anticipated benefits, federal officials delegated to IRB members the authority to interpret what risks are reasonable. The Common Rule requires that IRBs include as members nonscientists and persons not affiliated with the research institution (U.S. Department of Health and Human Services, 1991:28,015). By requiring such members, officials sought to ensure that reasonableness will be evaluated not just by researchers and their colleagues, but by persons who might have a different perspective on research harms and benefits. Reform proposals to increase the number of nonscientist and unaffiliated members are intended to increase the chance that a diversity of perspectives will be represented when research harms and benefits are balanced (NBAC, 2001:63).

Besides requiring IRBs to decide whether research risks are reasonable, the Common Rule and the federal regulations addressing research involving vulnerable populations direct IRBs to determine when research risks are minimal. According to the Common Rule, study interventions present minimal risk if "the probability and magnitude of harm or discomfort anticipated in the research are not greater in and of themselves than those ordinarily encountered in daily life or during the performance of routine physical or psychological examinations or tests" (U.S. Department of Health and Human Services, 1991:28,013–28,014).

As observed in the section on respect for persons in research, the Common Rule permits investigators to withhold certain information from prospective participants, or to forgo consent altogether, only if research interventions present no more than minimal risk. In addition, the NBAC proposed that research interventions presenting greater than minimal risk and no prospect of direct benefit should be allowed only with an incapable individual's prior competent consent or after review and approval by a special standing panel of diverse experts and community representatives convened by the Secretary of the Department of Health and Human Services (NBAC, 1998:54, 61).

The above approaches require IRBs and other reviewers to apply the Common Rule's minimal risk definition. Not everyone is satisfied with the regulatory definition, however. Some argue that its reference to the risks of everyday life is problematic. These critics say that IRB members are unlikely to know enough about the nature, probability, and degree of everyday risks to make comparisons with research risks (Kopelman, 1995). Furthermore, empirical studies have shown variations in the research interventions clinicians and others classify as minimal risk (Dresser, 1999:22).

Another problem is that the Common Rule's definition of minimal risk fails to clarify whether research risks should be compared to everyday risks faced by people in the general population or by subjects individually. Federal regulations issued in 1981 were accompanied by a preamble stating that "the risks of harm ordinarily encountered in daily life means those risks encountered in the daily lives of the subjects of the research" (U.S. Department of Health and Human Services, 1981:8373). But this interpretation is contested by the NBAC (2001:83) and other advisory groups (National Human Research Protections Advisory Committee, 2001), which take the position that minimal risk should be tied to daily risks faced by members of the general population. If everyday risks were individualized, higher research risks could be labeled minimal risk for participants facing higher-than-average daily risks due to illness or poor living situations. As a result, less ethical scrutiny could be devoted to studies involving people already at relative disadvantage. For example, a waiver of informed consent might be obtained in a study presenting higher risk because it involved participants living in high-crime areas. And as the NBAC noted, the individualized standard for minimal risk "would impose disproportionate burdens of research on the ill and provide weaker protections for them than for healthy individuals" (2001:83). Such an approach would thus disregard the ethical principle of justice, discussed below.

In applying the Common Rule's minimal risk and consent waiver provisions, the focus should be on whether research participation exposes older persons and caregivers to risks greater than those present in ordinary life and routine medical and social services encounters. For example, consider an interview study of family members caring for older individuals. If the study would expose participants to more detailed scrutiny than they would encounter in their usual interactions with the health care and social services systems, and if investigators planned to report suspected maltreatment to protective services authorities, the study would present more than minimal risk to study participants. The higher risk would exist because study participation would expose family members to reporting risks greater than those present in routine clinical and social services activities. If, however, data would be collected in interviews conducted as part of the ordinary activities of a social services agency, and the agency's ordinary reporting practices would be followed, the research risks would appear not to exceed the minimal risk threshold. In the first situation, the Common Rule would appear to rule out a consent waiver; in the second, the minimal risk requirement for a waiver would be satisfied.

An appropriate balance of risks and expected benefits is central to the ethical conduct of research on elder abuse and neglect. Specific challenges in determining what constitutes such a balance are discussed below in the section on confronting major ethical conflicts.

JUSTICE IN RESEARCH ON ELDER ABUSE AND NEGLECT

The Belmont Report's final ethical principle is justice. Justice in research involves the fair distribution of risks and benefits associated with research. The principle advises against relying too heavily on disadvantaged individuals or groups to bear the burdens of acting as research participants. On the other hand, the justice principle holds that individuals and groups should receive a fair share of the benefits available through study participation and the improved health and social interventions research makes possible.

The justice principle has several applications to research on elder abuse and neglect. One is that investigators observing the principle will not seek study participants solely from economically and socially disadvantaged populations simply because of "their easy availability, their compromised positions, or their manipulability" (National Commission for the Protection of Human Subjects of Biomedical and Behavioral Research, 1979:5). Similarly, vulnerable populations such as decisionally incapable adults should not be involved in research if adequate data can be obtained by studying adults able to make their own choices about participation. Instead, there must be sound scientific and policy justifications for targeting disadvantaged or vulnerable populations in research.

Three additional applications of the justice principle pertain to the distribution of benefits available through research on elder abuse and neglect. One such application is to give individuals and groups fair access to studies that offer potential direct benefit to participants. Thus, investigators ought not exclude certain people from studies simply because it is more inconvenient or costly to recruit them (Institute of Medicine, 1994:82).

Another application of the justice principle involves ensuring that the improved interventions publicly funded research makes possible are reasonably available to research participants and to those in the general population who would benefit from them (National Commission for the Protection of Human Subjects of Biomedical and Behavioral Research, 1979:5). Thus, when elder abuse and neglect studies yield health and social benefits, those benefits should be available to groups that participated in the studies and to others based on need rather than ability to pay.

Finally, the failure to implement a robust research program to study elder abuse and neglect can be seen as unjust, because it denies vulnerable older persons and their families the benefits that could flow from such a program. A fair system of research funding will allocate funds to studies of serious public health needs, including elder abuse and neglect (Dresser, 2001b).

CONFRONTING THE MAJOR ETHICAL CONFLICTS IN RESEARCH ON ELDER ABUSE AND NEGLECT

The societal importance of advancing knowledge and developing improved health and social programs addressing elder abuse and neglect is undeniable. At the same time, other important interests must be respected in the research process. Research ethics and policy recognize the interests of individuals (or their authorized representatives) in being informed about the studies they are asked to join. Research ethics and policy also deem important the protection of research participants from unnecessary and unreasonable risks. These ethical and policy considerations support certain restrictions on the conduct of research. Such restrictions reflect the judgment that advances in knowledge fail to justify compromising significant interests of the individual.

In research on elder abuse and neglect, the most serious ethical conflicts involve societal interests in gaining knowledge about elder abuse and neglect, participants' interests in being informed of research risks, and the interests of both participants and nonparticipants in being protected from harm. Below, I discuss the major conflicts that can arise and offer guidance on how to resolve them.

Conflicts Regarding Responses to Suspected Abuse and Neglect

The first set of conflicts concerns researchers' responses to suspected elder abuse and neglect. Here, a variety of interests may be at odds. Societal interests in advancing knowledge might be best served if researchers take no action in response to suspected harmful conduct. Relatives, professional caregivers, and older persons who prefer their current living situations might be more likely to enroll and supply accurate information if the information will be used purely for research purposes.

Though this approach promotes societal interests in generating high-quality research data, it gives little regard to older persons' interests in protection from harm. From a broader perspective, the approach overlooks the societal interest in preventing elder abuse and neglect, an interest explicitly recognized in laws requiring reporting of suspected maltreatment.

A researcher's complete failure to respond to suspected abuse and neglect is questionable on both legal and ethical grounds. Although state reporting laws vary, some have language that could apply to researchers (Garfield, 1991). As noted above, a federal certificate of confidentiality does not necessarily exempt researchers from state reporting requirements. Apart from statutory reporting mandates, some writers suggest that courts could hold investigators legally responsible for acting to minimize harm they discover in the course of research. The basis of this duty would be the decision in *Tarasoff v Board of Regents of the University of California* (529 P2d 334, 1976) and subsequent court decisions holding that professionals have duties to take reasonable measures to protect potential victims of their patients' or clients' violence. Paul Appelbaum and Alan Rosenbaum note that courts might deem certificates of confidentiality irrelevant to the investigators' duty to take some action on behalf of potential victims (1989).

Besides their possible legal obligations, researchers may have ethical responsibilities to respond to suspected neglect and abuse. Appelbaum and Rosenbaum suggest that "[o]n ethical grounds alone, . . . it may be reasonable for investigators to consider building provisions for the protection of potential victims into their protocols" (1989:889). Investigators in a consortium of longitudinal studies of child abuse and neglect known as LONGSCAN, as well as those conducting the MacArthur Risk Assessment Study of community violence in former mental patients, recognized an ethical responsibility to prevent harm to both study participants and third parties, although their exact responses varied due to the specific study circumstances and different philosophies of study teams and their reviewing IRBs (Knight et al., 2000; Monahan et al., 1993).[6]

The ethical and legal duties to report suspected abuse and neglect are strongest when researchers conclude that an older person is at risk of serious, imminent harm. If an older person appears to be in imminent danger, a report to protective services workers may be justified even if the older person refuses assistance (Garfield, 1991:870). Similarly, when investigators believe a decisionally impaired older adult is at risk of grave and immediate harm, they may have both legal and ethical responsibilities to report, despite a caregiver's refusal of assistance. As the probability, magnitude, and imminence of harm decrease, however, so does the justification

---

[6]Celia Fisher proposed that the views of the population of prospective research participants should be considered in formulating investigator responses to potential risky situations. In a study of high school students, Fisher and her colleagues elicited participants' opinions about what investigators should do if adolescents promised confidentiality in a study indicated they were in danger or engaged in high-risk conduct. Students were asked whether investigators should keep the information confidential, "talk to you first and let you get help," or notify a "parent or other concerned adult." According to Fisher and her colleagues, their most important finding was "that urban youth do not view the maintenance of confidentiality favorably in situations in which an investigator learns that a research participant is a victim of or engaged in behaviors adolescents perceive to be serious problems." Fisher and her colleagues also believe their findings suggest adolescent research participants promised confidentiality still expect assistance if they disclose abuse or involvement in high-risk conduct, including conduct presenting a serious risk to others (Fisher et al., 1996). Similar studies of older persons would indicate whether or not they hold beliefs resembling those of the adolescents Fisher's team studied.

for reporting. In the absence of a clear and serious threat, investigators may adopt alternative responses to the living situations of older persons and their caregivers.

One option is to furnish research participants with information on available community resources for individuals and families with various living difficulties. Investigators can also express any concerns they may have about a participant's living situation and urge the at-risk individual to obtain help. In planning their studies, investigators can identify an appropriate services agency and establish a referral process for participants expressing a wish for assistance (Appelbaum and Rosenbaum, 1989:892).

Investigators in the LONGSCAN studies adopted a variety of responses to participants in research on child abuse and neglect. In these studies, research team members are most likely to learn of possible maltreatment through interviews with 12-year-olds. Before their study participation, parents and children are told that children will be asked about abuse, neglect, or exposure to violence and that investigators will report children deemed to be at risk of serious harm. Children participate in a computer-administered interview that includes questions about various forms of abuse. A human interviewer is present but is unable to see the child's answers. The children are told that they may skip questions and stop the session at any time.

The LONGSCAN interviewers are trained to recognize and comfort children in distress, and interviewers may terminate the session when a child exhibits persistent distress. Interviews end with "a debriefing with each child that acknowledges that some of the questions may have been difficult, and all study participants are provided with a list of local family services agencies and how and why to contact these resources" (Knight et al., 2000:769). In two LONGSCAN studies, interviewers consult clinical staff if children appear distressed. In another study, interviews are conducted in schools and distressed children are asked to identify a counselor or teacher with whom they can discuss their problems.

Each LONGSCAN study has identified interview responses that could indicate abuse or neglect. Two LONGSCAN study teams report cases in which children give responses deemed to indicate they are at significant risk. Most interesting and controversial is the approach of two other LONGSCAN studies to a child's indications of possible maltreatment. When a child responds in this way, the computer asks whether the child wishes to discuss possible abuse with the interviewer or another person. If the child answers no, the interview ends without further inquiry into the threat. The interviewer is unaware of the child's responses, and the data are recorded in a manner that prevents other researchers from identifying the child (Kotch, 2000). Thus, the research team never obtains the information necessary to evaluate whether the situation should be reported. If the child answers yes, the interviewer or an adult the child designates asks follow-up questions to determine whether reportable abuse has occurred. If it has, the child is told how and why a report will be made. If the problem does not appear to be reportable abuse, the child meets with an appropriate adult to discuss personal problems and receives information on local resources and how to obtain future assistance (Kotch, 2000).

In commenting on this approach, ethicist N. King described its benefits and risks to children and their families. The approach protects children and families from the harm that could come from a more liberal reporting approach, including unjustified disruptions in home life and an inadequate or damaging social services intervention. At the same time, the two LONGSCAN studies' reporting model "privileges research over intervention," on the assumption that better data will produce better interventions in the future. Yet researchers may be biased in making this determination, she noted. Furthermore, King questioned whether 12-year-olds should be put in the position of deciding whether to discuss their situations with researchers. She asked, "is this a means for adolescents to adopt or respect the values and priorities within their families, or is it a way for LONGSCAN researchers to pass the buck to their adolescent subjects?" (1999:184).

The above LONGSCAN approach could be adapted to elder abuse and neglect studies involving older adults with full or mildly compromised decisional abilities. Investigators could devise measures that enabled them to avoid learning about indications of possible abuse or neglect when study participants refused to discuss these matters. Investigators proposing such a strategy could face opposition from IRBs and others evaluating the ethics of the research, however.

Related issues are presented when elder abuse and neglect research involves surveys or other methods in which participants remain anonymous or research team members are blinded to participants' responses. These approaches may be attractive because they allow investigators to guarantee confidentiality and avoid the need to devise measures to address suspected abuse and neglect. At the same time, such approaches have been challenged on ethical grounds. For example, the NBAC criticized the Common Rule's failure to cover anonymous surveys that ask sensitive questions (2001:37). Similarly, ethicists N. King and Larry Churchill raised the following questions about the use of investigator blinding in interview studies of child abuse and neglect: "Might such a research design increase the risk of wrongs or harms to the child subjects who expect to develop some relationship with the researcher who asks such intimate questions? Will anonymity obviate researchers' feelings of relationship with and obligations toward child subjects or just leave them with information on which they are powerless to act?" (2000:722).

The beneficence principle would support offering assistance to participants in research incorporating participant anonymity or investigator blinding. At minimum, investigators could supply to all prospective participants information on available health and social services for families and older persons. Research findings on the risk and prevalence of elder abuse and neglect in particular areas could also be shared with local protective services agencies and government officials, with the aim of increasing awareness of and services for at-risk individuals. Moreover, researchers should consider whether ethical principles would in some cases support alternatives to anonymity and blinding, alternatives such as "a thorough, thoughtful, nondeceptive, informed consent process in an ongoing research relationship, and a commitment to honor confidentiality unless grave harm appears imminent." (King and Churchill, 2000:722).

Conflicts Regarding Information Disclosure

The second major conflict pits the interests of participants in being informed of research risks against societal interests in advancing knowledge. Sometimes withholding information from prospective participants would allow investigators to collect the most accurate data. Two such situations may arise. One occurs when investigators studying relatives or professional caregivers plan to report or take other actions if a research team member comes to suspect elder abuse or neglect. In this case, the concern is that prospective participants aware of the investigators' plans will either refuse to enroll or if they do enroll, will provide inaccurate information. The other situation occurs when investigators are studying older persons. Here, the fear is that if investigators tell prospective participants (or their representatives) about plans to address suspected abuse or neglect, individuals opposed to protective interventions will refuse to enroll or, if they do enroll, will provide inaccurate information.

As indicated above, disclosure in both situations will often be required. The Common Rule permits exceptions to disclosure only when research presents no more than minimal risk to participants and when disclosure would make research impracticable. Underlying the narrowness of the exception is the ethical judgment that potential knowledge gains fail to justify depriving individuals of the freedom to refuse participation in research that exposes them to risks greater than those encountered in everyday life and routine health and social services practice (Beauchamp, 1996). Although failure to disclose reporting plans may be justified in clinical and social services programs designed to assist specific older persons, current policy deems such concealment unacceptable when data are collected for the purpose of advancing knowledge.

Current policy also recognizes that an investigator's failure to disclose plans for addressing suspicions of neglect and abuse could have negative long-term consequences for research, as well as the health care and social services systems. This is because research participants and community members who learn of the failure to disclose could lose trust in researchers, clinicians, and social workers (Bok, 1992).

At the same time, it should be recognized that the current policy requirements for disclosure could have negative consequences. The price of disclosure is a possible loss of societal benefits. This loss could occur if the disclosure requirements limit researchers' abilities to assess and understand the problem of elder abuse and neglect. Whether this occurs will depend in part on whether researchers are able to devise methods that avoid or compensate for possible underreporting and other problems related to the disclosure requirements.

The research ethics literature fails to address information disclosure in the specific context of research on elder abuse and neglect. This topic has been covered, however, in articles examining research on other forms of harmful behavior. Discussions of the ethics of research on child abuse and neglect generally support disclosure of investigators' plans to address suspected misconduct. For example, psychologist Celia Fisher argues for disclosure of all risks that could affect a child's and parent's willingness to enroll, including the possibility that suspected abuse will be reported (Fisher, 1999).

In the LONGSCAN studies of child abuse and neglect, investigators and reviewing IRBs favored disclosure as well. In these studies, parents, as well as children aged eight and older, are told that investigators will take various measures in response to suspected maltreatment, including reporting potentially serious harm to authorities. Parents also are given the option to review the questions their children will be asked. This represents a decision to give children and parents control over the information they provide, even though this may bias study results (Runyan, 1999). Study teams and IRBs in different LONGSCAN projects adopted different language to disclose reporting plans, however, with some disclosures more explicit than others. The language differences reflected differences in study responses to suspected abuse and neglect, which were discussed above.

A similar approach was adopted in the MacArthur Risk Assessment study of risk factors for community violence in former mental patients. In study consent forms, prospective participants were told that confidentiality would be preserved unless researchers believed the lives of participants or third parties were in danger or child abuse was discovered (Monahan et al., 1993). Thus, individuals had the option to refuse participation or to modify their response to investigators based on their awareness that reporting was possible.

In sum, if research participation will expose older persons or caregivers to risks greater than those present in ordinary encounters with health and social services personnel, both research policy and ethics support disclosure of such risks. Balancing the goals of advancing knowledge, respecting informed decision making, and protecting research participants from harm will never be easy. The investigator's overriding ethical obligation is to detect and evaluate potential conflicts in the initial phase of study planning. The appropriate ways to address conflicts will vary depending on the specific characteristics of the study. Often, there will be more than one ethically defensible option. What is most important is to develop approaches that are supported by a reasonable ethical analysis.

CONCLUSION: EXPANDING THE DELIBERATIONS

The Belmont Report principles and Common Rule requirements supply guidance on the appropriate conduct of research on elder abuse and neglect. Yet these principles and regulations are by necessity somewhat general. Every human research proposal presents its own issues; thus, careful deliberation by research teams, IRBs, and funding agency officials will always be essential.

These deliberations could be enriched by the views of people familiar with the actual situations of older persons, their families, and their caregivers. Since the Belmont Report and Common Rule were written, community consultation and representation have emerged as methods for making research more ethical. Indeed, the NBAC specifically advised that representatives of prospective research participants, including those from vulnerable populations, "should be encouraged to participate in the study design and oversight processes" (2001:91). By seeking information from members of the population of prospective research participants, investigators may learn of better ways to balance competing interests in their studies. As Celia Fisher and her colleagues have shown, people affected by research may have unexpected beliefs and attitudes about researchers' responsibilities to participants.

Elder abuse and neglect research seems especially suited to this approach. Several writers have endorsed the involvement of a panel of residents and others who will be affected by research to review proposals to conduct research in nursing homes (Sachs et al., 1993). This concept could be extended to support other forms of community involvement in research on elder abuse and neglect. Members of the relevant communities could help investigators determine the facts that should be disclosed to prospective research participants and create effective methods for conveying the information. They could help researchers discern the appropriate balance between protecting participants' privacy and preventing harm to vulnerable older persons. They could join researchers and social services workers in developing appropriate responses to suspected abuse and neglect discovered in the course of a study.

Awareness of the basic ethical and policy considerations, combined with insights from the community of research participants, will supply the most solid moral foundation for research on elder abuse and neglect. A research program built on this foundation is most likely to receive continued public support, as well. The need for increased knowledge about this serious social problem is great, but so is the need to respect and protect the individuals, families, and communities affected by research.

REFERENCES

Advisory Work Group on Human Subject Research Involving the Protected Classes
    1998   *Recommendations on the Oversight of Human Subject Research Involving the Protected Classes.* New York: New York State Department of Health.

Amaya-Jackson, L., R.R.S. Socolar, W.M.Hunter, and D.K. Runyan
    2000   Directly questioning children and adolescents about maltreatment. *Journal of Interpersonal Violence* 15:725–759.

Amdur, R., M. Speers, and E. Bankert
    2000   IRB triage of projects that involve medical record review. *IRB: A Review of Human Subjects Research* 22(January-February 2000):4–7.

Angell, M.
    2000   Is academic medicine for sale? *New England Journal of Medicine* 342:1516–1518.

Appelbaum, P., and T. Grisso
    1998   Assessing patients' capacities to consent to treatment. *New England Journal of Medicine* 319:1635–1638.

Appelbaum, P.S., and A. Rosenbaum
    1989   Tarasoff and the researcher: Does the duty to protect apply in the research setting? *American Psychologist* 44(6):885–894

Beauchamp, T.
    1996   Moral foundations. In *Ethics and Epidemiology*, S. Coughlin and T. Beauchamp, eds. New York: Oxford University Press.

Bellin, E., and N. Dubler
    2001   The quality improvement-research divide and the need for external oversight. *American Journal of Public Health* 91:1512–1517.

Berg, J.W.
    1996   Legal and ethical complexities of consent with cognitively impaired research subjects: Proposed guidelines. *Journal of Law, Medicine and Ethics* 24:18–35.

Bok, S.
    1992   Informed consent in tests of patient reliability. *Journal of the American Medical Association* 267:1118–1119.

Bonnie, R.
    1997   Research with cognitively impaired subjects. *Archives of General Psychiatry* 54:105–111.

Cassarett, D., J. Karlawish, and J. Sugarman
    2000   Determining when quality improvement initiatives should be considered research. *Journal of the American Medical Association* 283:2275–2280.

Centers for Disease Control and Prevention
    1999   Guidelines for Defining Public Health Research and Public Health Non-Research.
             Available: *http://www.cdc.gov/od/ads/opspoll1.htm* [Accessed November 28,
             2001].
Dresser, R.
    1996   Mentally disabled research subjects: The enduring policy issues. *Journal of the
             American Medical Association* 276:67–72.
    1999   Research involving persons with mental disabilities: A review of policy issues and
             proposals. In *Research Involving Persons with Mental Disorders That May Af-
             fect Decisionmaking Capacity,* vol. 2. Bethesda, MD: National Bioethics Advi-
             sory Commission.
    2001a   Dementia research: Ethics and policy for the twenty-first century. *Georgia Law
             Review* 35:661–690.
    2001b   *When Science Offers Salvation: Patient Advocacy and Research Ethics.* New
             York: Oxford University Press.
Fisher, C.
    1999   Relational ethics and research with vulnerable populations. In *Research Involv-
             ing Persons with Mental Disorders That May Affect Decisionmaking Capacity,*
             vol. 2. Bethesda, MD: National Bioethics Advisory Commission.
Fisher, C., A. Higgins-D'Alessandro, J.B. Rau, T.L. Kuther, and S. Belanger
    1996   Referring and reporting research participants at risk: Views from urban adoles-
             cents. *Child Development* 67:2086–2100.
Garfield, A.
    1991   Elder abuse and the states' adult protective services response: Time for a change
             in California. *Hastings Law Journal* 42:861–937.
Glantz, L,
    1992   The influence of the Nuremberg Code on U.S. statutes and regulations. In *The
             Nazi Doctors and the Nuremberg Code,* G. Annas and M. Grodin, eds. New
             York: Oxford University Press.
Hastings Center
    1987   *Guidelines in the Termination of Life-Sustaining Treatment in the Care of the
             Dying.* Bloomington: Indiana University Press.
High, D., P.J. Whitehouse, S.G. Post, and L. Berg
    1994   Guidelines for addressing ethical and legal issues in Alzheimer disease research:
             A position paper. *Alzheimer Disease and Associated Disorders* 4:66–74.
Hoffman, D., and J. Schwartz
    1998   Proxy consent to participation of the decisionally impaired in medical research—
             Maryland's Policy Initiative. *Journal of Health Care Law & Policy* 1:123–153.
Institute of Medicine
    1994   *Women and Health Research: Ethical and Legal Issues of Including Women in
             Clinical Studies,* vol. 1. A. Mastroianni, R. Faden, and D. Federman, eds. Wash-
             ington, DC: National Academy Press.
Kass, N., and J. Sugarman
    1996   Are research subjects adequately protected? A review and discussion of studies
             conducted by the Advisory Committee on Human Radiation Experiments.
             Kennedy Institute of Ethics Journal 6:271–282.
Keyserlingk, E.W., K. Glass, S. Kogant, and S. Gauthier
    1995   Proposed guidelines for the participation of persons with dementia as research
             subjects. *Perspectives in Biology and Medicine* 38:319–362.

King, N.
1995 Privacy and confidentiality in research. In *Encyclopedia of Bioethics*, W. Reich, ed. New York: MacMillan.
1999 Research in distressed families. In *Beyond Regulations*, N. King, G. Henderson, and J. Stein, eds. Chapel Hill, NC: University of North Carolina Press.
2000 Defining and describing benefit appropriately in clinical trials. *Journal of Law, Medicine & Ethics* 28:332–343.

King, N., and L. Churchill
2000 Ethical principles guiding research on child and adolescent subjects. *Journal of Interpersonal Violence* 15:710–724.

Knight, E., D. Runyan, H. Dubowitz, C. Brandford, J. Kotch, A. Litrownik, and W. Hunter
2000 Methodological and ethical challenges associated with child self-report of maltreatment. *Journal of Interpersonal Violence* 15:760–775.

Kopelman, L.
1995 Research Policy: Risk and Vulnerable Groups. In *Encyclopedia of Bioethics*, W. Reich, ed. New York: MacMillan.

Kotch, J.
2000 Ethical issues in longitudinal child maltreatment research. *Journal of Interpersonal Violence* 15:696–709.

Monahan, J., P.S. Appelbaum, E. Mulvey, P.C. Robbins, and C. Lidz
1993 Ethical and legal duties in conducting research on violence: Lessons from the MacArthur Risk Assessment Study. *Violence and Victims* 8:387–396.

National Bioethics Advisory Commission (NBAC)
1998 *Research Involving Persons with Mental Disorders That May Impair Decisionmaking Capacity*, vol. 1. Bethesda, MD: National Bioethics Advisory Commission.
2001 *Ethical and Policy Issues in Research Involving Human Participants: Report and Recommendations*, Bethesda, MD: National Bioethics Advisory Commission.

National Commission for the Protection of Human Subjects of Biomedical and Behavioral Research
1975 *Research Involving Children: Report and Recommendations*, DHEW Publication No. (OS) 76-127. Washington, DC: U.S. Government Printing Office.
1978 *Research Involving Those Institutionalized as Mentally Infirm: Report and Recommendations*. Washington, DC: U.S. Government Printing Office.
1979 *The Belmont Report: Ethical Principles and Guidelines for the Protection of Human Subjects of Research*. Washington, DC: U.S. Government Printing Office.

National Human Research Protections Advisory Committee
2001 Children's Workgroup Report Draft. Available: *http://ohrp.osophs.dhhs.gov* [Accessed December 5, 2001].

Office of Protection from Research Risks
1993 *Protecting Human Research Subjects: Institutional Review Board Guidebook*. Washington, DC: U.S. Government Printing Office.

O'Sullivan, C., and C. Fisher
1997 The effect of confidentiality and reporting procedures on parent-child agreement to participate in adolescent risk research. *Applied Developmental Science* 1:185–197.

Pritchard, I.
2000 Searching for research involving human subjects. *IRB: A Review of Human Subjects Research* 22(January-February):4–7.

Ratzan, R.
  1985   Technical aspects of obtaining informed consent from persons with senile demen-
          tia of the Alzheimer type. In *Alzheimer's Dementia: Dilemmas in Clinical Re-
          search*, V. Melnick and N. Dubler, eds. Clifton, NJ: Humana Press.
Runyan, D.
  1999   Maltreatment in families: A research dilemma. In *Beyond Regulations*, N. King,
          G. Henderson, and J. Stein, eds. Chapel Hill: University of North Carolina
          Press.
  2000   The ethical, legal, and methodological implications of directly asking children
          about abuse. *Journal of Interpersonal Violence* 15:675–681.
Sachs, G., and C. Cassel
  1990   Biomedical research involving older human subjects. *Law, Medicine & Health
          Care* 18:234–243.
Sachs, G., J. Rhymes, and C. Cassel
  1993   Biomedical and behavioral research in nursing homes: Guidelines for ethical
          investigations. *Journal of the American Geriatrics Society* 41:771–777.
U.S. Department of Health and Human Services
  1981   Final Regulations Amending Basic HHS Policy for the Protection of Human Sub-
          jects. *Federal Register* 46:8366–8391.
  1991   Federal Policy for the Protection of Human Subjects (Common Rule). *Federal
          Register* 56:28,012–28,018.
  1999   Additional Protections for Children Involved as Subjects in Research, *Code of
          Federal Regulations* 45:§ 46.408(c).
U.S. Food and Drug Administration
  1999   Protection of Human Subjects. *Code of Federal Regulations* 21: Parts 50 and 56.
Wendler, D., and K. Prasad
  2001   Core safeguards for clinical research with adults who are unable to consent.
          Annals of Internal Medicine 135:514–523.
World Medical Association
  2000   Declaration of Helsinki: Ethical principles for medical research involving human
          subjects. *Journal of the American Medical Association* 284:3043–3045.

12

The Clinical and Medical Forensics of Elder Abuse and Neglect

Carmel Bitondo Dyer, Marie-Therese Connolly, and Patricia McFeeley*

The medical forensic aspects of elder abuse and neglect are largely unexplored and undocumented. Those who work in the field of elder abuse and neglect believe that the state of medical knowledge and forensic science regarding elder abuse and neglect is approximately equivalent to that of child abuse and neglect three decades ago and domestic violence 10 to 15 years ago (Elder Justice Roundtable Report, 2000). Within the relevant victimized populations there are similarities and differences among the factors contributing to their vulnerability and victimization. Similarities include feared retaliation, perceived stigmatization at having been victimized, desire not to leave home, desire to protect the

*Carmel Bitondo Dyer, M.D., is an assistant professor of medicine at Baylor College of Medicine, Houston, Texas, and the Director of the Harris County Hospital District Geriatrics Program; Marie-Therese Connolly, J.D., is a senior trial counsel in the Civil Division, Department of Justice; Patricia McFeeley, M.D., is an associate professor in the Office of the Medical Investigator at the University of New Mexico.

The views expressed in Marie-Therese Connolly's contributions to this paper are her own and do not necessarily reflect those of the Department of Justice.

The authors would like to acknowledge Samuel Riley and Rosa Torres for their technical assistance, and Jill Callahan for her editorial assistance. They are also grateful for review of the manuscript by Drs. Kenneth L. Minaker and Constantine G. Lyketsos and members of the National Academy of Sciences Panel on Risk and Prevalence of Elder Abuse and Neglect.

wrongdoer, other emotional harm, and as in some cases involving persons with diminished capacity, difficulties in communicating what transpired.

Perhaps the starkest difference is that whereas children and younger victims of domestic violence are generally healthy and not expected to die, older people often have numerous underlying medical problems, and functional dependencies and are assumed to be more vulnerable to stressors causing death. Thus, when a younger person dies of unexplained causes, the cause of death is almost always carefully analyzed. The death of an older person, however, is rarely as carefully scrutinized, if at all, regardless of risk factors or indications of possible abuse or neglect. In addition, old age often brings medical conditions and physiological attributes that may mimic or mask the markers of elder abuse and neglect, further complicating the analysis and detection.

Despite these many complexities, a recent study—one of the few in the area—most clearly underscores the importance of increasing our understanding of these phenomena. That study (Lachs et al., 1998) demonstrates that elder abuse and neglect significantly shorten older victims' lives, even controlling for all other factors. Incidents of mistreatment that many would perceive as minor can have a debilitating impact on the older victim. A single episode of victimization can "tip over" an otherwise productive, self-sufficient older person's life. In other words, because older victims usually have fewer support systems and reserves—physical, psychological, and economic—the impact of abuse and neglect is magnified, and a single incident of mistreatment is more likely to trigger a downward spiral leading to loss of independence, serious complicating illness, and even death.

Unfortunately, there is a paucity of primary data relating to forensic markers of elder abuse and neglect, or even regarding the phenomena themselves. The ensuing discussion describes several potential forensic markers of elder abuse and neglect, including: abrasions, lacerations, bruising, fractures, restraints, decubiti, weight loss, dehydration, medication use, burns, cognitive and mental health problems, hygiene, and sexual abuse. We also are including financial fraud and exploitation because they often coexist with physical and emotional abuse and neglect. Some of the markers discussed are actual observations (such as bruises or fractures), whereas others are descriptions or conclusions based on underlying observations (for example, sexual abuse is a conclusion that might result from the observation of a vaginal tear or abdominal bruise, and a conclusion of neglect might result from the observation of poor hygiene and burns). Some of the markers are also potential risk factors (for example, self-neglect, cognitive and mental health problems, and financial abuse). But the current evidence regarding risk factors does not tell us the amount of risk conferred or by what mechanism.

Where evidence-based data or other studies were found relating to the forensic markers discussed in this paper, they are referenced. But the majority of information on this topic currently is derived from working hypotheses based on the experience of clinicians and pathologists. Discussion of each factor includes (a) a definition of the phenomenon, (b) a discussion of how it is affected by age-related changes, and (c) what we currently know of clinical and forensic markers indicating abuse and neglect.

The term forensic is defined as pertaining to the law or employed in legal proceedings. Thus, medical forensic markers of elder abuse and neglect are factors that are relevant to medical and legal determinations of whether elder abuse or neglect has occurred. Consistent evidence-based medical definitions are urgently needed to assist health care and social service professionals in detecting, treating, responding to, referring, and better understanding this grave and increasingly important public health problem. Coherent legal definitions are needed for legal and public safety professionals to determine when the law may have been broken, what types of criminal, civil, or administrative cases may be pursued, and for lawmakers to determine what new laws should be proposed or enacted. Defining appropriate forensic markers will lead to more effective prevention strategies and medical, legal, social service, and public safety interventions.

Expanding our medical forensic knowledge base is vital to all the myriad ways in which the law is expected to address elder abuse and neglect. Potential legal interventions include the following: federal, state, and local law enforcement entities (including prosecutors, investigators, and police) may pursue criminal and civil cases relating to allegations of elder abuse and neglect. The government generally pursues such cases in its *police power* capacity—to punish, deter, remediate, and/or redress wrongdoing. Government also may use the law in its *parens patrie* capacity—pursuing guardian and commitment cases, primarily intended to protect those who cannot care for themselves. Almost all cases brought by government entities in this field rely on medical forensic evidence. Some government entities (such as the Departments of Justice and Health and Human Services) have resources to fund projects relevant to medical forensic issues. Private plaintiffs may file civil suits against health care providers depending on available medical forensic evidence. Federal and state legislative bodies can enact laws that provide for funding, create new entities, establish civil and criminal causes of action, and provide for other measures to address the problem. Federal and state regulatory bodies determine and/or enforce reimbursement, licensure, and administrative enforcement rules. Each legal aspect of this issue would benefit from being informed by more and better research.

Elder abuse and neglect are often not detected or diagnosed, precluding any intervention, including prosecution. Thus research aimed at improving detection is crucial to law enforcement. Furthermore, even when there is detection or diagnosis, cases will not be prosecuted unless the suspected abuse or neglect is reported (which often is not the case even where there are mandatory reporting laws). Criminal and civil elder abuse and neglect prosecutions are pursued for many reasons, including to stop, redress, punish, and deter the wrongdoing, and to recoup government monies provided for care that was not rendered. However, the current state of legal, social science, and medical knowledge does not include an evaluation of which types of prosecution and which remedies and punishments best address these goals. By providing the tools necessary to detect and prove these cases, research on the forensic markers of elder abuse and neglect can help law enforcement make appropriate cases a priority.

DETECTING ABUSE AND NEGLECT IN ELDERS

The American Medical Association (1996) has defined *physical abuse* as an act of violence that may result in pain, injury, impairment, or disease. *Neglect* is the failure to provide the goods or services necessary for functioning or to avoid harm. A *caregiver* may be a family member, a friend, or an employee of the elder or of a nursing or other type of facility, or it may be the entity responsible for providing care. Definitions and intent standards may vary depending on discipline, entity, location, or jurisdiction, as well as the relationship of the victim and the perpetrator. Furthermore, intent in a legal proceeding is the province of the fact finder (judge or jury) and therefore opened to argument by both the plaintiff/prosecutor and the defendant. Thus, the above-provided descriptions are intended as a general guide and a way to frame the discussion, but not as specific legal definitions.

Actual abuse or neglect is rarely directly observed by medical, legal, or protective service professionals. In the absence of eyewitness testimony, law enforcement must rely on other circumstantial evidence to prove the existence of abuse or neglect. In most instances the experience of other direct observers is sought or the circumstances are deduced through investigation or physical examination. The state of current knowledge, however, does not always allow health care and social science professionals to link physical signs with a diagnosis of abuse or neglect. Further research will help identify and define useful forensic markers to help practitioners detect and treat elder abuse and neglect victims.

How, when, why, and by whom injuries have been inflicted on elderly victims are all important questions to be answered before actors in the legal system take any affirmative action to protect the victim and deter future wrongdoing. Thus, a fractured bone may heal and a bruise may resolve regardless of whether a practitioner can identify the cause. And yet, the cause of the break or the bruise is the starting point for any legal action. Thus, even where there are clear bad outcomes (harm to an older person), absent a causal link and evidence to support a hypothesis of illegal abuse or neglect, the law will provide no remedy or accountability.

The most extreme cases of abuse and neglect are not diagnostic dilemmas. In some cases—gunshot wounds, knife wounds, or rope burns, for instance—it is clear that the older person has been abused. In other cases multiple large decubiti or starvation may indicate severe neglect. Bite marks, too, are established evidence of abuse (Rawson et al., 1984; American Board of Forensic Odontology, 1986). But most cases fall into a gray area where abuse and neglect are not so nearly clear-cut, often because of subtle physiologic and psychological changes that occur in old age.

No gold standard test for abuse or neglect exists, and those working with abused or neglected elderly victims rely on forensic markers. The difficulty with this approach is that there is often a great overlap among the markers of disease and neglect (and sometimes abuse). Although abuse often is considered to require an overt act, whereas neglect is considered to require an omission, it sometimes is difficult to distinguish between the two. There are cases in which neglect is so profound and widespread, and the caretaker is knowledgeable of what was needed but not provided, that many would consider it abuse. For example, if a case includes apparently preventable decubiti, neglect may be indicated. The line between abuse and neglect becomes murkier, however, when a person presents with multiple serious decubiti, and the caregiver was aware of the decubiti and of what care was needed but still failed to render adequate care. The ambiguity between abuse and neglect is similarly demonstrated in scenarios where caregivers, particularly those who know better, either withhold necessary medication or fail to perform needed care (for example, fail to change a bandage and cause the loss of part of a limb and/or sepsis, or cause illness and death by not giving needed insulin).

The absence of clear and consistent legal definitions of neglect limit our ability to address the phenomenon. Liability for neglect is dependent on the ability to assign blame, and blame is easier to assign with acts of commission than acts of omission (Phillips, 1988). Definitional (and legal) distinctions also are necessary in determining when self-neglect evolves into caregiver neglect. This is a combined medical-legal inquiry: Is the person physically or mentally incapacitated? At what point does the legal responsibility for the care of that person shift from self to another? What are the legal responsibilities of a caregiver under law such that failure to render such care in a home or community setting subjects the caregiver to civil or criminal liability? What types of documentation must exist to justify a failure by caregivers to intervene in the face of self-neglect (e.g., refusal to eat) in an institutional setting? The answers to these questions, to the extent that such answers exist, vary from state to state, and sometimes from community to community, complicating the analysis and any research of the issue.

Resolution of these difficult distinctions is beyond the scope of this paper. It is worth noting, however, that whether elder abuse and neglect has occurred is a conclusion drawn from a constellation of factors—some are medical (the individual's medical condition), and some are legal (the jurisdiction's definition of caregiver neglect). Developing consistent definitions and laws relating to elder abuse and neglect is critical to (a) developing useful forensic markers, (b) effective detection and diagnosis by health care professionals, (c) law enforcement's determination of a violation of law and of what cases to prosecute, and (d) researchers' and policy makers' determination of the scope of the problem and of what new laws (including causes of action and remedies) and other measures are needed to adequately address it.

To the extent that the term forensic is defined as "pertaining to the law," medical forensic markers also are relevant to guardianship, involuntary commitment, power of attorney, and other types of *parens patrie* cases. Because this panel is examining abuse and neglect, however, those applications of forensic markers are not specifically discussed in this paper.

Abuse and neglect may occur in community or institutional/residential settings. For most of the markers described, there is no literature describing the relevance of various settings to the medical forensic analysis. This, too, is a topic in need of study.

POTENTIAL MARKERS OF ABUSE AND NEGLECT

Fourteen potential markers of elder abuse and neglect are discussed below, including for each a brief definition, a description of age-related changes, and a review of what is known about each as a medical forensic marker of elder abuse and neglect. Most of the forensic markers discussed in this section apply both to living persons and to postmortem evaluations. Factors pertaining peculiarly in the postmortem context are discussed in the next section.

Abrasions and Lacerations

Abrasions are superficial injuries involving the outer layer of skin; lacerations are characterized by full-thickness splitting of the skin. Abrasions are caused by movement of the skin over a rough surface; lacerations are the result of blunt force (Crane, 2000). Skin tears are a very common type of laceration seen in the elderly and are defined as a splitting of the epidermis (superficial layer of the skin) from the underlying connective tissue resulting in a flap of skin (Malone et al., 1991).

Age-Related Changes

Skin thickness and elasticity decrease with age. Tensile strength also declines, increasing the susceptibility to shearing-force trauma (Griffiths, 1998). Abrasions can occur in older persons with minor trauma. Common lacerations in elderly persons are the skin tears that occur most frequently on the forearms and occasionally on the legs. Persons usually have no more than one or two skin tears at a time, and skin tears often heal completely without scarring.

A primary data study revealed that the annual incidence of skin tears in a large nursing home was a little less than one per year per resident. The majority of tears were approximately 0.75 inches in length, though nearly 6 percent were 1.6 inches or longer. Eighty-five percent of the lacerations occurred on the arms. A known cause was identified in less than half the cases (47 percent), and most known causes were attributed to falls or bumping into something; wheelchairs accounted for 30 percent of the injuries (Malone et al., 1991). In cases in which the cause was unknown (53 percent), the skin tears may have occurred accidentally and may not have been noticed or may have been forgotten by the elder, or they could have been due to rough handling or worse by staff members and others. This study included no analysis of the cases with known causes as compared to those with unknown causes.

Clinical and Forensic Markers Indicating Abuse or Neglect

Abrasions retain the pattern of the causative agent better than any other type of injury, and careful documentation by health care personnel is important for identification of the mode of injury. Skin tears in sites other than the arms and legs or multiple tears or abrasions should raise suspicion. Lacerations often heal with scarring (Knight, 1997), as opposed to skin tears, which heal without scarring. Abrasions or lacerations are most commonly seen in cases involving physical abuse, although they can occur in cases of caregiver neglect.

Bruises

A bruise is the result of blunt force with concomitant rupture of small blood vessels under the skin. Blood escapes to the surrounding tissues propelled by the muscular contractions of the heart. Bruises are most commonly seen in physical abuse but can be a result of caregiver neglect. Bruises can surface hours to days after an initial insult, depending on the depth of the wounds. Blood can track through fascial planes and result in bruises distant from the site of injury. The eyelids, neck, and scrotum are very susceptible to bruising.

Age-Related Changes

Bruises often occur more frequently and resolve much more slowly in older persons than in younger persons and can last for months instead of the usual one to two weeks (Knight, 1997; Crane, 2000). Langlois and Gresham (1991) prospectively studied bruising by collecting over 200 photographs of bruises occurring in persons over the age of 65. They concluded no bruises less than 18 hours old demonstrated yellow coloration (p < 0.001). The opposite was, however, not true; some bruises did not develop a yellow color until much later. This primary data study is included in the Appendix to Chapter 1.

Clinical and Forensic Markers Indicating Abuse or Neglect

The pattern of the bruise may suggest the cause of the injury. Bruises may retain the shape of knuckles or fingers. Parallel marks, called tramline bruising, indicate injury from a stick (Knight, 1997; Crane, 2000). The site of the injury may also indicate abuse. The most common locations for nonaccidental injury are the face and neck, the chest wall, the abdomen, and the buttocks (Crane, 2000). Intentional injury was determined in a retrospective review of random charts in New Zealand to be 13 times more likely to involve the head than other areas of the body. In this study internal injuries were two times as common in the assault victims (Fanslow et al., 1998). Bruising on the palms and soles may serve as forensic markers since the tissue at those sites is made of tough fibrous tissue and is not usually injured accidentally (Knight, 1997).

The color of the bruise is usually unhelpful for dating because two bruises in the same person may heal at different rates. Reddish blue, blue, or purplish bruises are more likely to be recent while bluish green, greenish yellow, and brown bruises are more likely to be in some stage of healing (Crane, 2000). Multiple bruises in various stages of healing may indicate physical abuse (Knight, 1997).

Bruises are common sequelae of falls, the most common cause of injury in older persons. Abusive or neglectful caregivers often attribute intentional bruises to a fall. Falls, however, cannot always be prevented and have multiple causes, such as poor vision and transient ischemic attacks. The causes of any given fall in an elder should be evaluated and the results of the fall, such as the type of bruising or fracture, may be forensic markers worthy of study and provide useful information about whether abuse or neglect was involved.

Fractures

Fractures are broken bones and include a frank severing of the bone or a compression of intact bone.

Age-Related Changes

The bones of older persons are thinner and less dense, making them more susceptible to fractures as the result of bone disease or injury. Poor nutrition, vitamin D deficiency, alcoholism, and age-related sex hormone deficiencies also contribute to an increased propensity to fractures (Francis, 1998). Other bone diseases such as osteoporosis and all its causes, such as chronic steroid use, osteomalacia, and Paget's disease, make the bones more brittle. Any type of cancer that invades bone weakens the osseous structure, making the patient more prone to fractures—these are called pathological fractures. The most common sites of fracture are the hip in those over the age of 75 and the distal wrist in persons younger than 75 (Francis, 1998). The wrist is a common site of fracture with falls in older individuals because many use their hands to help break the fall. Older women in particular are susceptible to vertebral fractures. Alcoholics are prone to multiple falls with resulting fractures of the arms, legs, and ribs.

Two types of bone fractures are known to occur spontaneously: vertebral fractures in osteoporotic older women, and hip fractures. There are two series that report cases of hip fracture in which abuse was suspected but subsequently attributed to medical causes (osteomalacia or soft bones, prolonged bed rest, Paget's disease) (Kane and Goodwin, 1991; Connolly et al., 1995). Prolonged bed rest, chronic limb paralysis, or non-weight-bearing status put elderly persons at increased risk for spontaneous fracture (Kane and Goodwin, 1991).

Clinical and Forensic Markers Indicating Abuse or Neglect

A sizable literature on the resolution of fractures in abused children exists, but there are little or no data on fracture resolution in elders. Elders' bones, however, heal at much slower rates, making the child abuse data on fracture resolution invalid for older adults. Also, 30 percent of community-dwelling older persons and 50 percent of nursing home patients fall; therefore, falls alone should not necessarily increase suspicion of abuse. Most persons who fall experience one to three falls per year. A person who falls once has joined a grouping prone to frequent falls. A detailed examination of the patient, records, and/or collateral history from caregivers is needed to determine if fractures in frail elders constitute physical abuse.

Dentists and oral surgeons often see physically abused patients with fractured, subluxed, or avulsed teeth or fractures of the zygomatic arch (the bony structures around the eyes) or the mandible and maxilla (jaw bones) (Fenton et al., 2000). Fanslow and colleagues (1998) showed in a retrospective chart review that fractures of the head, spine, and trunk are more likely to be assault injuries than limb fractures, sprains or strains, or musculoskeletal injuries in adults. A spiral fracture of a large bone with no history of gross injury is diagnostic of abuse, as are fractures with a rotational component (*Medical Tribune*, 1995). Fractures in nonalcoholics at sites other than the hip, wrist, or vertebrae should raise suspicions of abuse.

Restraints

Restraints are means of controlling the behavior of older persons, especially in hospitals and nursing facilities. There are two forms of restraints, mechanical and chemical. The following discussion refers to mechanical restrains, such as Posey vests, and wrist and ankle restraints made of leather, plastic, or cloth.

Standards of Care for Elders

The only acceptable reason for restraining an elder is to prevent significant harm (Knight, 1997). Appropriate restraints help stop the agitated patient from pulling out a tube that is a conduit for life-saving treatments such as an endotracheal intubation for mechanical ventilation, oxygen replacement, or intravenous fluids and medications.

Clinical and Forensic Markers Indicating Abuse or Neglect

Abuse or neglect occurs whenever a person is restrained in a noncritical situation and without a concomitant evaluation by a medical practitioner. If restraints are determined to be necessary, the restrained patient must be monitored closely and frequently. The restraints must not be so tight as to completely restrict movement. Proper bedding must be used to prevent decubiti (bedsores).

In many studies, physical restraint is very strongly associated with increased injury and death (Miles, 1996; Mohr and Mohr, 2000). Restraints, in fact, often do not control behavior and instead may result in a worsening of behavioral problems. Despite this evidence, many health professionals still believe that restraints will help prevent injury due to falling. Restraints can be a form of neglect when used in lieu of adequate caretaking because they render persons "easier" to care for. They can be a form of physical abuse, for example, when they leave scars or result in wrist wounds or decubiti.

Decubiti

The breakdown of skin integrity resulting in an ulcer is known as a decubitus, or bedsore. Decubiti are the result of circulatory failure due to pressure; shearing forces cause thrombosis of the microcirculation (clotting or blockage of blood in small blood vessels), resulting in tissue necrosis (Barton and Barton, 1981). Most decubiti occur over the sacrum; the hip and the heels are also common locations. Although decubiti may be divided into four stages, in general they are either deep or superficial.

Age-Related Changes and Standards of Care

Normal aging skin has relatively well-preserved blood flow. The elderly are more susceptible to decubiti because of disease states and not on the basis of age alone (Bennett and Bliss, 1998). Decubiti most often occur in medically ill or cognitively impaired individuals. Intrinsic causes such as acute illness, neurological disease, peripheral vascular disease, incontinence, and poor nutritional status place individuals at higher risk (Bennett and Bliss, 1998). Although poor nutrition is a risk factor, improving nutritional status doesn't always reverse or prevent the process (Henderson et al., 1992; Finucane et al., 1999). The healing may take weeks to months, depending on the underlying comorbidities and the extent of the decubiti. Risk factors for decubiti were found not to be predictive where appropriate care was provided; however, when the standard of care was not met, risk factors were found to be predictive (Berlowitz et al., 2001).

The standard of care for decubitus ulcers is to prevent them from occurring, particularly in high-risk patients. Prophylactic measures include turning patients regularly, range-of-motion exercises, appropriate nutritional supplementation, and bedding. New therapies available for treatment including hydrocolloid dressings and hydrogel preparations, are superior to wet-to-dry dressings and the use of povidone iodine in wounds (Patterson and Bennett, 1995).

Clinical and Forensic Markers Indicating Abuse or Neglect

There are divergent views regarding which decubiti are due to illness and which are due to neglect or even abuse. The failure to adhere to the standard of care could be due to medical, institutional, or caregiver neglect.

Deep decubiti in multiple sites also may indicate neglect (Schor et al., 1995). Failure to provide proper care to high-risk persons may indicate neglect; if a foul-smelling or necrotic ulcer is not brought to the attention of a physician and not appropriately cared for, neglect is almost always present. Preventable decubiti are usually considered to be due to caregiver neglect, although the number, severity, and lethal result may cause some to ascribe the findings to abuse.

Malnutrition

Malnutrition is defined as poor health status due to the decreased intake of necessary nutrients.

Age-Related Changes

Old age results in a decline of both smell and taste, which decreases appetite. Many patients with cancer lose weight regardless of efforts to maintain nutritional status. Poor health, including poor dentition, depression, dementia, and malabsorption syndromes, also may contribute to weight loss and undernutrition (Thomas, 1998). Numerous other disorders can lead to malnutrition, including strokes, Parkinson's disease, amyotrophic lateral sclerosis, and disorders of the esophagus.

Clinical and Forensic Markers Indicating Abuse or Neglect

Malnutrition often is a marker of caregiver neglect, especially in institutional settings. More than 40 percent loss of body weight can result in death (Knight, 1997). Inappropriate prescribing of such medications as anticholinergic drugs (nerve blocking drugs, which cause excessive dry mouth and confusion), psychotropic drugs, and other medications that impair mentation or appetite may constitute neglect. Caregivers may fail to maintain oral hygiene, which can lead to the loss of teeth and poor nutritional intake. Nursing home residents may decline to eat when institutions do not recognize cultural food preferences. However, the most frequent cause of malnutrition due to neglect in an institutional setting appears to be an inadequate number of staff to assist those who need help with eating (Harrington et al., 2000).

Similarly, such improper feeding techniques as forceful assistance or other inappropriate feeding may lead to choking, aspiration, pneumonia, or death. It may also lead to food revulsion, refusal to eat, and depression, catalyzing a downward spiral. Appropriate documentation is required where the explanation for malnutrition is refusal to eat. Malnutrition may be an important predisposing factor for other illness or death and may be due to mismanagement of persons living in nursing homes (Hood, 2000).

Dehydration

Dehydration, inadequate level of water in the body, is caused by decreased fluid intake or excessive water loss seen commonly in persons living in very warm climates or in athletes such as marathon runners.

Age-Related Changes

The elderly are much more prone to dehydration with minimal provocation than are younger people. Dehydration is a common reason for emergency department visits by older persons (Lowenstein et al., 1986). Older persons have decreased body water reserves and thirst drive; their thirst drive may remain depressed even after 12 to 24 hours of water deprivation. The central nervous system regulation of water is altered; although antidiuretic hormone (ADH) is secreted properly in response to volume depletion, the older kidney responds less well to changes in ADH and continues to excrete water in the face of dehydration (American Geriatrics Society Review Syllabus, 1998). Hydration status is particularly difficult to monitor in older persons who can experience very rapid changes in their fluid status without much in the way of symptomatology.

Clinical and Forensic Markers Indicating Abuse or Neglect

In general, in moderate climates, the loss of water results in death within 10 days (Knight, 1997), this time frame is likely to be much shorter in the case of older persons.

Although most commonly caused by a medical illness, dehydration and volume depletion can serve as forensic markers for abuse or neglect when withholding food and water or insufficient care is part of the history.

Confusion and somnolence are common signs of volume depletion or dehydration, but they are nonspecific indicators and occur in many other disease states in the elderly. Sometimes the mental changes attributable to dehydration are subtle, especially in very demented persons. Neglect may be present if inadequate fluids are offered or provided or if dehydration goes unrecognized for a long period of time by medical or nursing personnel. Neglect also may be present in cases in which caregivers, home or facility, fail to seek help when problems are apparent. Obvious changes in the weight or mental states of persons residing in nursing homes and other care facilities should be assessed carefully. Weight changes or changes in vital signs should be brought to the attention of a clinician or otherwise promptly evaluated. Where the explanation for dehydration in an institutional setting is a refusal of fluids, this should be historically and appropriately documented. As with malnutrition, inadequate staff support may lead to neglectful, inadequate hydration.

Medication Use

Proper medication use is among the most important strategies for maintaining good health and preventing adverse side effects in the older individual

Age-Related Changes

Older patients use three times the number of medications that younger patients use (Monane et al., 1997). They do not respond as predictably to most medications as younger patients, and they have an increased risk of adverse side effects. A number of physiologic changes complicate the prescribing of effective yet safe drug regimens in older persons. Older persons have decreased hepatic metabolism (clearance of drugs through the liver) and decreased plasma protein binding, which increase drug levels. Older persons have decreased gastrointestinal absorption, and their bodies, due to age-related changes in body water, fat, and lean muscle, distribute drugs differently (Zubenko and Sunderland, 2000). In general, there is more fat and less water, leading to longer time of action of fat-soluble drugs and higher abrupt drug concentrations for water-soluble medications.

Drug regimens in older people are complicated by the fact that often they include multiple medications, which may interact. In addition, approximately one-half to one-third of patients do not take their medications properly (Monane et al., 1997). Patient noncompliance occurs for a variety of reasons. Some elders may not understand the instructions given. Some take their neighbors' medication or overdose on alternative therapies. Others may not have the resources (funds, transportation) to obtain needed medication. The most common form of noncompliance is failure to take or to renew needed prescriptions.

Polypharmacy in the elderly, as described by Monane and colleagues (1997), is the use of any unnecessary medication regardless of the total number of pills consumed. Conversely, needed medications, such as cancer chemotherapy, are withheld from older people for fear of side effects. Standards of care for specific disease states, such as a three-drug regimen for persons with heart failure or a two-drug regimen for Alzheimer's disease, have been established.

Clinical and Forensic Markers Indicating Abuse or Neglect

Misuse of medication, for example, giving a patient too much or too little of an indicated drug, withholding a necessary medication altogether, or administering unnecessary or inappropriate medication, may constitute either neglect or abuse, depending on whether the misuse or withholding was intentional or an excusable error.

The forensic markers for abuse or neglect as the result of misuse or withholding of medication may present in many different ways. In general, older persons should receive medications in doses smaller than those received by younger patients; and thus, in general, a prescription for an older person of a standard dose of medication may be an indicator of abuse. The signs and symptoms of medication side effects should be monitored, and the failure to do so may constitute neglect. Nongeriatricians may not be as attuned as geriatricians or geriatric nurse practitioners to the signs of drug overdose in elders because they often use the same drug dosages with impunity in younger adults. Increasing credentialing for medical practitioners requires proof of age-reliant continuing education and certification during the licensing procedures. Failure to obtain appropriate training for the population one is caring for is a potential cause of professional neglect.

The reasons for adverse side effects are complex and varied. They may be due to improper dosing, noncompliance, drug-drug interactions, the different presentation of disease states in the elderly (especially demented patients), or the particular constellation of disorders in a given patient. Failure to follow the standards of care indicates abuse or neglect. The determination of neglect due to medication misuse is best made by a practitioner other than the prescribing doctor.

Elders may misuse prescription drugs because they lack the capacity to handle this task or they reject efforts by medical professionals to help them. Abusive or neglectful caregivers may withhold necessary drugs, use the elders' drugs themselves, or overdose patients to keep them quiet and manageable. Insufficient staffing in facilities may result in increased medication errors and insufficient time to administer medication properly or at all. Depletion of institutional resources may result in failure to keep reliable and unexpired stores of necessary medications on the premises, including, for example, insulin for insulin-dependent diabetics.

Burns

A burn results from tissue injury following exposure to heat above 50° C (Knight, 1997). Burns are categorized by the body surface affected and the depth of tissue destruction.

Age-Related Changes

Data from the National Fire Protection Association show that persons over the age of 65 have twice the national average death rate due to burns. This risk triples at age 75 and quadruples at age 85. At the U.S. Army Institute of Surgical Research, at the renowned burn unit of Fort Sam Houston in Texas, persons over the age of 60 represent 8 percent to 12 percent of all admissions (Bird et al., 1998). In addition, although burn survival has improved for most age groups, there have been relatively few gains in burn survival for elderly persons in the past decade.

Clinical and Forensic Markers Indicating Abuse or Neglect

The association of burns and child abuse or neglect is well documented (Bowden et al., 1988; Andronicus et al., 1998; Evasovich et al., 1998; Hultman et al., 1998). Burns in older people also may result from abuse or neglect. Bowden and colleagues (1988), from the University of Michigan Burn Center, examined the relationship of adult abuse and neglect to burns. Seventy percent of the cases were deemed due to neglect and abuse. In a later study, Bird and colleagues (1998), at the Fort Sam Houston Burn Unit, found that 40 percent of burn cases occurring in persons over 60 were due to abuse or neglect, with 36 percent of the cases due to neglect. (See Appendix to Chapter 1).

These two studies were conducted retrospectively with relatively small numbers of patients. Nonetheless, their data are intriguing and suggest that burns in elders might be a forensic marker for self-neglect and caregiver neglect as well as abuse. White (2000), in a paper about forensic nurses, also recommends that burns be considered a marker for elder neglect.

Cognitive and Mental Health Problems

Cognitive and mental health disorders are some of the most pervasive and clinically challenging problems of old age. The Texas Elder Abuse and Mistreatment (TEAM) Institute has treated over 300 abused or neglected elders; the most common cognitive and mental disorders noted are depression, dementia, psychosis, and alcohol abuse (Dyer and Goins, 2000). Preliminary data from an ongoing cross-sectional research study of neglect clients not referred to a medical team revealed similar results (Dyer et al., unpublished data).

Dementia is a progressive impairment of memory and other areas of cognition which results in an eventually reduced ability to care for oneself. Patients suffering from dementia frequently experience anxiety and depression early in the disease and delusions and hallucinations in the later stages.

Depression is characterized by sadness, decreased appetite, insomnia, and loss of interest in hobbies. Psychosis is an altered mental state characterized by delusions and hallucinations. Alcohol abuse exists if the intake of alcohol impairs social functioning. Substances other than alcohol may be abused, but in elderly populations, alcohol abuse is most common.

Self-neglect often accompanies dementia and mental health problems in older people. It is an important issue that requires additional research, but it is not addressed in this paper except to the extent that it constitutes a risk factor for or sign of elder abuse and neglect inflicted by others—in effect, a forensic marker. Self-neglect may be a risk factor in that it makes victims more vulnerable to and less able to ward off mistreatment by others who might prey on them. Similarly, as capacity for self-care decreases, dependence on others increases, and if potential caregivers are either unable or unwilling to provide assistance, then the risk for being abused and neglected by caregivers increases. Conversely, someone who has been victimized by abuse or neglect may become depressed and in turn lose the desire or capacity for self-care. Thus, self-neglect also may be a forensic marker that abuse or neglect has been committed by another person.

Age-Related Changes

Dementia. Dementia is present in 15 percent of persons over the age of 65 and 50 percent of persons over the age of 80 (Abrams et al., 1995a). Dementia is by definition a loss of function that often results in increased reliance on others for care. Many with the dementia syndrome refuse needed care, and/or their children are uneasy with becoming caregivers.

Depression. Depression affects from 15 to 50 percent of older persons. Institutionalized elders and those with medical illness have the highest incidences of depression, which can be as high as 70 percent following a stroke. Elderly persons with depression are more prone to psychosis than are younger persons with depression (Abrams et al., 1995b).

Psychosis. Four to five percent of older adults experience psychosis (Abrams et al., 1995b). It is most commonly associated with depression, but elders can experience acute and chronic episodes of paranoid ideation (formation of paranoid ideas).

Alcohol Abuse. Alcohol abuse is present in up to 5 percent of older persons and is more common in men than in women. Older adults can become inebriated at lower levels of alcohol intake than younger adults and are more susceptible to its ill effects, including malnutrition, gastritis, and alcohol dementia (Abrams et al., 1995c).

Clinical and Forensic Markers Indicating Abuse or Neglect

Cognitive and mental health disorders affect a large number of aging persons and can lead to impairment of thinking, memory, functional ability, and ultimately decision-making capacity. They can prevent persons from seeking help, advocating on their own behalf, or extricating themselves from abusive situations, and they make elders more prone to exploitation by others. Dementia itself and its management can be a stimulus for abusive action when the family feels or is unprepared or unsupported in the care of an affected dependent. Ability to serve as a witness or provide testimony is diminished. Ultimately, the mental states of demented elders can progress to a point at which they are unable to meet even their most basic needs.

Most statistics on this topic are derived from adult protective services (APS) databases. The definition of mental disorders varies from state to state, as do the training requirements of APS workers, many of whom are not health care professionals. Some elders with impairments have otherwise well-developed social skills and, without formal testing, can escape notice by physicians and other professionals who care for them. The National Elder Abuse Incidence Study asked nonmedical volunteers to comment on depression and dementia based on their opinions. They found 59.5 percent incidence of dementia and 43.6 percent incidence of depression. Because the reporters were not health professionals nor did they have any mental health training, the data are estimates and not representative of actual diagnoses (National Center on Elder Abuse, 1998).

Self-neglect usually but not always is associated with either dementia or some type of mental health problem. Individually, and particularly in combination, these conditions may constitute risk factors for, as well as signs of, abuse and neglect. In a preliminary analysis by the Texas Department of Protective and Regulatory Services, self-neglect and medical neglect (failure to obtain or have obtained appropriate medical care) cases were more likely to be associated with other types of elder mistreatment than were cases of physical or sexual abuse (Dyer et al., 2000a). Self-neglect may very well represent a part of the continuum where older persons who are initially declining either functionally, mentally, or both try to care for themselves. If they can no longer meet their needs themselves, then they need help from others. Progressive functional decline may result in physical decline and in some instances institutionalization.

Dementia. Dementia is related to elder abuse and neglect (Benton and Marshall, 1991; Aravanis et al., 1993; Coyne et al., 1993; Lachs and Pillemer, 1995). Two primary data studies demonstrated that dementia was an independent risk factor for abuse and neglect (Lachs et al., 1998; Dyer et al., 2000a). In the study by Dyer and colleagues (2000a), dementia was noted in 51 percent of neglected or abused patients and only 30 percent of patients referred to geriatric clinic for other reasons.

Depression. Depression is a significant finding in abused or neglected patients (Benton and Marshall, 1991; Aravanis et al., 1993; Lachs and Pillemer, 1995; Dyer et al., 2000a). Dyer and colleagues found an even greater prevalence of depression than dementia in patients referred for mistreatment: 62 percent of neglected or abused patients had depression compared with 12 percent of patients referred for other reasons. Lachs and coworkers found the same clinical phenomenon using data from Connecticut (personal communication, 2001).

Psychosis. Persons with psychotic disorders are likely to neglect themselves and to be unable to care for themselves as a result of their delusions and hallucinations (Lachs and Pillemer, 1995; Dyer and Goins, 2000).

Alcohol Abuse. Alcohol abuse can lead to a failure to fulfill major role obligations, to alcohol use in situations that are physically hazardous, and to social or interpersonal problems (American Psychiatric Association, 1994). This pattern of behaviors puts persons at risk of perpetrating or being the victim of abuse and neglect, especially neglect (Goodyear-Smith, 1989; Fanslow et al., 1998; Marshall et al., 2000). Abuse of substances other than alcohol may have similar consequences.

Hygiene

Medical practitioners consider hygiene, defined as the ability to maintain cleanliness, an important component of good health and disease prevention.

Age-Related Changes

There are no changes in one's hygiene that occur strictly with age. Occasionally, impaired eyesight may make it more difficult to keep one's home or clothes clean; however, if cognitive ability remains normal, elders are able to perform the activities of daily living and maintain appropriate hygiene. Demented or psychotic individuals, on the other hand, often lack the ability to care for themselves, and depressed individuals may become less inclined to care for themselves and display poor personal hygiene.

Clinical and Forensic Markers Indicating Abuse or Neglect

Many have suggested that a decline in hygiene is a marker of neglect (Aravanis et al., 1993; Lachs and Pillemer, 1995; Butler, 1999; Marshall et al., 2000). Individuals may present with dirty clothes that reek of animal excrement; multiple insect bites due to mosquitoes, scabies, or fleas; or other signs of poor hygiene. For some persons, poor personal care is a matter of lifestyle or choice, and should not be blamed on age. Thus, this finding requires investigation of previous habits and any recent decline as well as screening for dementing or psychotic illness.

Sexual Abuse

Sexual abuse is characterized by sexual contact or exposure without the person's consent, including those cases in which persons are not able to consent (American Medical Association, 1996). Mickish (1993) categorized sexual abuse as the least perceived, acknowledged, detected, and reported type of elder abuse. Although the least frequently reported type of elder mistreatment (Tatara, 1993; Pavlik et al., 2001), it is nonetheless heinous. Several studies have demonstrated that the overwhelming majority of victims have cognitive impairment (75 percent to 77 percent) and/or have functional limitations (67 percent to 92 percent) (Ramsey-Klawsnik, 1991; Holt, 1993; Teaster et al., 2000). In the study by Teaster and colleagues (2000), which includes APS reports from 1996 to 1999, the most common form of sexual abuse was sexualized kissing and fondling but ranged from unwelcome sexual interest to rape.

Age-Related Changes

Women experience a number of physiologic changes in the genital tract as they age. Both progesterone and estrogen levels decline with aging (American Geriatrics Society Review Syllabus, 1998). Decreased estrogen levels result in changes in the shape of the vagina, increased vaginal dryness, and thinning of the vaginal walls. These changes may cause pain and bleeding during sexual intercourse. Such age-related changes as altered acidity of the vaginal secretions and decreased estrogen levels make older women more prone to spontaneous vaginal and bladder infections (Butler and Lewis, 1998). Note, however, that there is never a situation in which sexual abuse is considered normal, regardless of the age or functional status of the individual.

Clinical and Forensic Markers Indicating Abuse or Neglect

Victims of sexual abuse may present oral venereal lesions. Bruising of the uvula (Marshall et al., 2000) and bruising of the palate and the junction of the hard palate may indicate forced oral copulation (Fenton et al., 2000). Bleeding and bruising of the anogenital area as well as difficulty in sitting and walking may indicate sexual abuse in elderly women (Fulmer et al., 1984).

A retrospective descriptive study of reported cases of sexual assault from New Zealand looked at women and children, including some elderly women ranging in age from 60 to 83 years. One-third of women were assaulted in their homes, and one-third were intoxicated at the time of the assault. Fifty percent were restrained, and 75 percent had evidence of trauma. The most common site of bruising, inflammation, tenderness, abrasions, or trauma was the anogenital area (41 percent of cases). The remainder of the cases involved other parts of the body, with no particular site injured more frequently than another (Goodyear-Smith, 1989). Other types of bruising, for example, on the abdomen, might be suggestive of sexual abuse (Burgess, 2000). New diagnoses of sexually transmitted disease in nursing home residents or other elders may indicate abuse. Urinary tract infections in nursing home residents may indicate sexual abuse if several cases occur in a cluster. Behavioral signs indicating potential sexual abuse may include withdrawal, fear, depression, anger, insomnia, increased interest in sexual matters, or increased sexual or aggressive behavior.

Financial Fraud and Exploitation

Financial exploitation is the inappropriate use of an elderly person's resources for personal gain (American Medical Association, 1996). Financial fraud and abuse make up 12.3 percent of reports to protective service agencies (National Center on Elder Abuse, 1996).

Age-Related Changes

There is never a situation in which financial exploitation is considered normal, regardless of the age or functional status of the individual.

Clinical and Forensic Markers Indicating Abuse or Neglect

Paveza and his colleagues (1997) have studied the types of financial exploitation and the associated variables. They have determined that risk factors vary with the type of financial abuse; however, in general the victims are often widows or widowers, often in the seventh or eighth decade of life, and living in the community.

Financial exploitation includes credit card and telemarketing fraud, predatory lending, and theft or extortion. Such activities are usually targeted at vulnerable older adults and may leave them unable to pay for medications, health care, food, and the other necessities of life. Evidence of signing over of deeds or changes in wills should raise suspicion of exploitation as should the transfer of personal belongings or material goods without consent (Fulmer and Birkenhauer, 1992). The level of suspicion for this type of abuse should be increased for persons with cognitive impairment, which predisposes the victim to be trusting of caregivers, relatives, and acquaintances (Tueth, 2000). It is believed that many cases of financial exploitation go unrecognized and occur in conjunction with other types of abuse and neglect.

SPECIAL CONSIDERATIONS IN THE POSTMORTEM ANALYSIS

The mandate of the medical examiner or coroner is to determine the cause and manner of death. Determining the cause and manner of death involves not only a physical examination and/or autopsy in many cases but also extensive investigation, review of medical records, toxicology testing, and such special studies as radiology, cultures, or serology.

Postmortem Evaluation

Many of the same potential markers for elder abuse and neglect set forth above in the context of evaluation of living persons also apply in a postmortem evaluation but are limited by inability to interview the patient and evaluate such things as mental status and capacity. External examination should include an objective evaluation of the state of nutrition, including evaluation of markers for hydration, utilization of vitreous electrolytes to confirm visual evaluation, and documentation of cleanliness. A body with crusted fecal material and secretions or dirt in creases, which is clad in very clean or new-appearing clothing should suggest an attempt to disguise poor hygiene and living conditions. Documentation of decubiti, if present, should include measurements of size, depth, and location. Documentation of bruising, skin lacerations, and fractures should include a detailed description of the size, color, extent, and location of these injuries.

The lessons learned in the examination of child abuse may also apply here. Locations, extent, type, and multiplicity of injuries may suggest nonaccidental mechanisms or repetitive abuse. Explanations for multiple rib fractures such as, "She falls a lot," are not adequate and may be inaccurate. Explanations of how injuries occurred must be elicited and compared with the injuries observed. Tendency to multiple falls should be verified (or refuted) through medical records or objective observations if possible. Although abrasions and skin tears are common in the elderly, large skin tears or excessive scarring from more serious lacerations without an adequate explanation is suggestive of inflicted injuries or rough handling by caretakers.

Bruising also occurs frequently and may resolve more slowly in older than in younger persons. Color changes may occur slowly and may persist for weeks or longer. Loose, thin skin not only may bruise readily, but bruises can also spread through fascial planes to more distant areas, especially in such locations as the eyelids, neck, and scrotum. Medical conditions and medications (such as the blood thinners Coumadin and heparin) may greatly expand the extent of the bruise site. Patterned bruising or abrasions, when present, may be useful in determining the object(s) causing the injury. For example, a line of circular bruises on the inner aspects of the upper arms, especially if present bilaterally, may represent finger marks from forcibly lifting or pulling a person by the upper arms, such as moving a person onto or from a bed or a stretcher. Other patterns, such as the parallel lines caused by impact by a rounded or cylindrical object or an unusual pattern may be attributable to a specific object.

Internal examinations may obtain additional evidence relating to potential markers or findings of abuse and neglect. Internal organ examinations should include evaluation of the state of nutrition and hydration, and evidence of natural disease such as cardiovascular disease, chronic lung disease, infections, or malignancies. Stomach and bowel contents should be documented grossly and microscopically. Bones should be evaluated for osteoporosis and other changes, grossly, microscopically, and radiologically as indicated. The medical examiner or coroner should perform inspection of the external and internal genitalia to evaluate for sexual assault. Age-related and hormonal changes make the internal and external genitalia more susceptible to injury by penetration.

Child abuse protocols are by and large not applicable to adults; however, protocols for an adequate elder abuse examination could, like that for child abuse, include total-body x-rays. A complete neuropathology examination, preferably in conjunction with an experienced neuropathologist, is necessary to correlate clinical dementia or paralysis with documented gross and microscopic changes in the brain.

How Postmortem Forensic Markers May Differ from Those Applicable to Living Persons

Postmortem examination in many cases provides less information than would a complete physical examination in a living person. For example, a postmortem blood gas evaluation (measuring pH, oxygen, and carbon dioxide levels) provides scant if any information, whereas the same test in a living person may be quite valuable in determining the care needed and the extent of underlying disease. On the other hand, some postmortem examination procedures yield more information than physical examination and laboratory testing of a living patient. Antemortem computerized tomography and magnetic resonance imaging scans have significant limitations in detecting and evaluating such lesions as small central nervous system parenchymal or surface hemorrhages or pulmonary nodules. However, utilization of radiologic expertise to help document the number and location of fractures at autopsy can be quite valuable. Although these determinations in an elderly person with osteoporosis are complex, careful documentation of such findings along with estimates of age or time of occurrence are useful. As in evaluations of other types of domestic violence, maxillofacial (jaw and face) injuries should prompt suspicion of abuse, and estimates of age or time of occurrence are useful. As in evaluations of other types of domestic violence, maxillofacial injuries should prompt suspicion of abuse.

Injuries suggestive of defensive maneuvering, such as those on the back of the arms and hands, and injuries related to grasping, squeezing, or forcible restraint should also prompt suspicion (Brogdon, 1998). However, little is known and there are few studies, if any, that document the type and location of fractures relative to mechanism and degree of force required in the elderly. Such studies and published information would also be of great use to forensic pathologists testifying in court in criminal and civil cases.

Even if the cause of death may be obvious (for example, pneumonia), the manner of death (i.e. natural, accident, suicide, homicide, or undetermined) may vary depending on the contributions of other factors to the pneumonia. For example, if the pneumonia is secondary to rib fractures, the death could be accidental if the fractures were sustained in an accidental fall. However, if the rib fractures were numerous and serious enough that the patient should have received medical attention but no referrals or attempts to get treatment were made, the subsequent death could be considered the result of neglect and potentially considered a homicide. If the fractures were sustained in a beating, the manner would clearly be homicide.

Forensic Psychiatry

Some cases may necessitate a postmortem psychological or psychiatric evaluation. Although the performance of a psychological or psychiatric autopsy has been described in some instances of suspected suicides, the utilization of these somewhat specialized investigative tools has not been specifically described in investigation of elder deaths. The demonstrated associations of dementia, depression, and self-neglect to elder abuse and neglect, however, make such autopsies potentially critical tools. Whether used in their fully developed form by a forensic psychiatrist or incorporated into a series of extensive death investigation interviews by someone else, understanding the degree of cognitive impairment or decision-making capacity, even retrospectively, may be critical in investigating and classifying a death. The limitations would be that the most important informants might be those who were perpetuating the abuse or neglect, making them the least likely to give honest, objective responses. Similarly, indications of financial exploitation may provide valuable corroborating evidence during a death investigation.

OTHER FORENSICS CONSIDERATIONS

Three additional tools could be tremendously useful in developing and/ or identifying forensic markers of elder abuse and neglect: (1) consistent, validated screening tools, (2) forensic centers, and (3) multidisciplinary teams.

Screening Tools

There is general consensus that elder abuse and neglect are significantly underreported and underidentified, and that validated, uniform tools should be developed and tested to enhance detection. As set forth below, many different types of tools currently exist. But absent validation, uniform standards, and implementation, such tools will not gain general use, provide an accurate picture of the phenomena, or supply a useful base of data to be used in research.

It is essential to screen for elder mistreatment, particularly in older persons who are either unable, due to cognitive impairment, or unwilling, due to fear, to report it. Another confounder is that details about alleged abuse or neglect are derived through proxy interviews and in some circumstances the proxy might be the perpetrator. Jones and colleagues (1988) reported that 72 percent of elder abuse victims did not complain of the abuse at the time of presentation to an emergency center. The American Medical Association recommends screening of geriatric patients regardless of whether they complain of abuse, if physical signs are present (1996). The U.S. Department of Health and Human Services recommends that hospitals have protocols for screening patients for abuse or neglect. In a 1997 survey of emergency department physicians by Jones and colleagues, 31 percent worked in a department that had protocols, 33 percent worked in departments without protocols, and 36 percent were unsure. The Joint Commission on Accreditation of Health Care Organization's 1992 stan-

dards require screening protocols for elder abuse as well as domestic violence and child abuse (Aravanis et al., 1993). Others recommend that
screening for elder mistreatment be a part of the routine health assessment
for all older persons (Fulmer and Birkenhauer, 1992; Mouton and Espino,
1999).

A number of factors have limited the development of screening tools
for elder mistreatment. The low level of knowledge regarding the phenomena makes it difficult to develop a comprehensive and accurate tool. There
is no gold standard test for elder abuse or neglect. Legal definitions, clinical
experience, and standards relating to elder abuse and neglect vary from
state to state and even from entity to entity. As a result, many cases of elder
abuse and neglect go undetected and unreported, and some benign cases are
reported to involve abuse or neglect (Loue, 2001). Moreover, the process
of substantiating the validity and reliability of such tools is time-consuming, rigorous, and expensive (Wolf, 2000).

Current Screening Tools

Numerous types of screening tools relevant to elder abuse and neglect
exist, but most professionals collect information on the observations of
others and assess risk factors. The very proliferation of different types of
tools amidst the paucity of evidence-based data is evidence both of the
desire to improve detection and measurement and of the lack of uniformity
among the approaches to this issue. Some of the existing tools will be
briefly described. A few, with special relevance to forensic analysis, will be
described in greater detail.

Comprehensive Geriatric Assessment. Several authors have suggested that
the Comprehensive Geriatric Assessment (CGA) is an ideal tool for evaluation of abused or neglected individuals (Aravanis et al., 1993; Lachs and
Pillemer, 1995; Dyer and Goins, 2000). CGA, an integrated approach to
the screening of conditions in a variety of domains (Siu et al., 1994), requires obtaining a comprehensive history and physical examination, and
the use of validated instruments to quantify measures of psychosocial health
and functional ability. CGA has been shown to be an effective procedure in
at least eight randomized trials in Sweden and the United States (Alessi et
al., 1997). CGA can be performed efficiently in a variety of settings (hospital, outpatient clinic, nursing home, and private home). A multidisciplinary
team usually conducts the CGA because of the depth and breadth of the
evaluation. The team members always include geriatricians, geriatric nurse
practitioners, and gerontologic social workers and often include therapists,
pharmacists, chaplains, and a variety of other specialists.

AMA Assessment Protocol for Physicians. This assessment protocol does not incorporate any type of screening procedure.

APS Protocols. Eighteen state APS programs have screening protocols for use by APS specialists, but only four agencies performed any tests of validity or reliability on their tool (Wolf, 2000).

Risk Factor Checklists. Such checklists have been developed in a variety of settings (Canadian Task Force on Periodic Health Examination, 1994). These questionnaires are mostly based on descriptive studies and not on empirical data. They often do not assess for neglect or address the difference between disease and abuse.

The Mount Sinai/Victim Services Agency Elder Abuse Project Questionnaire. This tool (1998) developed in New York, is made up of nine closed-ended direct questions. It is short and easy to administer. Responses, however, rely on the subjective evaluation of the possible victim, who may not be forthcoming with or have the cognitive capacity to provide the personal information it requests. Positive responses should trigger further evaluation of potential abuse or neglect. This type of tool may be the best for quick screening in busy emergency centers or clinics.

Elder Assessment Instrument (EAI). This instrument first was developed in 1981 and now includes a checklist assessing five domains, a summary, a disposition, and a narrative if the examiner is so inclined (Fulmer and Wetle, 1986). The EAI has a content validity index of 0.83 (Fulmer et al., 1984) and a reliability index of 0.83 (Fulmer and Wetle, 1986). This instrument is comprehensive and precise and can be used for serial assessments. Fulmer and colleagues (2000) demonstrated that the sensitivity and specificity were 71 percent and 93 percent, respectively, when compared with a panel of experts. The EIA has been used successfully by emergency department nurses and appears to be ideal for research. The time required to complete the form's detailed inquiries make it less likely to be used by physicians in busy, acute medical settings (such as emergency departments) and more likely to be used in settings such as geriatric outpatient clinics.

Brief Abuse Screen for the Elderly (BASE). This tool contains five brief questions that take only a minute to complete (Reis and Nahmiash, 1998). It is coupled with training and designed to screen elders who are either caregivers or care receivers. Reis and Nahmiash (1998) report a 86 percent to 90 percent agreement by trained practitioners and a correlation between abusive and nonabusive caregivers. The BASE may be useful in busy clinical settings.

Indicators of Abuse Screen (IOA). This tool began as a 48-item checklist and has been reduced to a 29-item list (Reis and Nahmiash, 1998). It is a subjective measure that requires an experienced and trained administrator and two to three hours to complete. A multidisciplinary committee consensus panel reviewed the initial subsample. Cronbach alpha tests demonstrated an internal consistency of 0.92 and 0.91 on two separate samples (Reis and Nahmiash, 1998). According to Wolf (2000), the IOA identified 78 percent to 84 percent of senior abuse cases seen by a health and social service agency. It appears to have great potential as a research tool but is too lengthy to be used by most medical, social service, APS, or ombudsman personnel.

Hwalek-Sengstock Elder Abuse Screening Test (H-S/EAST). This test initially pooled and distilled over 1000 items into a 15-item tool to measure physical abuse, vulnerability, and potential abusive situations (Wolf, 2000). The tool was further trimmed to six items based on discriminant analysis (Neale et al., 1991). Based on an additional study (Scofield et al., 1999), the researchers suggested six questions suitable for a brief screening tool.

Special Issues Relating to Screening Tools

Several specific factors make development of appropriate tools to screen for markers of elder abuse and neglect simultaneously vital and very complex.

Dementia, Depression, Psychosis, and Substance Abuse. Several authors recommend screening for dementia, depression, psychosis, and substance abuse in older people to assess the risk of abuse and neglect. The TEAM Institute Battery includes the Mini-Mental State Examination, the Geriatric Depression Scale, the Clock Drawing Test, the Brief Psychiatric Rating Scale, and the CAGE questionnaire for their ease of administration during house calls and in busy clinics and for the interrater reliability (Dyer and Goins, 2000; Marshall et al., 2000). Failure to rule out reversible causes of these cognitive and mental health disorders also may indicate neglect.

Assessment of Decision-Making Capacity. The factors listed above, alone or in combination, may diminish the elder's capacity to participate fully in his or her own decision making. In addition, acute illness can reduce an older person's ability to make rational and informed decisions. Diminished decision-making capacity is a complex factor faced by law enforcement, adult protective service specialists, and medical personnel who deal with abused or neglected older persons, for example, when a patient with diminished capacity decides against hospital transport, resulting in inadequate medical care, worsening suffering, exacerbation of an illness or injury, or even death (Persse, unpublished data). In our society, patients have the legal right to be presumed competent, and evidence to the contrary must be presented before that right can be curtailed or removed. A competent individual has the right to be a fully informed participant in all aspects of decision making and, of course, has the right to refuse treatment. It is important to honor the choices of elders with capacity without abandoning those who lack capacity and whose expressed choices may lead to harm or even death. The determination of neglect versus poor choices hinges on an elder's capacity to participate in his or her own care, a situation on which statutes do not provide clear guidance (Loue, 2001). Aravanis and colleagues (1993) along with Benton and Marshall (1991) recommend capacity assessment for mistreated elders.

There are no easily administered standard tools that assess capacity. The gold standard is psychiatric interview, which is a process that takes hours and requires a specialist, rendering it impractical. A shorter, but still accurate and sufficiently sensitive, screening tool is needed to assist in assessing capacity and identifying those at highest risk.

Assessment Tools for Different Living Situations. Screening tools that presume normal or near-normal cognition are not useful in environments where many or most individuals do not have normal cognition. Screening tools designed for use in nursing homes and other care facilities (where the onus is less on family and friends and more on health professionals and institutional culture) have a different focus from screening tools for those cared for at home. Three care options exist: (a) provide care for oneself in one's home, (b) obtain care from a caregiver in the community, and (c) move to an institution or alternative setting such as a nursing home where basic daily needs can be met (Loue, 2001). Studies are needed to evaluate whether the assessment should differ based on whether the individual lives in a nursing home, at home, or in a community setting (assisted living home, group home, etc.).

Assessment of the environment is one of the key indicators for abuse by APS specialists (Toronjo et al., unpublished data). In a study of abused or neglected children, Watson-Perczel and colleagues (1988) found homes with large amounts of garbage, dirty clothes, spoiled food, and feces. They used the Checklist for Living Environments to Assess Neglect (CLEAN) home assessment tool to measure home conditions and to monitor subsequent clean-up efforts. Perhaps such an evaluation could be modified for cases of elder neglect.

Screening tools are not acid tests for mistreatment. As Fulmer and colleagues point out in a 1984 publication, without knowledge of the specific situation, judgment about abuse or neglect cannot always be rendered.

In any screening tool the context and the social situation of each individual case must be explored.

Postmortem Screening Tools. Injuries leading to morbidity or mortality in the older population should be investigated to determine whether the severity of the injury is compatible with the reported mechanism of injury. Screening tools that have been and are being developed for evaluating injuries in living populations are useful in some cases of suspected fatal abuse or neglect but are not always applicable in the postmortem evaluation. Developing and evaluating a standardized tool for performing a psychological autopsy, especially one directed toward determining the degree of dementia, cognitive impairment, and decision-making capacity before death, are worthwhile goals.

In sum, although many instruments and protocols exist, they are a disparate group, and do not, taken together, achieve the uniformity necessary to support an effective and coherent response from the medical, social service, public safety, and legal communities. These communities must work together to encourage and support research into, and development of, uniform, validated screening tools. (See recommendations below.)

Forensic Centers

Overview of Forensic Centers

Forensic centers have been developed to address and study numerous categories of illegal conduct usually associated with complex social problems as diverse as child abuse and neglect, sexual abuse, terrorism, food tampering, and computer crime. These centers are intended to bring together multidisciplinary groups of leading experts in their fields; to use state-of-the-art science, analytic tools, and techniques; to identify wrongdoing; to support law enforcement; to provide diagnostic resources; to conduct research and training; and to advance understanding in the specific field.

As such, forensic centers can be and have been a very useful tool in bringing a specialized multidisciplinary approach (and dedicated funding) to addressing, understanding, and redressing various vexing issues. The authors uncovered no forensic center in this country dedicated to elder abuse and neglect. As the discussion above demonstrates, elder victimization involves complex phenomena. A forensic center, where expertise, attention, and new funding could be focused, could advance understanding, treatment, and research as well as detection, intervention, and prosecution of elder abuse and neglect. It could also provide concentrated expertise, which others could use as a resource until more information is better distributed among the relevant practitioners.

Potential Models for Elder Abuse and Neglect Forensic Centers

National Forensic Center. A national forensic center would bring together leading experts in geriatrics, gerontology, forensic pathology, nursing, law enforcement, and other relevant fields. Time and funding would be dedicated to the diagnosis of and response to elder abuse and neglect, to research and training in its related fields, and to its prosecution. The center would conduct postmortem evaluations, consultations with living patients (using videoconferencing, if necessary), and interviews to answer questions relating to elder abuse or neglect. Medical records, samples, and other relevant data could be sent to the center for evaluation.

Regional Forensic Center. A regional center would be similar to the proposed national center, except it would be organized on a regional basis.

Local Forensic Center. The local forensic center model would be much more localized. It could consist of a mobile unit or team, including a physician, an APS specialist, and possibly a forensic or law enforcement specialist, that could be dispatched to the home or facility where the potential victim was located to do an on-site evaluation. Data could be collected and analyzed from several sites as part of a pilot project as well.

Multidisciplinary Teams

Multidisciplinary Screening Teams

While not an instrument per se, multidisciplinary team assessment and treatment has been suggested by many as the ideal approach to elder abuse and neglect (Fulmer, 1989; Dyer and Goins, 2000). Mount Sinai Hospital has had a multidisciplinary elder abuse team for over 10 years (Fulmer et al., 2000). Baylor College of Medicine's team has been in place for over 6 years. Other sites, including the University of California at Irvine and the Robert Wood Johnson Medical School of New Jersey, also have well-developed teams. Interdisciplinary comprehensive geriatric assessment (CGA) teams are available in most regions throughout the United States and employ a well-validated, well-accepted approach to frail elders. It only makes sense that these gerontological experts care for neglected elders, who are the frailest of the frail. Although there is no published outcome study of CGA and elder abuse, Dyer and colleagues (unpublished data) have preliminary data that showed that CGA reduced the prevalence of elder abuse and neglect at six months and greatly increased the assessment of self-related health by the victim.

Multidisciplinary Forensics Teams

A handful of locations around the country have created multidisciplinary teams to review and respond to suspected cases of elder abuse and neglect. These teams are not only capable of providing a better coordinated intervention and response than unaffiliated professionals working outside a team structure, but they also are developing experience and expertise in supplying a more sophisticated forensic analysis than was previously available, thereby increasing the likelihood that legal action is pursued and successful in appropriate cases. Multidisciplinary forensic teams may be employed to useful end in a variety of other contexts, for example as elder fatality or serious injury review teams. Because there are so few such teams and because the data are so scarce, multidisciplinary efforts dedicated to addressing elder abuse and neglect should be studied, encouraged, and supported.

RECOMMENDATIONS FOR RESEARCH

As a supplement to primary research in this area, it is critical to ensure that a validated evaluative component is built into all promising practices, innovative programs, and other efforts, so that results can be measured and others have ready access to outcome data. Given the nascent state of the field, the areas for potential research are plentiful. Only a sampling of potential areas of study are discussed here.

Research to Establish Forensic Markers

The need for research to develop medical forensic markers of elder abuse and neglect is urgent. That research is the threshold to detection and diagnosis, without which reporting, intervention, and prosecution are impossible. Unless we develop benchmarks giving practitioners the tools to recognize elder abuse and neglect, we cannot measure or address the problem. Such research should result in data that provide guidance to health, social service, and public safety professionals on the location, pattern, color, marking, severity, natural history, and other characteristics of injuries associated with elder abuse and neglect. Some of these factors (for example, medication misuse and cognitive and mental health problems) should be evaluated both as forensic markers and in terms of whether and to what extent they constitute risk factors for being a victim or a perpetrator of elder abuse and neglect. Mortality rates associated with each marker also should be evaluated.

This research, among other things, should determine in a scientific manner the difference between age and unavoidable disease-related changes versus abuse and neglect. Very few studies of any of the 14 factors listed below have been done; more are needed. For example, descriptive studies of skin tears are needed that compare those with known causes to those with unknown causes. Burnight (2000) has suggested a national database of witnessed injuries. Many forms of trauma could be studied, beginning with witnessed falls, which occur commonly in hospitals and nursing homes. Research protocols should be designed to provide information applicable to minority populations and to both genders. The study by Langlois and Gresham (1991) was limited to whites; a study of bruising is needed for people of color. A few suggestions (there are many more) for research needed relating to the markers discussed in this paper include the following:

Fractures

The significance of type and location of fractures is not well understood relative to mechanism and degree of injury. Objective documentation of the degree and ensuing impact of osteoporosis is needed. Research into osteoporosis to determine its objective documentation postmortem and how it affects fracturing, mechanisms (i.e., degree of force required) would be useful to the forensic analysis.

Burns

The findings on burns and elder abuse or neglect are intriguing and could be further studied at U.S. burn centers. The high incidence of burns in cases of self-neglect raises the question: When does a history or propensity of an elder to set fires give rise to a duty by a caregiver to intervene? This inquiry would benefit from research to develop forensic markers to guide the analysis. The high mortality rates in elders as a result of burns make this public health issue a compelling research topic.

Cognitive and Mental Disorders

The existing data on cognitive and mental disorders raise many research questions. What is the impact of cognitive and mental disorders in cases of abuse or neglect? What is the prevalence of dementia, depression, and psychosis in abused or neglected individuals or perpetrators? Are mortality and morbidity higher in persons with cognitive or mental disorders? Because dementia and alcoholism are treatable and depression and psychosis are curable, interventions derived from trials may decrease or even reverse some cases of elder abuse and neglect.

Elder Sexual Abuse

To improve recognition of elder sexual abuse, researchers need to develop precise anatomic diagnostic criteria, something that is yet to be determined for child sexual abuse (Kerns, 1998). Studies are needed comparing anogenital examination findings and psychological characteristics in sexually abused elders with findings in examinations of those who participate in consensual sexual relations.

Studies in each of the additional categories below should be conducted to determine what physical and behavioral signs should catalyze further examination, inquiry, and possible reporting by caregivers. The categories include: abrasions and lacerations, bruises, restraints, decubiti, malnutrition, dehydration, medication use, self-neglect, and financial fraud and exploitation. Additional studies should be conducted to determine what other markers should be added to the list (for example, contractures).

Research on Distinctions in Medical Forensic Markers in Home Versus Residential Settings

The study of these forensic markers in caregiver neglect is difficult because so many variables are involved. Some caregivers may neglect patients because of a lack of knowledge, resources, training, assistance, and available time due to competing responsibilities. Others may neglect intentionally or sadistically. In the institutional context, a corporate decision maker may order cutbacks that result in neglect. Research is needed to develop appropriate standards of care for caregivers that are meaningful and achievable regardless of socioeconomic status.

Most of the adverse events that happen to frail elders are not the result of abuse or neglect. Tracking of data on adverse and unexpected events is important in determining standards for such incidents and is already performed by state and federal agencies. Intermingled with data on, for example, falls, may be data on bruises and fractures that occurred because of abuse or neglect unbeknownst to investigators. Gurwitz and colleagues (1994) have collected data on adverse and unexpected events in long-term care settings. A study in which investigators collect a single stream of data, screen data for abuse and neglect, and compare positive cases to negative cases may give results that are more accurate.

Assessment Tools

The lack of statutory or well-studied screening instruments can result in highly subjective standards by mandated reporters, leaving prosecutors with very little hard evidence on which to base their cases (Loue, 2001). Health care providers and social services agencies may not reach the people who need them most if cases of abuse and neglect cannot be adequately identified.

Research is vital to creating validated, uniform screening tools. The lack of a gold standard requires using alternative methods for validating tools, such as a lead standard. One lead standard might be an expert consensus panel. Consideration should be given to developing (a) a form with a short format for busy environments, such as emergency centers, with questions applicable to all elders; (b) a form applicable to community-dwelling elders; and (c) a form suited to residents of institutions. These various forms are required because we do not know what risk different settings confer.

A second form with a long format, also validated and uniform, should be developed with a structure similar to that of a, b, and c above. The long form would be intended to be used by those who historically take a lengthy interview, such as protective service specialists or ombudsmen. The long form could serve as a research tool in conjunction with the short form if the individual appears to be at high risk for abuse or neglect. Screening for all elders, coupled with targeted comprehensive assessment in high-risk populations, may be the most practical and fruitful approach.

Finally, comprehensive geriatric assessment is already a well-validated procedure for assessing and intervening in the care of frail elders and merits study in populations of abused or neglected individuals.

Just as in the evaluation of potential abuse and neglect in living persons, there is a need for development of screening or evaluation tools that are specifically useful in the postmortem setting. For example, research could compare the number, location, and type of fractures incurred in documented accidental situations versus those encountered in the setting of inflicted injury. It is intriguing to think that there might be biological markers of elder abuse or neglect. While the need for epidemiological research on screening and assessment tools is clear, it does not preclude searching for other objective laboratory measures.

Mortality Data for Abused and Neglected Elders

Although a 100 percent autopsy rate, including proper investigation, review of medical records, consultation with specialists, including geriatricians, odontologists, radiologists, and other specialists would be ideal to obtain baseline information, it is not practical financially and would over-whelm most medical examiner/coroner systems. Consideration should be given to a pilot study using statistically selected cases for investigation and autopsy to determine the prevalence of abuse and neglect and their contri-bution to death in an autopsied elderly population.

Medical examiners and coroners should exchange information with geriatricians and others, including being active members of multidisciplinary teams to review deaths, review reporting mechanisms, and identify system issues that work for and against adequate reporting and intervention. De-velopment of additional scientific literature on all markers would be useful to support a medical examiner's diagnoses and conclusions when chal-lenged in court. It would be useful to study what number or percent of cases of elder abuse and neglect contributing to death are not investigated or autopsied. This research likely will require predicate research into the markers to enhance detection in the first instance.

Research Regarding Certification of Elder Deaths

To ensure better certification of elders' deaths, researchers should docu-ment aspects of aging that are natural and compare them with features of injury due to accidental mechanisms and to malevolence. Training in rec-ognizing signs and typical features of abuse and neglect is important for medical examiners, coroners, death investigators, law enforcement, and those who first respond to emergency calls reporting deaths, and should be enhanced. Policy makers should consider expanding elder death manda-tory-reporting laws beyond institutional cases. Development of standard-ized protocols for examination of deaths in elders, particularly when there is a suspicion of abuse or neglect, is fundamental and could benefit from the expertise of all health care professionals concerned about fatal abuse and neglect of the elderly.

Legal Issues for Study

Research is needed to determine what types of criminal, civil, and administrative cases best protect elders in all settings. To date, there has been no research on the efficacy of current laws and existing remedies or how to develop more effective ones.

Reporting

There is a wide divergence of views regarding whether reporting of elder abuse and neglect should be mandatory, whether mandatory-reporting laws should be aggressively enforced, and regarding the efficacy, in general, of mandatory reporting. In addition, some states have specific reporting requirements, such as the Arkansas law requiring immediate reporting of deaths of nursing home residents. Research protocols should be developed that inform this debate and to track the impact and efficacy of reporting laws.

Developing Experts in Forensic Geriatrics

Development of a group of forensic pediatricians has reportedly improved detection, diagnosis, reporting, and prosecution of child abuse and neglect. Pilot programs to train a group of forensic geriatricians, and to identify what types of programs are most effective, should be developed and tested.

Screening Tools, Forensic Centers, and Multidisciplinary or Interdisciplinary Teams

As discussed earlier in this paper, each of these potential tools should be the subject of study to determine how best to construct screening tools, forensic centers, and multidisciplinary/interdisciplinary teams (including fatality and serious-injury review teams), likely including several pilot or demonstration projects in several sites. A predicate for such research would be to examine and evaluate what is known about screening tools, forensic centers, and multidisciplinary/interdisciplinary teams used in other areas, such as child abuse and neglect, sexual abuse, and domestic violence.

There are many more areas of needed study and many more recommendations could be made. The reader is directed to Elder Justice Roundtable Report (2000).

CONCLUSION

Evidence-based forensic markers of elder abuse and neglect have attracted little research interest and therefore remain largely unidentified. No data exist regarding the number of documented forensic markers or prosecuted cases. A comprehensive research agenda should be developed that will provide the information needed to help derive accurate clinical and forensic markers for elder abuse and neglect in both living and deceased persons, in home and residential settings alike.

The significantly increased mortality rate for elder victims of abuse and neglect underscores the pressing need for a national research agenda and extensive study by the relevant disciplines to address this growing issue.

REFERENCES

Abrams, W.B., M.H. Beers, R. Berkow, and A.J. Fletcher, eds.
   1995a   Cognitive failure: Delirium and dementia. In *The Merck Manual of Geriatrics, Second Edition.* Whitehouse Station, NJ: Merck & Co.
   1995b   Depression. In *The Merck Manual of Geriatrics, Second Edition.* Whitehouse Station, NJ: Merck & Co.
   1995c   Alcohol abuse and dependence. In *The Merck Manual of Geriatrics, Second Edition.* Whitehouse Station, NJ: Merck & Co.

Alessi, C.A., A.E. Struck, and H.U. Aronow
   1997   The process of care in preventive in-home comprehensive geriatric assessment. *Journal of the American Geriatrics Society* 45:1044–1050.

American Board of Forensic Odontology
   1986   Guidelines for bite mark analysis. *Journal of the American Dental Association* 112:383–386.

American Geriatrics Society Review Syllabus
   1998   A Core Curriculum in Geriatric Medicine, Fourth Edition 1999-2001. E.L. Cobbs, E.H. Duthie, Jr., and J.B. Murphy, eds. Dubuque, IA: Kendall/Hunt Publishing.

American Medical Association (AMA)
   1996   Diagnostic and Treatment Guidelines on Elder Abuse and Neglect. AA25:96-937:4M:12/96.

American Psychiatric Association (APA)
   1994   *(DSM-IV) Quick Reference to the Diagnostic Criteria from Diagnostic and Statistical Manual-IV.* Washington, DC: American Psychiatric Association.

Andronicus, M., R.K. Oates, J. Peat, S. Spalding, and H. Martin
   1997   Non-accidental burns in children. *Journal of the International Society for Burn Injuries* 24(6)(September):552–558.

Aravanis, S.C., R.D. Adelman, R. Breckman, T.T. Fulmer, E. Holder, M. Lachs, J.G. O'Brien, and A.B. Sanders
   1993   Diagnostic and treatment guidelines on elder abuse and neglect. *Archives of Family Medicine* 2:371–388.

Barton, A., and M. Barton, eds.
   1981   *The Management and Prevention of Pressure Sores.* London: Faber and Faber.

Bennett, G.C.J., and M.R. Bliss
   1998   Pressure sores: Etiology and prevalence. In *Brocklehurst's Textbook of Geriatric Medicine and Gerontology, Fifth Edition,* R. Tallis, H. Fillit, and J.C. Brocklehurst, eds. London: Harcourt Brace & Co.

Benton, D., and C. Marshall
   1991   Elder abuse. *Clinics in Geriatric Medicine* 7(4):831–845.

Berlowitz, D.R., G.H. Brandeis, J.J. Anderson, A.S. Ash, B. Kader, J.N. Morris, and M.A. Moskowitz
   2001   Evaluation of a risk-adjustment model for pressure ulcer development using the Minimum Data Set. *Journal of the American Geriatrics Society* 49(7):872–876.

Bird, P.E., D.T. Harrington, D.J. Barillo, A. McSweeney, K.Z. Shirani, and C.W. Goodwin
   1998   Elder abuse: A call to action. *The Journal of Burn Care & Rehabilitation* 19(6):522–527.

Bowden, M.L., S.T. Grant, B. Vogel, and J.K. Prasad
   1988   The elderly, disabled and handicapped adult burned through abuse and neglect. *Burns, Including Thermal Injury* 14(6):447–50.

Brogdon, B.G.
   1998   *Forensic Radiology.* Boca Raton, FL: CRC Press.

Burgess, A.W.
  2000 Elder Justice: Medical Forensic Issues Concerning Abuse and Neglect. Paper presented at the Department of Justice medical forensic roundtable discussion, Washington, D.C., October 18, 2000. Available at: *http://www.ojp.usdoj.gov/nij/elderjust.*

Burnight, K.
  2000 Elder Justice Roundtable: Medical Forensic Issues Concerning Abuse and Neglect. Paper presented at the Department of Justice medical forensic roundtable discussion, Washington, D.C., October 18, 2000. Available at: *http://www.ojp.usdoj.gov/nij/elderjust.*

Butler, R.N.
  1999 Warning signs of elder abuse: The family physician may be the patient's only protection from family violence. *Geriatrics* (March); 54(3):3–4.

Butler, R.N., and M.I. Lewis
  1998 Sexuality in old age. In *Brocklehurst's Textbook of Geriatric Medicine and Gerontology, Fifth Edition*, R. Tallis, H. Fillit, and J.C. Brocklehurst, eds. London: Harcourt Brace & Co.

Canadian Task Force Periodic Health Examination
  1994 Periodic health examination, 1994 update: 4. Secondary prevention of elder abuse and mistreatment. *Canadian Medical Association Journal* 151:1413–1420.

Connolly, V., A.A. McConnell, and G. McGarrity
  1995 Battered granny or spontaneous fractures? A legal dilemma. *Postgraduate Medical Journal* 71(840):630–632.

Coyne, A.C., W.E. Reichman, and L.J. Berbig
  1993 The relationship between dementia and elder abuse. *American Journal of Psychiatry* 150:643–646.

Crane, J.
  2000 Injury interpretation. In *Forensic Science: A Physician's Guide to Clinical Forensic Medicine*, M. M. Stark, ed. Totowa, NJ: Humana Press.

Dyer, C.B., and A.M. Goins
  2000 The role of the interdisciplinary geriatric assessment in addressing self-neglect of the elderly. *Generations* 23–27.

Dyer, C.B., V.N. Pavlik, K.P. Murphy, and D.J. Hyman
  2000a The high prevalence of depression and dementia in elder abuse and neglect. *Journal of the American Geriatrics Society* 48:205–208.

Dyer, C.B., V.N. Pavlik, and N.A. Festa
  2000b Elder mistreatment: Analysis of allegation types and variables associated with multiple allegations from a statewide database. Published abstract. The annual meeting of the American Geriatrics Society, May 20, 2000.

Dyer, C.B., V.N. Pavlik, N.A. Festa, D.J. Hyman, M. Vogel, and E.L. Poythress
  2001 *Outcomes of Comprehensive Geriatric Assessment.* Baylor College of Medicine, Houston, TX.

Elder Justice Roundtable Report: Medical Forensic Issues Concerning Abuse and Neglect
  2000 The Department of Justice medical forensic roundtable discussion, Washington, DC, October 18, 2000. Available at: *http://www.ojp.usdoj.gov/nij/elderjust.*

Evasovich, M., R. Klein, F. Muakkassa, and R. Weekley
  1998 The economic effect of child abuse in the burn unit. *Journal of the International Society for Burn Injuries* 24(7):642–645.

Fanslow, J., R. Norton, and C. Spinola
  1998 Indicators of assault-related injuries among women presenting to the emergency department. *Annals of Emergency Medicine* 32:341–348.

Fenton, S.J., J.E. Bouquot, and J.H. Unkel
    2000   Orofacial considerations for pediatric, adult, and elderly victims of abuse. *Emergency Medical Clinic of North America* 18(3):601–617.
Finucane, T.E., C. Christmas, and K. Travis
    1999   Tube feeding in patients with advanced dementia: A review of the evidence. *Journal of the American Medical Association* 282(14):1365–1370.
Francis, R.M.
    1998   Metabolic bone disease. In *Brocklehurst's Textbook of Geriatric Medicine and Gerontology, Fifth Edition*, R. Tallis, H. Fillit, and J.C. Brocklehurst, eds. London: Harcourt Brace & Co.
Fulmer, T.
    1989   Mistreatment of elders: Assessment, diagnosis, and intervention. *Nursing Clinics of North America* 24(3):707–716.
Fulmer, T., S. Street, and K. Carr
    1984   Abuse of the elderly: Screening and detection. *Journal of Emergency Nursing* 10(3):131–140.
Fulmer, T., and T. Wetle
    1986   Elder abuse screening and intervention. *Nurse Practitioner* 11(5):33–38.
Fulmer, T., and D. Birkenhauer.
    1992   Elder mistreatment assessment as a part of everyday practice. *Journal of Gerontology Nursing* (March):42–45.
Fulmer, T., G. Paveza, I.I. Abraham, and S. Fairchild
    2000   Elder neglect assessment in the emergency department. *Journal of Emergency Nursing* 26:436–443.
Goodyear-Smith, F.A.
    1989   Medical evaluation of sexual assault findings in the Auckland region. *The New Zealand Medical Journal* 102(876):493–495.
Griffiths, C.E.M.
    1998   Aging of the skin. In *Brocklehurst's Textbook of Geriatric Medicine and Gerontology, Fifth Edition*, R. Tallis, H. Fillit, and J.C. Brocklehurst, eds. London: Harcourt Brace & Co.
Gurwitz, J., M. Sanchez-Cross, M. Eckler, and J. Matulis
    1994   The epidemiology of adverse and unexpected events in the long-term care setting. *Journal of the American Geriatrics Society* 42(1):33–38.
Harrington, C., C. Kovner, M. Mezey, J. Kayser-Jones, S. Burger, M. Mohler, R. Burke, and D. Zimmerman
    2000   Experts recommend minimum nurse staffing standards for nursing facilities in the United States. *The Gerontologist* 40(1):5–16.
Henderson, C.T., L.S. Trumbore, S. Morharban, R. Benya, and T.P. Miles
    1992   Prolonged tube feeding in longterm care: Nutritional status and clinical outcomes. *Journal of American College of Nutrition* 11:309–325.
Holt, M.G.
    1993   Elder sexual abuse in Britain: Preliminary findings. *Journal of Elder Abuse and Neglect* 5(2):63–71.
Hood, I.
    2000   Elder Justice: Medical Forensic Issues Concerning Abuse and Neglect. Paper presented at the Department of Justice medical forensic roundtable discussion, Washington, D.C., October 18, 2000. Available at: *http://www.ojp. usdoj.gov/ nij/elderjust.*
Hultman, C.S., D. Priolo, B.A. Cairns, E.J. Grant, H.D. Peterson, and A.A. Meyer
    1998   Return to jeopardy: The fate of pediatric burn patients who are victims of abuse and neglect. *Journal of Burn Care and Rehabilitation* 19(4):367–376.

Jones, J., J.D. Dougherty, D. Schelbie, and W. Cunningham
 1988 Emergency department protocol for the diagnosis and evaluation of geriatric abuse. *Annals of Emergency Medicine* 17:1006–1015.
Jones, J.S., T.R. Veenstra, J.P. Seamon, and J. Krohmer
 1997 Elder mistreatment: National survey of emergency physicians. *Annals of Emergency Medicine* 30(4):473–479.
Kane, R., and J. Goodwin
 1991 Spontaneous fractures of the long bones in nursing home patients. *American Journal of Medicine* 90:263–266.
Kerns, D.L.
 1998 Triage and referrals for child sexual abuse medical examinations: Which children are likely to have positive medical findings? *Child Abuse & Neglect* 22(6):515–18;519–522.
Knight, B., ed.
 1997 *Simpson's Forensic Medicine, Eleventh Edition.* New York: Oxford University Press, Inc.
Lachs, M.S.
 2000 Elder Justice Roundtable: Medical Forensic Issues Concerning Abuse and Neglect. Paper presented at the Department of Justice medical forensic roundtable discussion, National Institute of Justice, Washington, D.C., October 18, 2000. Available at: *http://www.ojp.usdoj.gov/nij/elderjust.*
Lachs, M.S., and K. Pillemer.
 1995 Abuse and neglect of elderly persons. *New England Journal of Medicine* 332(7):437–443.
Lachs, M.S., C. Williams, S. O'Brien, L. Hurst, and R. Horwitz
 1996 Older adults: An 11-year longitudinal study of adult protective service use. *Archives of Internal Medicine* 156:449–453.
Lachs, M.S., C.S. Williams, S. O'Brien, K.A. Pillemer, and M.E. Charlson
 1998 The mortality of elder mistreatment. *Journal of the American Medical Association* 280(5):428–432.
Langlois, N.E.I., and G.A. Gresham
 1991 The ageing of bruises: A review and study of the colour changes with time. *Forensic Science International* 50:227–238.
Loue, S.
 2001 Elder abuse and neglect in medicine and law. *Journal of Legal Medicine* 22:159–209.
Lowenstein, S.R., C.A. Crescenzi, D.C. Kern, and K. Steel
 1986 Care of the elderly in the emergency department. *Annals of Emergency Medicine* 15:528–535.
Malone, M., N. Rozario, M. Gavinski, and J. Goodwin
 1991 The epidemiology of skin tears in the institutionalized elderly. *Journal of the American Geriatrics Society* 39(6):591–595.
Marshall, C.E., D. Benton, and J.M. Brazier
 2000 Elder abuse: Using clinical tools to identify clues of mistreatment. *Geriatrics* 55(2):42–53.
Medical Tribune
 1995 Radiological screens improve detection of domestic violence in patients of all ages. December.
Mickish, J.
 1993 Abuse and neglect: The adult and elder. In *Adult Protective Service: Reach and Practice,* B. Byers and J. Hendricks, eds. Springfield, IL: Charles C. Thomas.

Miles, S.
    1996   A case of death by physical restraint: New lessons from a photograph. *Journal
            of the American Geriatrics Society* 44(3):291–292.
Mohr, W.K., and B.D. Mohr
    2000   Mechanisms of injury and death proximal to restraint use. *Archives of Psychiat-
            ric Nursing* 14(6):285–295.
Monane, M., S. Monane, and T. Semla
    1997   Optimal medication use in elders: Key to successful aging. *The Western Journal
            of Medicine* 167(4):233–237.
The Mount Sinai/Victim Services Agency Elder Abuse Project
    1988   Elder mistreatment guidelines for health care professionals: Detection, assess-
            ment and intervention. New York: Mount Sinai/Victim Services Agency Elder
            Abuse Project.
Mouton, C.P., and D.V. Espino
    1999   Health screening in older women. *American Family Physician* 59(7):1835-1842.
National Center on Elder Abuse
    1996   Elder abuse Information Series No. 1: Type of elder abuse in domestic settings.
            Washington, D.C. [Online.] Available at: *http://www.elderabusecenter.org.*
    1998   *The National Elder Abuse Incidence Study.* Washington, DC: National Center
            on Elder Abuse.
Neale, A.V., M.A. Hwalek, R.O. Scott, and C. Stahl
    1991   Validation of the Hwalek-Sengstock elder abuse screening test. *Journal of Ap-
            plied Gerontology* 10(4):406–418.
Patterson, J.A., and R.G. Bennett
    1995   Prevention and treatment of pressure sores. *Journal of the American Geriatrics
            Society* 43:919–927.
Paveza, G.J., C. VandeWeerd, and V. Hughes-Harrison
    1997   Financial exploitation of the elderly: A descriptive study of victims and abusers
            in an urban area. Paper presented at the 50th Annual Scientific Meeting of the
            Gerontological Society of America, Cincinnati, Ohio, November 14–18.
Pavlik, V.N., D.J. Hyman, N.A. Festa, and C.B. Dyer
    2001   Quantifying the problem of abuse and neglect in adults: Analysis of a statewide
            database. *Journal of the American Geriatrics Society* 49:45-48, 2001.
Persse, D.
    no   Patient refusal of transport by emergency medical services. Unpublished data.
    date   Houston Emergency Medical Services, Houston, Texas.
Phillips, L.R.
    1988   The fit of elder abuse with the family violence paradigm, and the implications of
            a paradigm shift for clinical practice. *Public Health Nursing* 5(4)(December):222–
            229.
Ramsey-Klawsnik, H.
    1991   Elder sexual abuse: Preliminary findings. *Journal of Elder Abuse and Neglect*
            3(3):73–90.
Rawson, R.D., R.K. Ommen, K.G. Johnson, and A. Yfantis
    1984   Statistical evidence for the individuality of the human dentition. *Journal of Fo-
            rensic Sciences* 29:245.
Reis, M., and D. Nahmiash
    1998   Validation of the indicators of abuse (IOA) screen. *Gerontologist* 38(4):471–
            480.

Schor, J.D., A. Selby, and C.A. Bertone
   1995   Geriatric assessment in the diagnosis and treatment of elder abuse. *New Jersey Medicine* 92(2):108–110.
Scofield, M., R. Reynolds, G. Mishra, P. Powers, and A. Dobson
   1999   Vulnerability to abuse, powerlessness and psychological stress among older women. (Unpublished report). Callaghan, NSW, University of Newcastle: Women's Health Australia Study.
Siu, A.L., D.B. Reuben, and A.A. Moore
   1994   Comprehensive geriatric assessment. In *Principals of Geriatric Medicine and Gerontology*, W.R. Hazard, E.L. Bierman, and J.P. Blass, eds. New York: McGraw-Hill.
Tatara, T.
   1993   Understanding the nature and scope of domestic elder abuse with the use of state aggregate data: Summaries of the key findings of a national survey of state APS and aging agencies. *Journal of Elder Abuse and Neglect* 5(4):35–51.
Teaster, P.B., K.A. Roberto, J.O. Duke, and M. Kim
   2000   Sexual abuse of older adults: Preliminary findings of cases in Virginia. *Journal of Elder Abuse & Neglect* 12(3/4):1–16.
Thomas, A.J.
   1998   Nutrition. In *Brocklehurst's Textbook of Geriatric Medicine and Gerontology, Fifth Edition*, R. Tallis, H. Fillit, and J.C. Brocklehurst, eds. London: Harcourt Brace & Co.
Toronjo, C., V.N. Pavlik, D.J. Hyman, E.L. Poythress, M. Keith, N.A. Festa, and C.B. Dyer
   no   How adult protective service specialists validate cases of elder neglect. Unpub-
   date   lished paper. Texas Elder Abuse and Mistreatment Institute, Houston, TX.
Tueth, M.J.
   2000   Exposing financial exploitation of impaired elderly persons. *American Journal of Geriatric Psychiatry* 8(2):104–111.
Watson-Perczel, M., J. Lutzker, B. Greene, and B. McGimpsey
   1988   Assessment and modification of home cleanliness among families adjudicated for child neglect. *Behavior Modification* 12(1):47–81.
White, S.W.
   2000   Elder abuse: Critical care nurse role in detection. *Critical Care Nursing Quarterly* 23(2):20–25.
Wolf, R.
   2000   Risk Assessment Instruments. National Center on Elder Abuse Newsletter, September.
Zubenko, G.S., and T. Sunderland
   2000   Geriatric psychopharmacology: Why does age matter? *Harvard Review of Psychiatry* 7(6):311–333.

13

Financial Abuse of the Elderly in Domestic Settings

Thomas L. Hafemeister*

In some ways financial abuse is very similar to other forms of elder abuse in that it can be devastating to the victim and is frequently traced to family members, trusted friends, and caregivers. But unlike physical abuse and neglect, financial abuse is more likely to occur with the tacit acknowledgment and consent of the elder person[1] and can be more difficult to detect and establish. As a result, financial abuse requires a distinct analytical perspective and response. Unfortunately, these differences are often overlooked.

Little empirical research has been conducted that directly addresses financial abuse of the elderly, and in general it has received less attention than other forms of elder abuse (Nerenberg, 2000b). Although the amount of attention given to it has increased in recent years, most commentary rests

---

*Thomas L. Hafemeister, J.D., Ph.D., is Director of Legal Studies at the Institute of Law, Psychiatry, and Public Policy, University of Virginia. He is indebted to Lori Stiegel, Carla VandeWeerd, and Richard Bonnie, who read and provided valuable comments on an earlier draft of this report.

[1]There is some controversy over whether this population should be referred to as elder persons (the elderly) or as older persons (older people). This dispute tends to focus on conflicting views regarding which terminology is the most descriptive and the least likely to perpetuate inappropriate stereotypes. Resolving this dispute, however, is tangential to the focus of this report. "Elder persons" and "the elderly" are used throughout this report primarily because they are widely used terms and appear routinely in related legislation and legislative hearings (see U.S. Congress, 2000).

on a relatively thin empirical base and draws heavily on anecdotal observations and relies (perhaps inappropriately) on research and analysis addressing other forms of elder abuse, child abuse, and spouse/partner abuse. Because financial abuse is frequently addressed in conjunction with other forms of elder abuse, a brief overview of elder abuse in general is provided before turning specifically to financial abuse of the elderly.

PREVALENCE OF ELDER ABUSE IN GENERAL

Elder abuse, at least to some degree, has probably always existed. Only in the past few decades, however, has it been recognized as a major societal problem. Attention to elder abuse followed the "discovery" of child abuse in the 1960s and spouse abuse in the 1970s. Today, elder abuse is widely characterized as both a pervasive problem and a growing concern (Dessin, 2000; Heisler, 2000; Moskowitz, 1998b).

The National Elder Abuse Incidence Study (NEAIS), which was described as the first national study of the incidence of elder abuse in the United States,[2] estimated that nearly a half million persons aged 60 and over in domestic settings were abused or neglected during 1996 (National Center on Elder Abuse, 1998).[3] Furthermore, this study determined that for every reported incident of elder abuse or neglect, approximately five incidents were unreported (National Center on Elder Abuse, 1998), supporting a wide consensus that elder abuse is greatly underreported (Choi and Mayer, 2000; Dessin, 2000; U.S. General Accounting Office, 1991; Kleinschmidt, 1997; Moskowitz, 1998b; National Center on Elder Abuse, 1996). The NEAIS confirmed a general view that state agencies established to receive such reports, such as Adult Protective Services (APS) agencies, receive reports of the most visible and obvious occurrences of elder abuse, but that there are many other incidents that are not reported. Nevertheless,

---

[2] It should be noted that the methodology employed in the NEAIS study has been questioned (Comijs et al., 2000; Thomas, 2000). However, methodological limitations are associated with virtually all elder abuse research. The goal of this report is not to provide a methodological critique of elder abuse research in general or financial abuse in particular. In addition, regardless of any methodological limitations, the NEAIS study provides useful comparisons across categories of elder abuse. There is, however, a need for more rigorous research on both elder abuse in general and financial abuse of the elderly in particular.

[3] An earlier and frequently cited report from the House Select Committee on Aging suggested that between 1 million and 2 million older Americans experience mistreatment each year (U.S. Congress, 1991). Recent review articles have estimated the number of elderly individuals victimized each year as 2 million (Moskowitz, 1998a), 1.5 million (Dessin, 2000), 1 million (Marshall et al., 2000), and 818,000 (Coker and Little, 1997). It has also been estimated that 5 percent of elder persons suffer some form of abuse each year and that one out of every four will experience abuse or neglect at some time (Dessin, 2000).

the number of APS elder abuse reports substantially increased over the past 10 years, an increase that exceeded the growth in the elderly population during this period (National Center on Elder Abuse, 1998).

FORMS OF ELDER ABUSE

What constitutes elder abuse is defined by state law, and state definitions vary considerably (U.S. General Accounting Office, 1991; Kapp, 1995; National Center on Elder Abuse, 2001; Moskowitz, 1998b; Roby and Sullivan, 2000).[4] Not surprisingly, researchers have also used many different definitions in studying the problem (Choi and Mayer, 2000; Kleinschmidt, 1997; Macolini, 1995; National Center on Elder Abuse, 2001; Pillemer and Finkelhor, 1988).[5] The variation in definitions has been cited as a significant impediment to elder abuse recognition, management, research, and analysis (U.S. General Accounting Office, 1991; Kleinschmidt, 1997; Lachs and Pillemer, 1995; Moskowitz, 1998b; Nerenberg, 2000a; Roby and Sullivan, 2000; Rosenblatt et al., 1996).

Elder abuse in domestic settings (i.e., within the older person's own home or in the home of a caregiver) is often differentiated from elder abuse within institutional settings (i.e., within residential facilities for older persons such as nursing homes) (Brandl and Meuer, 2000; National Center on Elder Abuse, 1996, 2001). Domestic elder abuse has been asserted to be more prevalent than institutional elder abuse (Kosberg and Nahmiash, 1996; Marshall et al., 2000; Moskowitz, 1998b), in part because it has been estimated that 80 percent of the dependent elders in this country are cared for at home (National Center on Elder Abuse, 1996). However, research directly substantiating this assertion is lacking.[6] Another dichotomy frequently used distinguishes between elder abuse by individuals who have a special relationship with the elder person (e.g., spouses, children, other relatives, friends, or caregivers providing services within the

---

[4]These variations include whether elder abuse is addressed as a separate category or whether it is grouped with the abuse of adults with a disability of any age, the age cutoff used to define an elder person, the definitions of various types of abuse, and whether elder abuse encompasses self-neglect or sexual abuse (Dessin, 2000; Lachs and Pillemer, 1995; Mehta, 2000).

[5]The little research that has been conducted has been criticized for conceptual and methodological weaknesses, including reliance on underinclusive or nonrepresentative samples of cases brought to the attention of social agencies or reporting authorities, unclear definitions of elder abuse, reliance on professional reports rather than victim interviews, and failure to use rigorous research designs, such as random-sample surveys and case-comparison studies (Pillemer and Finkelhor, 1988; Schiamberg and Gans, 2000).

[6]Data on institutional elder abuse are so scarce that it is not possible to make any national estimates of its incidence or prevalence" (National Center on Elder Abuse, 1996:2).

elder person's home) and individuals with whom such a preexisting special relationship does not exist (Kosberg and Nahmiash, 1996; Marshall et al., 2000; National Center on Elder Abuse, 1996, 2001).[7] Within domestic settings, it has been reported that the perpetrators of elder abuse are much more likely to be family members (National Center on Elder Abuse, 1996).

Although conceptualizations of what elder abuse encompasses vary considerably, the National Center on Elder Abuse (2001) identifies six major categories of elder abuse. They include physical abuse, sexual abuse, emotional or psychological abuse, neglect, abandonment, and financial abuse. Among these categories, financial abuse has received limited attention and is often not assessed in studies of elder abuse (Choi et al., 1999; Kleinschmidt, 1997; Tueth, 2000). Nonetheless, financial abuse is increasingly viewed as both sufficiently important to necessitate its inclusion in studies of elder abuse in general and sufficiently distinct to justify addressing it separately (Choi and Mayer, 2000).

PARAMETERS OF FINANCIAL ABUSE OF THE ELDERLY

The remainder of this report focuses on financial abuse of the elderly within a domestic setting by individuals relatively well known to the elder person. This focus encompasses financial abuse by family members, friends, and caregivers of the elder person and excludes financial abuse within institutional settings or by strangers. Domestic settings are not only a frequent setting for this abuse,[8] but their tendency to involve complex family dynamics and deep-seated conflicts tends to make them particularly challenging. Although financial abuse of the elderly within institutional settings (e.g., within nursing homes) and by strangers (e.g., in the course of consumer fraud) are serious concerns in their own right and in need of systematic study (of which little has been generated to date),[9] they are not the foci of this report.

To address financial abuse of the elderly, its parameters should first be defined. Variously referred to as financial mistreatment; exploitation; or fiduciary, economic, or material abuse, this type of abuse encompasses a

---

[7]The latter would encompass most incidents of consumer fraud.

[8]About 80 percent of the estimated 6 million dependent elders in this country are cared for at home" (National Center on Elder Abuse, 1996:11–12). Furthermore, although little research has been conducted on financial abuse within institutional settings, recent studies identifying the top 10 deficiencies in long-term care facilities identified physical abuse or neglect more frequently than financial abuse (Menio and Keller, 2000).

[9]For a discussion of consumer fraud perpetrated on the elderly, see Deem (2000), McGhee (1983), Smith (1999), and U.S. Congress (2000).

broad range of conduct (National Committee for the Prevention of Elder Abuse, 2001). There have been widespread complaints that financial abuse of the elderly is poorly defined, in part because it is hard to define, which makes it difficult to identify, investigate, and prosecute (Dessin, 2000; Langan and Means, 1996; Marshall et al., 2000; Roby and Sullivan, 2000; Sanchez, 1996; Wilber and Reynolds, 1996). The absence of a uniform definition perhaps explains why it is often not included or is poorly addressed in research on elder abuse in general (Langan and Means, 1996).

Because elder abuse, like other domestic ills, has generally been considered a state concern rather than a federal concern, the absence of federal law pertaining to elder abuse has placed on the states the responsibility to define this activity. Forty-eight states and the District of Columbia are reported to specifically mention financial abuse in their elder abuse statutes (Roby and Sullivan, 2000; Wilber and Reynolds, 1996).[10] States' definitions, however, vary widely on what constitutes financial abuse and who can be held accountable for it (Roby and Sullivan, 2000; Sanchez, 1996).

One complicating factor is variations in the class of individuals targeted for protection from financial abuse. Three general approaches are employed. In some states all individuals who have reached a given age are specifically protected, in other states protection is provided to all vulnerable or incapacitated adults regardless of age, and a third group of states uses a hybrid approach that protects vulnerable or incapacitated adults of any age and all adults over a certain age (Dessin, 2000; Roby and Sullivan, 2000). The last two approaches can make it difficult for researchers to distinguish reports of elder abuse from reports of adults in general (Coker and Little, 1997). The first approach, however, has been criticized for perpetuating the unfounded stereotype that all elderly persons are vulnerable and in need of protection (Roby and Sullivan, 2000). Also, some states require diminished decision-making capacity by the elder person before financial abuse is considered to occur, while other states do not impose such a requirement (Tueth, 2000). States even vary on the age when someone becomes "elderly" (Coker and Little, 1997; Paveza, 2001).

Other variations in state definitions are associated with who can be held accountable for financial abuse. Some states require dishonest tactics by perpetrators, such as the use of force, duress, misrepresentation, undue influence, or other illegal means, to take advantage of the elder person. Other states do not require a showing of such tactics if the perpetrator knew or should have known that the elder person lacked the cognitive

---

[10]As of 1995, New York and Oregon were purported to be silent on financial abuse (Wilber and Reynolds, 1996).

capacity to make financial decisions (Tueth, 2000). Similarly, some states limit financial abuse to an intentional improper use of the elder's resources, while other states encompass negligent, or at least reckless, advice or conduct, such as failing to use income effectively for the care of the older person (Dessin, 2000; Roby and Sullivan, 2000).

Generally the victim must experience some disadvantage as a result of the transaction, but some states also require that the perpetrator gain some advantage from the transaction (Dessin, 2000). The latter would not penalize actions that merely wasted the elder person's assets (Dessin, 2000). States also vary on whether abuse is limited to the abuse of the elder person's money and real property or also encompasses other resources such as the elder person's goods and services (Roby and Sullivan, 2000). Finally, some states limit financial abuse to those in a "position of trust" to an elder person (Roby and Sullivan, 2000).

It is widely recognized that it is difficult, even for experienced professionals, to distinguish an unwise but legitimate financial transaction from an exploitative transaction resulting from undue influence, duress, fraud, or a lack of informed consent (Tom, 2001).[11] The seasoned professional can also be tested by the complex and varied nature of these transactions (Dessin, 2000). It may also be difficult to distinguish abusive conduct from well-intentioned but poor, confused, or misinformed advice and direction (Dessin, 2000; Langan and Means, 1996). Evaluating whether financial abuse has occurred has been characterized as a complex and often subjective determination (Bernatz et al., 2001).

Further complicating efforts to establish the parameters of financial abuse of the elderly are that both the elder person and the perpetrator may feel that the perpetrator has some entitlement to the elder person's assets (Dessin, 2000). Elder persons may feel a desire to benefit their heirs or to compensate those who provide them with care, affection, or attention (Dessin, 2000; Langan and Means, 1996). It can be difficult to discern a transfer of assets made with consent from an abusive transfer (Dessin, 2000; Wilber and Reynolds, 1996).

Also, conduct that began in the elder person's best interests may become abusive over time, as when perpetrators initially provide helpful advice regarding financial investments but take on greater control and ulti-

---

[11]Wilber and Reynolds (1996) provide a framework for distinguishing financial abuse of the elderly from acceptable exchanges, while Tueth (2000) identifies transactions needing careful scrutiny before concluding that financial exploitation has occurred. Roby and Sullivan (2000) argue that definitions of financial abuse should be broad enough to provide sufficient flexibility to address the range of financial abuse and offenders, yet specific enough to protect individuals acting in the best interests of the elder person.

mately misappropriate funds for themselves as the elder person's cognitive abilities decline (Dessin, 2000). Typically, financial abuse in a domestic setting reflects a pattern of behavior rather than a single event and occurs over a lengthy period of time (National Clearinghouse on Family Violence, 2001; Wilber and Reynolds, 1996). Determining when financial abuse began can be very difficult (Smith, 1999).

Finally, a number of commentators have asserted that whether financial abuse is considered to have occurred should reflect the elder person's perception of the purported abuse and the cultural context in which it takes place (Moon, 2000; Nerenberg, 2000a; Sanchez, 1996; Wolf, 2000; see generally Tatara, 1999). For example, attitudes about the legitimacy of a transfer may reflect expectations within a given culture that elderly persons will share their resources with family members in need, while other cultures reject this notion (Brown, 1999; Moon, 2000; Nerenberg, 2000a). Studies have shown considerable variation in what constitutes financial abuse across cultural, racial, and ethnic groups (Brown, 1999; Hudson and Carlson, 1999; Moon, 2000; Nerenberg, 2000a), and it has been argued that a failure to take into account these differences undercuts efforts to assess financial abuse of the elderly (Sanchez, 1996).[12]

TYPES OF FINANCIAL ABUSE OF THE ELDERLY

In efforts to address financial abuse of the elderly, advocates for the elderly often delineate typical examples of this abuse.[13] Examples specifically relevant to a domestic setting and financial abuse by individuals relatively well known to the elder person include:

- taking, misusing, or using without knowledge or permission money or property (Dessin, 2000; National Center on Elder Abuse, 2001; National Clearinghouse on Family Violence, 2001; National Committee for the Prevention of Elder Abuse, 2001);
- forging or forcing an elder person's signature (National Center on Elder Abuse, 2001; National Clearinghouse on Family Violence, 2001; National Committee for the Prevention of Elder Abuse, 2001);
- abusing joint signature authority on a bank account (Rush and Lank, 2000);

---

[12]At the same time, the law places considerable weight on the importance of establishing requisite standards of behavior that are uniform, consistent, and predictable across groups of individuals.

[13]For a lengthy list of specific examples of financial exploitation, see U.S. Congress (1981).

- misusing ATMs or credit cards (New York State Department of Law, 2000);
- cashing an elder person's checks without permission or authorization (National Center on Elder Abuse, 2001);
- misappropriating funds from a pension (New York State Department of Law, 2000; Langan and Means, 1996);
- getting an elder person to sign a deed, will, contract, or power of attorney through deception, coercion, or undue influence (National Center on Elder Abuse, 2001; National Clearinghouse on Family Violence, 2001; National Committee for the Prevention of Elder Abuse, 2001);
- providing true but misleading information that influences the elder person's use or assignment of assets (Dessin, 2000);
- persuading an impaired elder person to change a will or insurance policy to alter who benefits from the will or policy (Central California Legal Services, 2001; Frolik, 2001; Smith, 1999);
- using a power of attorney, including a durable power of attorney, for purposes beyond those for which it was originally executed (Hwang, 1996; National Clearinghouse on Family Violence, 2001; Thilges, 2000);
- improperly using the authority provided by a conservatorship, trust, etc. (National Center on Elder Abuse, 2001);
- negligently mishandling assets, including misuse by a fiduciary or caregiver (Dessin, 2000);
- promising long-term or lifelong care in exchange for money or property and not following through on the promise (National Committee for the Prevention of Elder Abuse, 2001);
- overcharging for or not delivering caregiving services (Central California Legal Services, 2001); and
- denying elder persons access to their money or preventing them from controlling their assets (National Clearinghouse on Family Violence, 2001; Smith, 1999).

PREVALENCE AND IMPACT OF FINANCIAL ABUSE

Prevalence of Financial Abuse of the Elderly

The prevalence of financial abuse of the elderly (like elder abuse in general) is difficult to estimate because there is no national reporting mechanism to record and analyze it, cases often are not reported, definitions vary, and it is difficult to detect (Coker and Little, 1997; Deem, 2000; National Clearinghouse on Family Violence, 2001). However, the consensus is that it is a significant problem (Dessin, 2000).

The National Center for Elder Abuse found that financial abuse accounted nationally for about 12 percent of all substantiated elder abuse reports in 1993 and 1994 (National Center on Elder Abuse, 2000; Zimka, 1997). A subsequent more comprehensive study conducted by the same entity found that 18.6 percent of the 115,110 substantiated elder abuse reports submitted to APS agencies nationwide in 1996—which included reports of self-neglect—and were reports of financial or material exploitation (National Center on Elder Abuse, 1998). Excluding reports of self-neglect, this exploitation appeared in 30.2 percent of the substantiated reports. This represented the third largest category of reports, less than neglect (48.7 percent) and emotional or psychological abuse (35.41 percent), but more than physical abuse (25.6 percent).[14] A national survey in Canada found that financial abuse was the most common type of elder abuse in that country (Podnieks, 1992).[15]

Some parts of the country report an even greater prevalence of financial abuse.[16] Financial exploitation has been reported to be the most frequent form of perpetrator-related elder abuse in Illinois (Neale et al., 1996) and Oregon (U.S. Congress, 2000). It has been asserted that half of all abuse cases in New York state include financial exploitation and that in New York City 63 percent of abuse cases involve finances (New York State Department of Law, 2000). A study of APS reports in upstate New York between 1992 and 1997 that led to state intervention found that financial exploitation was present in 38.4 percent of the cases (Choi and Mayer, 2000). A study in Massachusetts found that almost one-half of the cases of elder abuse serious enough to require reporting to a district attorney involved financial exploitation (Dessin, 2000). A review of California reports from 1987 found that fiduciary abuse was the most prevalent type of exploitation and appeared in 41.5 percent of the cases, with the next most prevalent type of exploitation being physical abuse, which appeared in 33.3 percent of the cases (County Welfare Directors Association, 1988). In their review of older studies, Wilber and Reynolds (1996) determined that between 33 percent and 53 percent of an estimated 1 million elder abuse victims experienced financial abuse.

Financial abuse has also been reported to be greater among various minority populations. For example, exploitation was found to be the most commonly reported abuse in samples of Korean immigrant and black elders

---

[14]More than one substantiated type of abuse could be reported for an incident. The study did not, however, provide specific information about this overlap (e.g., how often financial abuse occurred in conjunction with another form of elder abuse).

[15]A British Columbia study is reported to have found that 8 percent of older adults had been financially abused, with an average loss of $20,000 each (National Clearinghouse on Family Violence, 2001).

[16]The variation in rates among states may be attributed in part to differing definitions and assessments of financial abuse (Lavrisha, 1997).

(Hall, 1999; Moon, 1999). It has also been suggested that in general financial abuse is particularly likely to be underreported (Coker and Little, 1997; Hwang, 1996; Wilber and Reynolds, 1996).

It has been asserted that financial abuse often occurs in conjunction with other forms of elder abuse (Choi et al., 1999; National Clearinghouse on Family Violence, 2001; Paris et al., 1995), although research generally does not establish how frequently this overlap occurs.[17] In a study of one county's investigated APS reports of financial exploitation Choi et al. (1999) found that caregiver neglect also occurred in 12.1 percent of the cases, self-neglect in 6.1 percent, physical abuse in 5.1 percent, and psychological abuse in 3.8 percent. In a later analysis, Choi and Mayer (2000) found that 33.7 percent of this county's investigated reports involved financial exploitation plus either neglect or abuse, while 37.6 percent involved only financial exploitation. However, in a Canadian national survey, only 19 percent of victims were victims of more than one form of maltreatment, although it was not reported how often financial abuse occurred in conjunction with other forms of elder abuse (Podnieks, 1992).

Financial exploitation has been described as the fastest growing form of elder abuse (New York State Department of Law, 2000), although empirical support for this assertion is scanty. Societal attention to elder abuse in general is a relatively recent phenomenon, and attention to financial abuse is even more nascent (Dessin, 2000). It has been suggested that an increase in reports reflects closer scrutiny by federal, state, and local officials rather than necessarily an increase in the prevalence of financial abuse (Lavrisha, 1997). Greater attention to this issue has been attributed to increases in the number of elderly people, an increased emphasis on care at home, and the substantial resources of the elderly (Langan and Means, 1996).

The Impact of Financial Abuse on the Elderly

One of the most frightening scenarios for an elder person is the possibility of financial ruin (Dessin, 2000). Although not systematically assessed, losing assets accumulated over a lifetime, often through hard work and deprivation, can be devastating, with significant practical and psychological consequences (Dessin, 2000; Nerenberg, 2000c; Smith, 1999). Financial abuse can have as significant an impact for an elder person as a violent crime (Deem, 2000) or physical abuse (Dessin, 2000).

Replacing lost assets is generally not a viable option for retired indi-

---

[17]Elder abuse examples provided in governmental reports often show a combination of financial abuse and physical or psychological abuse or neglect (County Welfare Directors Association, 1988; U.S. Congress, 1981).

viduals or individuals with physical or mental disabilities (Coker and Little, 1997; Dessin, 2000; Moskowitz, 1998b; Nerenberg, 2000c). Also, because of their age, the elderly will have less time to recoup their losses and often are solely dependent on their savings to meet subsequent expenses and needs (Smith, 1999). A depletion of assets is likely to result in a loss of independence and security for the elder person (Choi et al., 1999; Nerenberg, 2000c), which can have significant symbolic and practical ramifications. Such abuse may necessitate that the elder person become dependent on family members, inducing or adding to their financial burden and stress (Coker and Little, 1997). Alternatively, financial abuse may result in elder persons becoming dependent on social welfare agencies, with a significant decline in their quality of life (Coker and Little, 1997).

From a psychological perspective, a loss of trust in others has been identified as the most common consequence of financial abuse (Deem, 2000). In addition, victims may become very fearful, both of crime and of their vulnerability to crime, which in turn may lead to dramatic changes in lifestyle and emotional well-being (Fielo, 1987). Victims may also experience a loss of confidence in their own financial abilities, stress, and isolation from family or friends (Deem, 2000). Financial abuse may lead to depression, hopelessness, or even suicide (Nerenberg, 2000c; Podnieks, 1992).

In addition, it has been noted that, unlike physical and psychological abuse, the effects of financial abuse may not end with the death of the victim. Family members whose inheritance was reduced or depleted as a result of the financial abuse will suffer loss and may themselves feel abused, particularly if they felt entitled to inherit the victim's assets (Dessin, 2000).

WHY ELDER PERSONS ARE TARGETS FOR FINANCIAL ABUSE

Although empirical support is often not provided, many reasons have been identified for why the elderly are targeted for financial abuse. One set of reasons addresses the financial assets and acumen of the elderly. For example, one widely cited factor is that elder persons possess a large proportion of the nation's wealth (Central California Legal Services, 2001; National Committee for the Prevention of Elder Abuse, 2001), with 70 percent of all funds deposited in financial institutions controlled by persons age 65 and older (Dessin, 2000). Other explanations have been that older people may be more trusting than their younger counterparts (Central California Legal Services, 2001) or may be relatively unsophisticated about financial matters, particularly when they are unfamiliar with advances in technology that have made managing finances more complicated (National Committee for the Prevention of Elder Abuse, 2001). Also, they may not realize the value of their assets—particularly homes that have appreciated greatly in value (Central California Legal Services, 2001; National Committee for the Prevention of Elder Abuse, 2001). It has also been suggested that the difficulties of living on a fixed income may enhance their willingness to try a "get-rich-quick" scheme (Dessin, 2000).

Other reasons focus on characteristics of the elderly. One explanation is that elder persons may be easily identifiable and are presumed vulnerable (Central California Legal Services, 2001). In addition, elder persons may be more likely to have conditions or disabilities that make them easy targets for financial abuse, including forgetfulness or other cognitive impairments (Central California Legal Services, 2001; Choi and Mayer, 2000). Elder persons may also have a diminished capacity to rationally evaluate proposed courses of action (Dessin, 2000).

A third set of factors focuses on social isolation that the elderly may experience (Quinn, 2000). For example, elder persons may be more likely to have disabilities that make them dependent on others for help. These "helpers" may have ready access to elder persons' assets, documents, or financial information or be able to exercise significant influence over the elder person (National Committee for the Prevention of Elder Abuse, 2001; Nerenberg, 2000c; Quinn, 2000). In addition, seniors may be isolated due to their lack of mobility or because they live alone, which shields perpetrators from scrutiny and insulates victims from those who can help (Dessin, 2000; Nerenberg, 2000c). Also, the elderly may be lonely and desire companionship and thus be susceptible to persons seeking to take advantage of them (Hwang, 1996).

A fourth group of reasons suggests that perpetrators assume that financial abuse of the elderly is unlikely to result in apprehension or repercussions. Perpetrators may believe that elder persons are less likely to report abuse or take action against perpetrators, particularly if they have been victimized by family members or other trusted individuals (Central California Legal Services, 2001; Hwang, 1996; National Committee for the Prevention of Elder Abuse, 2001). The elder person may be afraid or embarrassed to ask for help or be intimidated by the abuser (Hwang, 1996). Perpetrators may also recognize that older people in very poor health may not survive long enough to follow through on lengthy legal interventions (Central California Legal Services, 2001; National Committee for the Prevention of Elder Abuse, 2001) or that they will not make convincing witnesses (National Committee for the Prevention of Elder Abuse, 2001).

RISK FACTORS AND CHARACTERISTICS OF VICTIMS

A number of conditions or factors have been identified as increasing the likelihood that an older person will be the victim of financial abuse in a domestic setting. However, there has also been limited systematic research on this issue.

Older women who are white and live alone are considered to be the most likely victims of this abuse, perhaps more so than for any other form of elder abuse. The national NEAIS report found that 63 percent of the APS reports from 1996 involved victims who were women, which was somewhat more than their percentage of the elder population at that time (57.6 percent) (National Center on Elder Abuse, 1998). However, when relying on the reports of their sentinels, which were asserted to be more comprehensive in scope and to include unreported incidents, the NEAIS report concluded that 91.8 percent of the victims of financial abuse of the elderly were women, the highest percentage for any form of elder abuse (the next highest proportion was 83.2 percent for physical abuse) (National Center on Elder Abuse, 1998). The NEAIS report also found that the targets of financial abuse tended to be the oldest old, with 48 percent of the substantiated APS reports and 25.3 percent of the sentinel reports involving victims 80 years of age or older, even though they only comprised 19 percent of the total elderly population (National Center on Elder Abuse, 1998). Finally, the NEAIS report found that 83 percent of the substantiated APS reports and 92.4 percent of the sentinel reports of financial abuse involved white victims (whites comprised 84 percent of the national population of elders in 1996) (National Center on Elder Abuse, 1998).

Another report concluded from the scant amount of research available and the authors' analysis of cases from Alabama that more than 60 percent of the victims of financial abuse of the elderly were likely to be elderly white females over the age of 70 (Coker and Little, 1997). A study of APS financial exploitation reports in an upstate New York county between 1989 and 1996 found that the elder victims were, on average, 78 years old, 68.7 percent of them were female, and 66.9 percent of them lived alone (Choi et al., 1999). A Canadian national survey found that 62 percent of elder victims of financial abuse were female, only 31 percent were married (the lowest percentage of any category of elder abuse—51 percent of elderly nonvictims were married), 54 percent were widowed, and 58 percent lived alone (the highest percentage of any category of elder abuse, with only 39 percent of elderly nonvictims living alone) (Podnieks, 1992). The widely cited profile of a target for financial abuse is generally a white woman over 75 who is living alone (Bernatz et al., 2001; Rush and Lank, 2000; Tueth, 2000).

A number of reasons are given for why most elder victims of financial abuse are women (Dessin, 2000). One is actuarial in nature; namely, women live longer than men and thus more women are available as targets for financial abuse of the elderly. Second, perpetrators may perceive women as weak and vulnerable in general. Third, many women have not handled their financial affairs because their husbands handled them. When their husbands die or lose the capacity to manage their finances, these women make particularly good targets for perpetrators who offer "help" but instead exploit available assets.

Regardless of gender, a lack of familiarity with financial matters in general or the means of conducting a particular financial transaction enhances the likelihood of financial abuse (Choi et al., 1999; Choi and Mayer, 2000; National Committee for the Prevention of Elder Abuse, 2001). Changes in and unfamiliarity with the means by which financial transactions are conducted, including electronic transactions, add to this vulnerability. The risk of financial abuse may also be increased when the elder person is uncomfortable speaking about financial issues (Rush and Lank, 2000). In general, elders who own a house, a substantial and visible asset, are more likely to be exploited (Choi et al., 1999; Choi and Mayer, 2000).

Other factors identified as increasing the likelihood of financial abuse focus on the social status of the elder person. Identified risk factors include an elder person's social isolation, loneliness, and recent loss of loved ones (Bernatz et al., 2001; Choi and Mayer, 2000; Hwang, 1996; National Committee for the Prevention of Elder Abuse, 2001; Podnieks, 1992; Quinn, 2000; Tueth, 2000; Wilber and Reynolds, 1996). Having family members who are unemployed or who have substance abuse problems have also been identified as placing an elder person at greater risk of financial abuse (National Committee for the Prevention of Elder Abuse, 2001). Similarly, when a relative is the elder person's only social support, the risk of financial exploitation may be increased (Choi et al., 1999). Conversely, having family members who are actively involved in good faith in assisting with or managing the financial affairs of the elderly has been determined to diminish the risk that the elderly will experience financial abuse (Rush and Lank, 2000). However, a combination of denial of a need for such assistance, busy lives, and a reluctance to confront difficult issues may keep many family members from such involvement (Rush and Lank, 2000). It has also been noted that little is known about the close bonds that develop naturally between the elderly and their caregivers, particularly when services are provided the elderly within their homes, and what leads to financial abuse (Quinn, 2000).

Physical or mental disabilities of elder persons have also been identified as risk factors, including medical problems that limit their ability to understand and comprehend financial issues and impairments that create dependency on others (Bernatz et al., 2001; Choi et al., 1999; Giordano et al., 1992; Hwang, 1996; National Committee for the Prevention of Elder Abuse, 2001; Podnieks, 1992; Tueth, 2000; Wilber and Reynolds, 1996). However, it has been argued that the extent to which older persons are vulnerable to financial abuse is more directly related to the circumstances in which they live than advanced age per se (Smith, 1999) and that age alone should not lead to a presumption of incapacity (Wilber and Reynolds, 1996).

SIGNALS OF FINANCIAL ABUSE

Relying primarily on anecdotal evidence, personal experience, or commonly shared beliefs, practitioners have compiled and circulated a number of indicators that suggest when financial abuse of an elder person may be occurring. These indicators have been distributed to bank employees, lawyers, and the public in general. It is recommended that no single indicator be taken as establishing the existence of financial abuse, as there may be other explanations for the occurrence of the indicator; instead reliance is placed on a pattern or cluster of indicators (National Committee for the Prevention of Elder Abuse, 2001). It has also been argued that it is almost impossible to detect financial abuse without considerable knowledge of the victim's financial affairs (Dessin, 2000). It has been suggested that bank tellers, personal bankers, officials responsible for registering deeds, family members, and neighbors are the most likely to observe the signs of financial abuse (Henningsen, 2001). The indicators can be grouped by the setting or circumstances in which they are most likely to be observed.[18]

For example, a number of indicators can be apparent during a visit to the home or residence of the elder person. A relatively obvious indicator is missing belongings or property (e.g., jewelry) (Hwang, 1996; National Center on Elder Abuse, 2001; National Clearinghouse on Family Violence, 2001; National Committee for the Prevention of Elder Abuse, 2001; Zimka, 1997). Financial abuse may be suggested by an absence of documentation about financial arrangements or transactions (e.g., pensions, stock, government payments, credit card charges) (Central California Legal Services, 2001; National Committee for the Prevention of Elder Abuse, 2001). Implausible or evasive explanations by the elder person or the caregiver about the elder person's finances, the elder person's unawareness of or confusion about recently completed financial transactions, or the elder person appearing to be afraid or worried when talking about money may serve as indicators (Carroll, 2001; Central California Legal Services, 2001; National Clearinghouse on Family Violence, 2001; National Committee for the Prevention of Elder Abuse, 2001). Alternatively, unpaid bills, eviction or foreclosure

---

[18]Wilber and Reynolds (1996) have developed a framework that organizes various indicators of financial abuse in such a way as to assist professionals to distinguish legitimate from illegitimate transactions.

notices, or notices to discontinue utilities despite the availability of adequate financial resources may suggest financial abuse (Carroll, 2001; Central California Legal Services, 2001; National Center on Elder Abuse, 2001; National Committee for the Prevention of Elder Abuse, 2001; Zimka, 1997).

Financial abuse may also be indicated by a lack of care or substandard care, a decline in personal grooming, or an absence of clothing, food, or other basic necessities when the older person can afford them (National Center on Elder Abuse, 2001; National Clearinghouse on Family Violence, 2001; National Committee for the Prevention of Elder Abuse, 2001; Zimka, 1997). Similarly, financial abuse may be suggested by complaints from the elder person about once having had money but not seeming to have much anymore (Carroll, 2001; Zimka, 1997) or a sudden inability to pay bills (Langan and Means, 1996). Additional signals may be provided by an unkempt residence when arrangements have been made for providing care or a failure to receive services for which payment has already been made (Central California Legal Services, 2001). Alternatively, the provision of services that are not necessary may also indicate financial abuse (National Center on Elder Abuse, 2001). Untreated medical or mental health problems may be an indication of financial abuse (Central California Legal Services, 2001; Hwang, 1996). In general, significant cognitive impairments suggest vulnerability to financial abuse (Choi et al., 1999; Choi and Mayer, 2000; Wilber and Reynolds, 1996).

Another widely cited indicator is social isolation of the elder person, including a discontinuation of prior relationships with family and friends (Central California Legal Services, 2001; Henningsen, 2001; National Clearinghouse on Family Violence, 2001; Wilber and Reynolds, 1996). Increased dependence on others, loneliness, loss of loved ones, and a reduced sense of self-worth can indicate vulnerability to financial abuse (Wilber and Reynolds, 1996). Relatedly, financial abuse may be suggested by new acquaintances or "best friends," particularly those who take up residence with the older person, who the elder person relies on totally, or who express overenthusiastic affection for the elder person (Carroll, 2001; Coker and Little, 1997; Hwang, 1996; National Committee for the Prevention of Elder Abuse, 2001). Financial abuse may be suggested by a noticeable increase in the spending of people living with or caring for the older person (Dessin, 2000; Henningsen, 2001) or by sudden heavy traffic in and out of the home (Hwang, 1996). Another warning signal may be caregivers or family members who express excessive interest in the amount of money being spent on the older person, who ask only financial questions, or who do not allow the elder person to speak (Carroll, 2001; Langan and Means, 1996; National Clearinghouse on Family Violence, 2001; National Committee for the Prevention of Elder Abuse, 2001; Tueth, 2000). Also a promise of lifelong care may be accompanied by an implicit or explicit expectation that the elder person's funds will be transferred to the caregiver (Hwang, 1996).

Family members who are addicted to alcohol or drugs or who indicate they feel entitled to the elder person's funds may suggest financial abuse (Hwang, 1996). Alternatively, a circle of mutual dependence or conflict that engulfs family members may engender financial abuse or leave family members blind to its possibility (Gold and Gwyther, 1989).

A second setting in which indicators of financial abuse may arise is associated with the conduct of banking transactions. For example, financial abuse may be suggested by withdrawals from or transfers between bank accounts that the older person cannot explain, unusual or unexplained sudden activity, including large withdrawals (particularly when the elder person is accompanied by another person), or frequent transfers or ATM withdrawals (Coker and Little, 1997; Commonwealth of Massachusetts, 2001; Henningsen, 2001; Hwang, 1996; National Center on Elder Abuse, 2001; National Clearinghouse on Family Violence, 2001; National Committee for the Prevention of Elder Abuse, 2001). Other indicators include having bank statements and canceled checks sent to an address that is not the elder person's residence, suspicious signatures on checks or other documents, and the inclusion of additional names on an elder person's credit card or bank signature card (Coker and Little, 1997; National Center on Elder Abuse, 2001; National Clearinghouse on Family Violence, 2001; National Committee for the Prevention of Elder Abuse, 2001; Zimka, 1997).

Related indicators focus on deviations from the elder person's usual banking behavior (Commonwealth of Massachusetts, 2001; National Center on Elder Abuse, 2001). They include suspicious activity on credit card accounts; bank activity that is erratic, unusual, or uncharacteristic; and bank activity inconsistent with the person's abilities (e.g., ATM withdrawals by someone who is homebound) (Central California Legal Services, 2001; Coker and Little, 1997; Dessin, 2000; Zimka, 1997). Another indication is provided when individuals have no awareness of the current state of their personal financial affairs (Rush and Lank, 2000). A signal may be provided when checks uncharacteristically begin to lack adequate funds to cover them, when the person is in debt and does not know why, when mostly smaller checks increase to larger checks for a variety of items, or an unusual number of checks are written to "cash" (Carroll, 2001; Dessin, 2000; Henningsen, 2001; National Clearinghouse on Family Violence, 2001).

A third cluster of indicators is associated with legal transactions involving the elder person and is directed largely at attorneys. They include the execution of legal documents or arrangements, such as powers of attorney, by an older person who is confused or who does not understand or remember the transaction (Carroll, 2001; Central California Legal Services, 2001; Hwang, 1996; National Clearinghouse on Family Violence, 2001; National Committee for the Prevention of Elder Abuse, 2001). Other signs are suspicious or forged signatures on documents and changes in the older person's property, titles, will, or other documents, particularly if the changes are unexpected, sudden, or favor new acquaintances (National Center on Elder Abuse, 2001; National Clearinghouse on Family Violence, 2001; National Committee for the Prevention of Elder Abuse, 2001; Zimka, 1997). Another signal can be the sudden appearance of previously uninvolved relatives claiming rights to an elder person's affairs and possessions (National Center on Elder Abuse, 2001).

A fourth cluster of signals is associated with visits to physicians or other health care providers. One such signal is a patient's unmet physical needs notwithstanding the availability of financial resources (Lachs and Pillemer, 1995). Other identified behaviors are missed medical appointments, dropping out of treatment, uncharacteristic nonpayment for services, declining physical and psychological health, defensiveness or hostility by the caregiver during visits or on the phone, and an unwillingness by the caregiver to leave the elder person alone during appointments (Tueth, 2000).

MOTIVATIONS AND CHARACTERISTICS OF PERPETRATORS

As is true of most aspects of financial abuse of the elderly, little research has been conducted on the motivations and characteristics of its perpetrators. Nevertheless, there has been considerable speculation about them by professionals interested in reducing this abuse.

One set of motivations widely identified tends to be associated with all forms of elder abuse. Frequently cited motivations include the perpetrator's substance abuse, mental health, gambling, or financial problems (Dessin, 2000; National Committee for the Prevention of Elder Abuse, 2001; Tueth, 2000). The perpetrator's actions may be based on "learned violence" or be modeled after the prior behavior of the elder person (Dessin, 2000). Where the perpetrator is a primary caregiver, caregiver stress has been cited as a cause of this abuse (Dessin, 2000).

There are also a number of characteristics linked relatively uniquely to financial abuse. For example, the perpetrator may stand to inherit assets and feel justified in taking an advance or in exercising control over assets that are perceived to be almost or rightfully the perpetrator's own (Dessin, 2000; National Committee for the Prevention of Elder Abuse, 2001). When the perpetrator is an heir, he or she may conclude that preemptive steps are necessary to prevent the inheritance from being exhausted in paying for medical or other expenses (National Committee for the Prevention of Elder

Abuse, 2001). Alternatively, negative attitudes toward persons identified as likely heirs may motivate the perpetrator to act to prevent them from acquiring the elder person's assets (National Committee for the Prevention of Elder Abuse, 2001). Because of a prior negative relationship with the elder person, the perpetrator may feel a sense of entitlement to these resources as payback for prior exploitation or abuse (Dessin, 2000; National Committee for the Prevention of Elder Abuse, 2001). The perpetrator may be motivated by a sense that he or she should be reimbursed for having carried a substantial care-giving burden for the elder person (Dessin, 2000). The perpetrator may conclude that the elder person has more assets than needed and the perpetrator has too few, and thus the perpetrator is entitled to a share of the elder person's assets (Quinn, 2000). Also, an intricate relationship may exist between elders and their caregivers. Older people, who may no longer place as great a value on their material possessions, may give gifts as a means of maintaining a power balance in their relationship with the caregiver. At the same time, the caregiver may indicate that such gifts are necessary if the elder person wishes to retain the caregiver's attention and assistance (Quinn, 2000).

When such motivations are present, a perpetrator may read into an elder person's words or behavior consent to a conveyance that a more objective perspective would not. The recipient of a gift may argue that the elder person provided implicit or explicit indications that the individual be given certain assets. When consent to a transfer of assets has been clearly provided and is not induced by fraud, duress, or undue influence, many assets can be transferred on a relatively informal basis.[19] Because of the informal and private setting in which such transfers were purportedly made, the transfers may be the subject of good faith disputes but not represent financial abuse. However, individuals with the motivations described above may report consent to a transfer by an elder person that was not given or was not clearly provided, or attempt to induce this consent by fraud, duress, or undue influence.

Nonrelative perpetrators have been found to include career criminals in the business of defrauding others in general and elders in particular, while others were overcome by greed under the circumstances (Choi et al., 1999). It has been observed that many exconvicts become paid caregivers for vulnerable individuals, a practice that goes unchecked because most states do not require criminal background checks and do not prohibit persons convicted of certain crimes from working with the elderly (Nerenberg, 2000c).

---

[19]Certain assets, including real property, require more formal means of conveyance such as written documentation of the transfer in ownership.

As for the characteristics of the perpetrators, the NEAIS report concluded that the relative youth of perpetrators of financial abuse was particularly striking compared to other types of abuse (National Center on Elder Abuse, 1998). This study found 45.1 percent of the perpetrators were age 40 or younger (versus 27.4 percent for all forms of elder abuse) and another 39.5 percent were 41 to 59 years of age. It also found 59 percent of the perpetrators were male (versus 52.5 percent for all forms of elder abuse).

In addition, people who financially abuse the elderly are often family members, particularly adult children and grandchildren (National Center on Elder Abuse, 1996; Quinn, 2000; Rush and Lank, 2000; Sklar, 2000). The NEAIS report found that 60.4 percent of the substantiated 1996 APS financial abuse cases involved an adult child (versus 47.3 percent for all forms of elder abuse) and only 4.9 percent involved a spouse (versus 19.3 percent for all forms of elder abuse). In addition, it has been asserted that "crimes [by the elders' offspring] go undetected or are discovered long after the assets have been depleted" (Sklar, 2000:21).

A study of one county's APS reports of financial exploitation found that roughly 40 percent of the perpetrators were the victim's sons or daughters, 20 percent were other relatives (only 1.5 percent were spouses), and 4 percent were not relatives (Choi et al., 1999). A related study found that spouses were perpetrators of financial exploitation in only 1.5 percent of cases as opposed to 13.8 percent of all other elder abuse cases (Choi and Mayer, 2000). This study also found, however, that nonrelatives were the perpetrators in 38.8 percent of the financial exploitation cases in contrast to only 14.7 percent of all other elder abuse cases (Choi and Mayer, 2000). Another report concluded that perpetrators are often relatives, particularly children or grandchildren of the victim, many of whom depend on the elderly victim for housing or other assistance, have substance abuse problems, and are represented almost equally by both genders (Coker and Little, 1997).

Tueth (2000) constructed from the literature two types of perpetrators of elder exploitation. The first type consisted of dysfunctional individuals with low self-esteem who may be abusing substances, psychosocially stressed, or suffering from caregiver burden. Such individuals will not seek out victims but instead passively take advantage of opportunities that present themselves. The second, more aggressive type methodically identifies victims, establishes power and control over them, and obtains the elder's assets by using deceit, intimidation, and other forms of psychological abuse. Such individuals may have an antisocial personality disorder and have little regard for the rights of others. In a typical sequence, the victim is identified as impaired and vulnerable; the victim's trust is secured by being friendly, helpful, and providing assistance; the victim is made passive

and comfortable and then isolated; and finally the perpetrator takes possession of assets by employing psychological abuse.

APPROPRIATENESS OF ADOPTING MODELS ADDRESSING CHILD AND SPOUSE ABUSE

Societal attention to child abuse and spouse abuse[20] predated the attention given to elder abuse. The rising awareness of child abuse in the 1960s
and that of spouse abuse in the 1970s have been cited as triggering societal
awareness of the existence of elder abuse (Dessin, 2000).[21]

Preventive measures, reporting systems, and interventions designed to
curtail child abuse frequently provided a model for efforts to address elder
abuse (Capezuti et al., 1997; Gilbert, 1986; Kapp, 1995; Macolini, 1995;
Nerenberg, 2000a; Wolf, 2000). As statutes were already in place that
mandated child abuse reports and established service systems to redress
such abuse when elder abuse was "discovered," many states found it expe-
dient to apply the same model to elder abuse as well (Anetzberger, 2000).
One reason for using the same model is that child and elder abuse, whether
physical or financial in nature, are difficult to detect because the victim may
be reluctant or unable to report the abuse (Dessin, 2000), in part because
the perpetrator is likely to be a family member (National Center on Elder
Abuse, 1996). Also, the victims of both forms of abuse are frequently
perceived as particularly vulnerable or sympathetic and in need of society's

---

[20]The phrase "spouse abuse" also encompasses actions associated with wife assault, partner abuse, battered women, and domestic violence; is intended to refer to abuse between
adults who live together in intimate relationships, regardless of their marital relationship and
the gender of the partners; and remains the terminology used in a number of reporting
statutes.

[21]Growing awareness of child abuse and the need for society to take steps to curtail it also
led to increased efforts to address spouse abuse. Initially it was suggested that there were
relatively direct parallels between child and spouse abuse in that in both the victims were
relatively helpless captives of the abuser (a relationship sometimes suggested for elder abuse
victims). Such a perspective led to legislation that mandates reporting by various individuals
of suspected spouse abuse. However, this "infantilizing" of spouses has met considerable
resistance. For example, the American Medical Association's Council on Ethical and Judicial
Affairs asserted that spouse abuse differs from child abuse in important respects and concluded that mandatory reporting of spouse abuse violated the ethical standards of confidentiality that physicians owe to their adult patients (Council on Ethical and Judicial Affairs,
AMA, 1992). Rather than imposing mandatory reporting of spouse abuse, a number of other
mandatory steps pertaining to spouse abuse have been suggested for treating physicians,
including mandatory intensive domestic violence training for various specialties as part of
medical education and requiring treatment plans and protocols that assist the medical team in
identifying and responding to abuse (Council, 1992; Jecker, 1993).

protection (Wolf, 2000; Anetzberger, 2000). Nevertheless, although a state may achieve a certain degree of efficiency when it builds on existing models and service delivery systems, as will be discussed, important distinctions caution against a whole-scale adoption of a child abuse model (AARP, 1993; Anetzberger, 2000; Brandl, 2000; Kapp, 1995; Kleinschmidt, 1997; Macolini, 1995; Vinton, 1991; Wolf, 2000), particularly when addressing the financial abuse of the elderly.

Alternatively, some commentators argue that a spouse abuse model is better suited for crafting responses to elder abuse (Macolini, 1995; Pillemer and Finkelhor, 1988). However, as will also be noted, financial abuse of the elderly may represent a sufficiently distinct form of abuse that caution should likewise be exercised before applying a spouse abuse model to address it (Kleinschmidt, 1997).

Means of Detecting Abuse

Because of compulsory education, children of school age interact with people outside their home on a routine basis. Even younger children may regularly attend preschool or day care. These contacts result in individuals outside the home frequently being aware of a child's health and well-being and being in a position to detect and report abuse. For many elder persons, such outside contacts may be sporadic and infrequent, which in turn reduces the likelihood that elder abuse will be detected and reported. Indeed, an abuser of an older person may intentionally discourage or limit such contacts to diminish the likelihood of detection. Thus, unlike child abuse, a naturally occurring circle of individuals may not exist who can be encouraged or required to watch for and report elder abuse (Choi and Mayer, 2000; National Center on Elder Abuse, 1998).

Also, child abuse models focus heavily on physical abuse. Financial abuse is rarely an issue when a child is involved (Dessin, 2000).[22] As noted, financial abuse is a frequent concern when the elderly are involved. Moreover, the manner in which financial abuse occurs and its manifestations are often very different from that of physical abuse. Rather than acting out of rage or a loss of self-control, the perpetrator of financial abuse often acts in a very calculated fashion specifically designed to avoid detection. Also, physical abuse is more self-evident and more readily subject to proof than financial abuse.

---

[22]The closest analogy with regard to children would probably be the depletion of a child's potential inheritance by a parent. However, unless a trust or similar fiduciary account established in the child's name is being abused, parents are generally free to spend their assets, wisely or unwisely, however they desire even if it results in their children not receiving an inheritance from them.

In addition, the nature of the relationship between perpetrators of financial abuse and their victims may create an expectation by third parties that at least some financial resources will flow from the victim to the perpetrator and this may obscure detection of abuse (Dessin, 2000). Indeed, the perpetrator may feel entitled to the elder person's assets and may point to the elder person's apparent tacit consent in attempting to establish the legality of a transfer. Such consent is unlikely to be forthcoming or is relatively easily dismissed as ineffectual when physical abuse is involved.

In general, third parties may be more likely to respond to and report instances of physical abuse than financial abuse. Within our society, victims of physical violence tend to receive greater attention, sympathy, and support than victims of financial exploitation. For example, the victims' rights movement, which in recent years has brought attention to the needs of victims of violent crime, has not similarly focused attention on the plight of victims of financial crimes (Nerenberg, 2000c). Also, children may elicit more sympathy and protection than the elderly and thus reports of their abuse may be more forthcoming.[23] These factors suggest that models for detecting and preventing financial abuse of the elderly may need to be more proactive than models used to respond to child abuse.

Decision-Making Capacity of Children and the Elderly

Another reason for adopting a model for addressing financial abuse of the elderly that is relatively distinct from that used to respond to child abuse is that issues associated with the decision-making capacity of the elderly are quite different from those associated with children (Nerenberg, 2000a). Unlike children, elder persons at some point generally possessed the capacity to handle their financial affairs and exercised control over these affairs. All adults are presumed to possess this capacity unless shown otherwise in a legal proceeding. Until an elder person is determined to lack decision-making capacity, the elder person has the right to make what may seem to be poor or foolish financial decisions (Gilbert, 1986; Macolini, 1995; Wilber and Reynolds, 1996).[24] In addition, to strip or limit the ability of elder persons to make such decisions can be psychologically devastating as it may represent for them the removal of the last vestige of independence and emphasize their physical and mental decline, which in turn may accelerate this decline (Dessin, 2000). As a result, many elder persons will actively

---

[23]It has been argued that 1 of 3 cases of child abuse is reported compared to 1 in 5 or 1 in 15 cases of elder abuse (Rosenblatt et al., 1996).

[24]As will be discussed below, an elder person, like all persons, is entitled to legal protection if a financial decision is the result of fraud or undue influence.

resent and resist any steps to limit their financial independence (Macolini, 1995). For example, in Massachusetts approximately one-fifth of the elder persons for whom a report of abuse was filed refused a resulting offer of state services (Dessin, 2000).[25] It should be noted that such reports are typically limited to relatively egregious incidents. Such data may suggest that intervention to address the financial abuse of the elderly should be limited to when there is fraud, duress, or undue influence or a clear lack of capacity to make an informed decision (Dessin, 2000).[26] At a minimum, any model to prevent or remedy financial abuse of the elderly needs to take into account the fact that elderly victims are adults who in general previously had complete autonomy over their financial transactions (Dessin, 2000).[27] In particular, any such model needs to address whether and how to proceed when the elder person denies a need for assistance or resents or resists intervention (Capezuti et al., 1997).

Second, determining when an elderly person lacks decision-making capacity can be a difficult matter. Even if an elderly person intermittently experiences diminished capacity, he or she may in general retain decision-making capacity. Decision-making capacity among children is quite clearly, even if somewhat arbitrarily, demarked by the age of majority.[28] For elder adults, decision-making capacity tends not to be an all-or-nothing concept. An individual with a cognitive impairment may have the capacity to make some decisions but lack capacity to make others. Also, this capacity may vary over time, with individuals having good days and bad days (Dessin,

---

[25]Macolini (1995) reported that 6 states and the District of Columbia require the consent of the elder person before commencing an investigation of a report of elder abuse and that 29 states and the District of Columbia specifically require the consent of the elder person before services can be provided. See also Shifcraw et al. (1994); in cases in which allegations of elder abuse were substantiated on investigation by APS staff and clients were offered protective services, 13 percent of the victims refused such services; Gilbert (1986); perhaps 40 percent of the older adults who health care professionals believed were abused refused intervention and services.

[26]Such refusals are honored in Massachusetts unless there appears to be coercion or a lack of capacity to make an informed consent (Dessin, 2000). Some may argue (although not without vigorous opposition) that physical abuse or neglect poses a more immediate threat to the well-being of the elderly and thus necessitates a more proactive model akin to that used for child abuse.

[27]For example, even if the cognitive capacity of elder persons has become limited, their personal involvement in these transactions may provide a valuable source of information that should not be ignored.

[28]There are certain circumstances defined by state law when a child who has not reached the age of majority is considered emancipated and is therefore considered to have capacity to make decisions on his or her own behalf. In addition, a few states have recognized a mature minor doctrine.

2000; Langan and Means, 1996).[29]   Also, the diminishment of decision-making capacity is often a gradual process. Determining when individuals no longer have the capacity to make financial decisions for themselves is often difficult (Nerenberg, 2000a).

The American legal system places great weight on the right of individuals to make decisions for themselves, whether they be good or bad decisions, and limits when someone who has experienced a diminishment of decision-making capacity can have these rights curtailed. Furthermore, the definitions and elements of decision-making capacity tend to vary considerably (Nerenberg, 2000c). A general consensus has developed that an evaluation of incapacity should be based on an appraisal of the functional limitations of the person. However, what comprises a functional limitation and what this appraisal should be based on is frequently poorly articulated and inconsistently applied.[30]

In addition, a wholesale adoption of a child abuse model can contribute to the infantalization of the elderly and the perpetuation of ageism as the elderly are mistakenly assumed to be like children and to lack decision-making capacity (Capezuti et al., 1997; Gordon, 1986; Kapp, 1995; Macolini, 1995; Nerenberg, 2000a; Tueth, 2000). Physical decline does not necessarily correspond to significant mental decline and there is no evidence that advanced years or physical disability alone render a person incapable of making decisions (Gilbert, 1986; Wilber and Reynolds, 1996). Many, if not most, elderly individuals retain their capacity to make financial decisions for themselves (Dessin, 2000). It has been noted that professionals, especially nonhealth ones, often jump to the wrong conclusion that elderly people have dementia or otherwise lack decision-making capacity (Langan and Means, 1996). Elder persons may justifiably resent the imposition of a paternalistic model that appears to presume their lack of capacity, imposes supervision of their decisions, and seeks to make financial decisions on their behalf or delegate their decision-making authority to others (Kapp, 1995).

---

[29]Medication levels alone may induce a significant fluctuation in an individual's decision-making capacity.

[30]This evaluation includes an appraisal of the individual's ability to provide for his or her financial needs, to understand the issues being addressed, to communicate about these issues, to obtain needed financial assistance, to participate in the decisions being made, to understand the ramifications of these decisions, and to provide ongoing oversight of them. See, e.g., Dessin (2000); "The Uniform Probate Code focuses on the ability to make choices by defining incompetence as 'lacking sufficient understanding or capacity to make or communicate responsible decisions.'"

Impact of Differences Between Child Abuse and
Financial Abuse of the Elderly

As a result of the differences between child abuse and financial abuse of the elderly, models for redressing financial abuse of the elderly may need to adopt a different approach from that used in child abuse models. In light of the scarce amount of research on the topic, it is difficult to determine how a child abuse model might be usefully applied to the financial abuse of the elderly. If financial abuse of the elderly is more difficult to detect than child abuse, financial abuse of the elderly could necessitate a model that is more proactive in detecting and responding to instances of such abuse. Similarly, if research indicates that large numbers of egregious incidents of elder financial abuse go unreported or unaddressed under a child abuse model, more expansive measures than established under a child abuse model may be necessary to enhance the filing of financial abuse reports and their subsequent investigation.

On the other hand, if research shows that victims of financial abuse find reports and subsequent interventions to be relatively invasive and re-pugnant, the reporting and investigation of financial abuse may need to be circumscribed more narrowly than is typical for child abuse. If research shows that most elderly persons resist or resent intrusion into their financial affairs, that most older persons have bona fide reasons for their resistance or resentment, or that most reports are not subsequently confirmed, argu-ably the criteria for reporting or undertaking an investigation of reported abuse should be narrowed from that applied to reports of child abuse. Under such circumstances, greater weight may need to be given to the wishes of purported victims and their right to enter into or remain in what appear to be abusive interactions (Dessin, 2000).

As current research, albeit relatively scanty, tends to show support for both of the above scenarios, a dichotomous model relatively unique to financial abuse of the elderly may be needed. A paternalistic model (similar to that used for child abuse) might be applied to elder persons for whom a determination can be made that there is a lack of financial decision-making capacity. However, a less paternalistic model would be used for those elderly persons for whom such a determination cannot be made. For the former, the *parens patriae* rationale associated with the child abuse model is arguably more fitting, justifying vigorous efforts to monitor their vulner-ability to financial abuse and to enhance the reporting and investigation of potential abuse. For the latter, our legal system dictates that such individu-als be presumed to know what is in their best interests. Even if a transfer of resources seems unjustified or inequitable to a third party, reporting and intervention would be limited to when there is an indication of fraud, duress, undue influence, or the like. Of course, determining when an individual lacks financial decision-making capacity can be a difficult matter (unlike for children, where age provides a blunt but clear dividing line) and additional research would be needed to establish how this can or should be done on a routine basis. Nevertheless, there are elderly persons for whom there is clearly a lack of financial decision-making capacity and for whom the dichotomy can clearly be applied.

Applicability of the Spouse Abuse Model to Financial Abuse of the Elderly

A number of commentators have argued that financial abuse of the elderly should be viewed as a form of domestic violence and that legislative models targeting spouse abuse better address its dynamics and serve its victims (AARP, 1993; Brandl, 2000; Brandl and Meuer, 2000; Heisler, 1991; Vinton, 1991, 1999; Vinton et al., 1997).[31] For empirical support, an elder abuse survey conducted by Pillemer and Finkelhor (1988) is primarily and widely cited (see AARP, 1993; Vinton, 1991, 1999; Vinton et al., 1997). Pillemer and Finkelhor (1988) asserted that their research on elder abuse indicates that spouse abuse provides a better model for understanding and addressing elder abuse than does child abuse.[32] They argued that a child abuse model has been widely, but inappropriately, employed in responding to elder abuse because it was initially believed that elder abuse is intergenerational in nature. They contested this assumption based on their research findings that spouses were more likely to be perpetrators of elder abuse than adult children of the victim (58 percent versus 24 percent,

---

[31]The following discussion focuses on the applicability of a spouse abuse model to financial abuse of the elderly. A similar debate has focused on whether this model provides a better fit for elder abuse in general. See AARP (1993); Brandl (2000); Brandl and Meuer (2000); Heisler (1991); Nerenberg (2000a); Vinton (1991, 1999); and Wolf (2000). Although the debate continues, a number of commentators have rejected sole reliance on both caregiver stress (which is cited as providing a rationale for adopting the child abuse model) and caregiver violence (which is cited as providing a rationale for adopting a spouse abuse model) in favor of an approach that views elder abuse as encompassing a range of factors that may or may not be present in any given case and that invokes different models depending on the specific circumstances involved (Anetzberger, 2000; National Center on Elder Abuse, 1996; Nerenberg, 2000a; Ramsey-Klawsnik, 2000; Wolf, 2000).

[32]Pillemer and Finkelhor (1988) argue that shifting from an underlying child abuse model to a spouse abuse model would (1) better inform service providers about situations in which elder abuse is likely to occur, (2) help educate elders that abuse by a spouse is inappropriate and encourage them not to accept it, and (3) better shape services provided in response to elder abuse along lines already provided to abused spouses, such as battered women's shelters and self-help groups.

respectively) and that there was no statistically significant difference in the seriousness of the abuse inflicted by these two groups of perpetrators.

However, Pillemer and Finkelhor did not include financial abuse in their definition of elder abuse. Thus, they did not examine its occurrence and did not determine whether spouses or adult children of the victims were more likely to be perpetrators of financial abuse. In contrast, as noted above, the NEAIS report found that 45 percent of the perpetrators of financial abuse were age 40 or younger and only 4.9 percent of the incidents involved a spouse (National Center on Elder Abuse, 1998). In addition, Choi and Mayer (2000) found that spouses were the perpetrators of financial exploitation in only 1.5 percent of all financial exploitation cases. It has been widely asserted that it is adult children and grandchildren of the elderly that are particularly likely to perpetrate financial abuse (Coker and Little, 1997; Quinn, 2000; Rush and Lank, 2000; Sklar, 2000).

In addition, the underlying dynamic provided by Pillemer and Finkelhor (1988) to explain the occurrence of the forms of elder abuse they studied (physical abuse, psychological abuse, and neglect) further suggests that a spouse abuse model may not be appropriate for addressing financial abuse of the elderly. They argued that an elder person is most likely to be abused by the individual with whom the elder person lives. They reasoned that the higher proportion of elder abuse committed by spouses reflected the fact that many more elders live with their spouses than with their children. However, as discussed, a frequently identified precursor of financial abuse of the elderly is their social isolation and, in particular, their living alone (Hwang, 1996; National Committee for the Prevention of Elder Abuse, 2001; Podnicks, 1992; Quinn, 2000; Rush and Lank, 2000). Victims of financial abuse are more likely to be widowed and to report they have no one to help them in the event of illness or disability, while victims of physical violence tend both to be married and to be living with their abuser (Choi et al., 1999; Podnieks, 1992). These findings further suggest that a spouse abuse model may be inappropriate when developing responses to financial abuse of the elderly.

Finally, spouse abuse models have focused heavily on curbing physical violence (Moskowitz, 1998b). Not surprisingly, these models center on the physical injuries such violence is likely to produce and the need to promote the safety of victims and means by which such injuries can be reduced (Brandl, 2000; Council, 1992; Klingbeil and Boyd, 1984; Vinton, 1991). The financial abuse of spouses has been a relatively minor concern. Although some commentators assert that financial abuse of the elderly almost always occurs in conjunction with physical abuse (Vinton, 1991), there is little research that has addressed this issue and what there is suggests the contrary (Podnieks, 1992). In general, the applicability of a spouse abuse model has not been tested with older women (Nerenberg, 2000a) and the "cycle of violence" that forms a foundation for the spouse abuse model may have limited applicability to the financial abuse of the elderly.

While a spouse abuse model may be appropriate when addressing the physical abuse of the elderly, as well as a subset of financial abuse cases when physical violence and financial abuse coexist, the spouse abuse model (like the child abuse model) does not appear to provide a comprehensive explanatory model for financial abuse of the elderly.[33] A more eclectic approach that focuses on the relatively unique aspects of financial abuse of the elderly may be more appropriate. Among the specific factors that such an approach might encompass are the intergenerational nature of this abuse and tensions likely to occur across generations; the impact of financial dependence on these tensions; whether and when physical abuse and violence tend to accompany financial abuse and their impact; the nature and impact of more subtle forms of influence than violence; whether elder victims of financial abuse perceive the perpetrators of this abuse differently than perpetrators of physical abuse; and whether financial abuse is more likely to reflect mismanagment, financial need, or greed rather than a desire for power and control and the influence they exert on the manifestations of financial abuse. At the same time, such a model (and accompanying research) should also attend to the potential influence of factors typically associated with spouse abuse models such as the impact of power and control on financial abuse, victims' incorporation of internalized messages that they are to blame for this abuse, victims' fear of retaliation if they disclose their abuse, and social contexts that may lead an elder person to fear disruption of the status quo (Vinton, 1999).

REPORTING STATUTES

Forty-four states and the District of Columbia have enacted statutes that mandate the reporting of elder abuse by certain individuals, with the other states providing for the voluntary reporting of such abuse (Stiegel, personal communication, October 2001).[34] Although virtually all states specifically mention financial abuse in their reporting statutes (Moskowitz, 1998b; Roby and Sullivan, 2000), they often do not establish special procedures for the reporting and subsequent processing of reports of financial

---

[33]Indeed, the American Medical Association's Council on Ethical and Judicial Affairs has asserted that spouse abuse differs from elder abuse (and child abuse) in opposing mandatory reporting of spouse abuse by physicians (Council on Ethical and Judicial Affairs, 1992).

[34]Reporting is voluntary in Colorado, New Jersey, New York, North Dakota, South Dakota, and Wisconsin (Brandl and Meuer, 2000).

abuse.[35] States with mandatory reporting generally impose penalties, such as fines, imprisonment, or license revocation, if reporting does not occur within a specified time period following discovery of the abuse (Capezuti et al., 1997; Kapp, 1995; Macolini, 1995; Marshall et al., 2000; Moskowitz, 1998b), although enforcement is generally lax (Heisler and Quinn, 1995; Roby and Sullivan, 2000). According to Roby and Sullivan (2000), almost half of these states have universal mandatory reporting, while the other states limit mandatory reporting to specifically identified categories of professionals. Reporting is frequently mandatory for certain professionals, such as police officers, social workers, welfare and mental health workers, nursing home employees, and licensed health care providers, and permissive for all others (Dessin, 2000). In several states, certain professionals who have a confidential relationship with the elder person (e.g., clergy, physicians, lawyers, and therapists) are exempt from reporting, while other states require reporting notwithstanding conflicting confidentiality rules (Roby and Sullivan, 2000). The professionals mandated to provide reports vary from state to state (Moskowitz, 1998b).[36]

States typically provide good faith immunity for the reporter, regardless of whether abuse is confirmed and regardless of whether the reports came from a mandatory or a voluntary reporter (Capezuti et al., 1997; Moskowitz, 1998a; Roby and Sullivan, 2000). In most states, professionals who report abuse are also protected by disclosure confidentiality laws that prohibit the disclosure of the identity of the person who provided the report without that person's written consent (Marshall et al., 2000; Moskowitz, 1998a). States vary as to when a report is required, with most states having a more stringent standard for individuals having contact with the elderly in their professional capacity and a generic standard for everyone else (Roby and Sullivan, 2000).

Reports are generally directed to an agency authorized to initiate an investigation, with this investigation to be started within a specified time period (Moskowitz, 1998b; Roby and Sullivan, 2000). If the agency that received the report is not a law enforcement agency, it will turn the matter over to a criminal justice agency if it determines that a crime might have been committed, although some states require that a competent victim give permission to proceed (Henningsen, 2001; Roby and Sullivan, 2000). In

---

[35]But see Wisconsin where investigations of reports of material financial abuse must begin within five business days, while investigations of other forms of elder abuse must begin with 24 hours (Henningsen, 2001).

[36]At least 20 types of professionals are listed as mandatory reporters in the various states, including ambulance drivers, attorneys, bank personnel, chiropractors, clergy, and dentists (Moskowitz, 1998b).

addition, typically an agency is empowered to coordinate the provision of services for the elderly person determined to be at risk and to intervene to protect endangered individuals (Moskowitz, 1998b).

Sources of Reports

Third parties, not the victims themselves, are the most likely to report elder abuse in general (Choi and Mayer, 2000; Lavrisha, 1997; Moskowitz, 1998b; Tueth, 2000). The NEAIS review of substantiated APS reports in 1996 found that 25.7 percent of the reports came from hospitals, physicians, nurses, and clinics, 20 percent came from family members, 14.8 percent came from in-home or out-of-home service providers, 11.3 percent came from the police or sheriff, 9.1 percent came from friends or neighbors, and only 8.8 percent came from the victims (National Center on Elder Abuse, 1998). Most mandatory elder abuse reports appear to come from health-care providers, including home health-care providers, and family, friends, or neighbors of the victim (Rosenblatt et al., 1996; Wolf and Pillemer, 1989).[37]

For financial abuse, the NEAIS review found that the three most frequent reporters were friends and neighbors (15 percent), hospitals (14.2 percent), and family members (14 percent). Choi et al. (1999) found that two-thirds of the reports of suspected financial exploitation to an APS agency were made by social service or health care providers and one-third were made by other individuals, including relatives, friends, neighbors, landlords, law enforcement agencies, and banks. Choi and Mayer (2000) in a subsequent analysis determined that only 1.4 percent of the reports of elder abuse came from the victims, a figure that did not significantly vary when the focus was only financial exploitation cases.

It has been claimed that health care providers, particularly practitioners involved in the long-term care of the elderly, are in a unique position, perhaps the best position, to detect the financial abuse of the elderly (Bernatz et al., 2001; Hwang, 1996; Tueth, 2000). For example, it has been suggested that such practitioners may have the best opportunity to meet privately with the elder person outside the presence of a caregiver; may be asked for financial help or advice; may be likely to learn about an inability to pay for important services such as medical care; may learn that patients

---

[37]But compare Shiferaw et al. (1994); in a study of all reports of elder abuse over a three-year period to a county APS unit in North Carolina, the most referrals came from service agencies (32 percent), followed by family members (26 percent); Kleinschmidt (1997); "Physicians infrequently report elder abuse, despite being 'in an ideal position to recognize, manage, and prevent elder mistreatment.'"

have been forced to sign documents, provide loans or gifts, or sign documents they did not understand; may determine the elder person executed a power of attorney when the person lacked the mental capacity to do so; may notice suspicious companions and their relationship with the elder person; or may detect neglect that reflects financial abuse (Bernatz et al., 2001; Hwang, 1996; Lachs and Pillemer, 1995). It has been suggested that health care providers affirmatively ask patients whether they are being taken advantage of in any way (Bernatz et al., 2001; Lachs and Pillemer, 1995).

It has also been asserted that adding financial institutions to the list of mandatory reporters could "prove a valuable weapon against [financial] abuse" (Coker and Little, 1997:4). Similarly, lawyers have been identified as having a central role to play in identifying and preventing financial abuse of the elderly (Moskowitz, 1998a).

On the other hand, a report by the U.S. General Accounting Office concluded that increasing public and professional awareness of the existence of elder abuse was more important in identifying cases of elder abuse than reporting requirements and, although reporting laws are moderately effective in case identification, these laws were not effective in preventing first occurrences of elder abuse or treating substantiated cases (U.S. General Accounting Office, 1991). The U.S. General Accounting Office concluded that focusing the debate on the relative effectiveness of mandatory versus voluntary reporting was of questionable value (U.S. General Accounting Office, 1991). The U.S. General Accounting Office did not specifically address financial abuse, but it did include "material or financial exploitation" within its definition of elder abuse (U.S. General Accounting Office, 1991). In general, although not typically posed in the context of financial abuse, controversy has raged over whether elder abuse should be subject to mandatory reporting (Capezuti et al., 1997; Gilbert, 1986; Kapp, 1995; Kleinschmidt, 1997; Macolini, 1995; Moskowitz, 1998b; Podnieks, 1992; Roby and Sullivan, 2000).

Barriers to Reporting

As discussed, there is a wide consensus that elder abuse in general is greatly underreported (Coker and Little, 1997; Dessin, 2000; Marshall et al., 2000; Moskowitz, 1998b; National Center on Elder Abuse, 1996, 1998; Pillemer and Finkelhor, 1988; Wolf, 2000).[38] Although little data are

---

[38]But see Reis (2000), "It is also true that a seeming abuse is sometimes revealed as more benevolent when examined closely" (p. 13).

available on this point, there seems to be a general view that financial abuse of the elderly is perhaps even more likely to go unreported and thus undetected (Hwang, 1996; Wilber and Reynolds, 1996). For example, although it is frequently asserted that bank employees are particularly well positioned to detect financial abuse of the elderly (Coker and Little, 1997), a survey of a small number of banks in New York City found that 43 percent of the banks said they never reported financial abuse of the elderly to APS and 14 percent reported it only sometimes (Heisler and Tewksbury, 1992).

Reporting statutes rely on and are designed to encourage reports of elder abuse. A number of reasons have been given for this underreporting.

One potential source of reports is the victims themselves. As noted, victims are relatively unlikely to report financial abuse (Choi and Mayer, 2000; Kleinschmidt, 1997; National Center on Elder Abuse, 1998; Podnieks, 1992), reportedly more so than for other forms of elder abuse (Podnieks, 1992). Not surprisingly, one set of reasons for underreporting focuses on the characteristics of the victimized elder person. For example, the elder person may be embarrassed at falling victim to financial exploitation and may desire to avoid looking like a person who was too trusting (Coker and Little, 1997; Dessin, 2000; Hwang, 1996; Nerenberg, 2000c; Wilber and Reynolds, 1996). Similarly, elder persons may not want to report the financial abuse for fear it will suggest that they are having problems managing their affairs and provide a rationale for placement in a nursing home or the institution of a guardianship (Hwang, 1996; Nerenberg, 2000c). The elder person may also fear change and prefer the status quo, regardless of its deleterious nature (Dessin, 2000).

Elder persons may hold a view that some level of abuse is normal. For example, they may have a self-identity that they are weak or undeserving or a burden to others and thus may expect to be taken advantage of by others (Dessin, 2000). Alternatively, they may have prior experience living in an abusive environment where they witnessed abuse, were abused, or abused others and thus do not consider it abnormal (Dessin, 2000).

Because victims are often induced to cooperate in their own exploitation, they may believe that they are fully or partially to blame for their victimization (Nerenberg, 2000c). Alternatively, if the financial abuse has an impact on other family members, elder persons may be blamed for or feel responsible for the consequences (Deem, 2000). They may also be concerned that they will become a burden to their family as a result (Hwang, 1996).

The elder person may not realize that abuse occurred or that financial abuse is a crime that can be reported (Coker and Little, 1997; Deem, 2000; Wilber and Reynolds, 1996). Elder persons may also have an impairment that prevents them from reporting the abuse or from recognizing its existence (Dessin, 2000; Gordon, 1986; Smith, 1999).

A second set of reasons traces underreporting to the nature of the interaction between the victim and the perpetrator of financial abuse. A widely cited reason is the reliance of the victim on the perpetrator for support and care, a notion often planted and nurtured by the perpetrator, and a fear of losing this support and care (Dessin, 2000; Smith, 1999). The elder person may also fear the perpetrator, including a fear of retaliation that is heightened the more abusive the relationship is (Deem, 2000; Gordon, 1986; Hwang, 1996; Smith, 1999). The elder person may be reluctant to turn in a family member or someone with whom they feel a close bond (Coker and Little, 1997; Dessin, 2000; Nerenberg, 2000c; Wilber and Reynolds, 1996). Even if abusive, there may be a close personal relationship between the victim and the perpetrator (Smith, 1999). The victim may be unwilling to report financial abuse because it tends to be the result of a relationship gone wrong or a betrayal of trust rather than outright theft (Coker and Little, 1997; Wilber and Reynolds, 1996). Also, the elder person may feel a sense of responsibility for the perpetrator's actions, particularly in the case of a family member (Dessin, 2000).

A third set of explanations for underreporting identifies barriers associated with the system designed to receive and respond to such reports. For example, the elder person may be unaware of where to turn for help and how to initiate a report (Deem, 2000; Dessin, 2000). Similarly, the elder person may lack access to these channels, as when a perpetrator prevents the victim from leaving a residence or using a telephone (Dessin, 2000). It is also widely considered difficult for outsiders to detect financial abuse and thus to discern a need for such a report (Choi et al., 1999; National Center on Elder Abuse, 1998). Abuse may be relatively invisible to outsiders, particularly as it may unfold slowly, involve elders who are socially isolated, and not leave immediate, visible signs (Choi et al., 1999; Gordon, 1986).

As discussed above, an alternative source of such reports are various professional groups. However, the members of these groups have also been slow to report financial abuse of the elderly (Hwang, 1996). A number of explanations for this reluctance have been provided. For example, detecting financial abuse can be difficult, particularly when interactions are brief or where the individual does not have an expertise in financial affairs. Moreover, professionals may resist reporting because of a fear of being incorrect, because definitions are vague and ambiguous, or because of a fear of liability for filing incorrect reports (Lachs and Pillemer, 1995; Marshall et al., 2000; Sugg and Inui, 1992). Also, they may be unfamiliar with the reporting system and the implications and impact of filing reports (Lachs and Pillemer, 1995). Outsiders may not report financial abuse of the elderly because of their fear of getting involved in the "opening of a Pandora's box" (Sugg and Inui, 1992) or because the victim denies abuse occurred (Marshall et al., 2000). Finally, the perpetrator may prevent the professional from spending time alone with the elder individual (Paris et al., 1995).

Health care providers are one professional group whose reluctance to report financial abuse of the elderly has received considerable attention (Kleinschmidt, 1997). Physicians have been found to be most likely to report physical abuse and the least likely to report financial abuse (Rosenblatt et al., 1996). Health care providers may fear that raising concerns will offend or insult the patient, perhaps by impugning their financial competence, or invade the patient's privacy (Marshall et al., 2000). They may consider it an inappropriate topic for them to raise or believe that it goes beyond the scope of the evaluation provided (Lachs and Pillemer, 1995; Marshall et al., 2000; Tueth, 2000). Also, they may cite their busy schedules, particularly when it requires addressing a relatively complicated topic in a short period of time, or their lack of expertise and the absence of reliable standardized protocols for discerning whether finanancial abuse is present (Marshall et al., 2000; Rosenblatt et al., 1996). Also, they may believe financial abuse of the elderly occurs relatively infrequently among their patients[39] or that they are being asked to do too much already within the relatively short time they meet with patients (Rosenblatt et al., 1996; Sugg and Inui, 1992). Furthermore, it has been suggested that health care providers do not report financial abuse because they are uncertain as to where to make a report, believe it will not make a difference, or rationalize away its existence (Beck and Phillips, 1984). Although, as noted, some argue that health care professionals are well situated to detect and report financial abuse (Lachs and Pillemer, 1995; Paris et al., 1995), others argue that considering the many barriers faced, there are better ways by which physicians can serve their patients (e.g., by recommending the establishment of a guardianship or power-of-attorney when they identify that funds are being misappropriated) (Tueth, 2000).

Reliability of Reports

At the same time, studies have indicated that a relatively high percentage of elder abuse reports in general and reports of financial abuse of the elderly in particular are not substantiated following investigation (i.e., they

---

[39]This may be the case for emergency rooms. Fulmer and colleagues (1992), in a six-month study of the charts of elders seen in a hospital emergency department, found 3.4 percent of the patients suffered from neglect, 2.3 percent from abuse, 0.4 percent from violent crime, 0.2 percent from abandonment, and only 0.05 percent from exploitation. Arguably, however, this may be an unlikely setting for detecting financial abuse in elders and if relevant questions were not asked such charts are unlikely to reflect its occurrence.

are false positives).[40] For example, the national NEAIS report found that financial abuse reports to APS agencies were relatively unlikely to be substantiated (National Center on Elder Abuse, 1998). Only 44.5 percent of these reports from 1996 were substantiated, as opposed to 61.9 percent of physical abuse reports, 56 percent of abandonment reports, and 54.1 percent of psychological abuse reports. Only neglect reports (41 percent) were less likely to be substantiated.[41]

There may be a discrepancy between how an elder person perceives an act and how a third party, including a professional, perceives it (Shiferaw et al., 1994). It has been suggested that individuals who report elder abuse may be influenced by circumstantial evidence that is not confirmed on investigation (Shiferaw et al., 1994). An elder person may consider a financial conveyance to be a reward to someone for services rendered or kindnesses provided, while an outsider may find the gift to be out of all proportion to the nature of the service or kindness. Because professionals are often assigned responsibility to report suspected instances of financial abuse of the elderly, it is important that a professional's classification of behavior as abusive correlate at least to some degree with that of the older person (Marshall et al., 2000). As discussed, elder persons often refuse to cooperate with investigations triggered by reports of elder abuse or refuse offered services (Dessin, 2000; Kleinschmidt, 1997; Gilbert, 1986; Shiferaw et al., 1994), with one possible explanation being that they do not agree that what occurred was abuse.[42] Financial disputes, particularly among family members, tend to involve complicated interactions in which there may be conflicting perspectives on the appropriateness of the actions taken. Professionals reporting elder abuse may fail to evaluate the elder person's situation adequately (Capezuti et al., 1997). Also, commentators have argued that cultural differences may result in misperceptions of whether a given financial transaction constituted abuse (Brown, 1999; Griffin, 1999; Hall, 1999; Hudson and Carlson, 1999; Marshall et al., 2000; Moon, 2000; Nerenberg, 2000a; Sanchez, 1996; Wilber and Reynolds, 1996).[43]

---

[40]In general, it has been argued that what seems to be elder abuse may be more benevolent in nature on close examination (Reis, 2000).

[41]Another study found that 76 percent of the reports of elder abuse referred to an APS unit were not confirmed and, although the exploitation of resources was the most likely type of abuse to be confirmed, only 46 percent of those reports were confirmed (Shiferaw et al., 1994).

[42]Other explanations provided, as discussed above, are shame or embarrassment over their abuse, fear of reprisals by the perpetrator, reluctance to get a family member in trouble, guilt for causing family tensions, or fear of institutionalization (Gilbert, 1986).

[43]For example, cultural differences have been found to exist for Mexican-American, Korean-American, African-American, and Native American communities (Brown, 1999; Moon, 1999; Nerenberg, 1999a).

When viewed in conjunction with the barriers discussed above that limit the filing of such reports, it is likely that the elder abuse reporting system results in both an overreporting (i.e., false positives) and underreporting (i.e., false negatives) of financial abuse of the elderly.

OTHER SYSTEMIC POST-ABUSE RESPONSES

In part because of the many forms financial abuse of the elderly can take, commentators have noted the difficulty of crafting a response system that adequately redresses such abuse and deters its subsequent occurrence (Dessin, 2000). Because there is no federal statute that deals directly with financial abuse of the elderly, the issue has instead been addressed seriatim by the various states. It is not surprising that legislative measures for responding to financial abuse have often been criticized as piecemeal (Dessin, 2000). There has also been little systematic evaluation of these various measures and virtually no comparisons of their relative effectiveness. As will be discussed, drawbacks and limitations for each of them have been identified by commentators reviewing them. It has also been noted that the legal system would likely be overwhelmed if it was seen as the primary means of handling the financial affairs of even elder persons who lack decision-making capacity (Langan and Means, 1996). Nevertheless, most states have a range of measures available for responding to financial abuse of the elderly and new measures are being instituted (Stiegel, 2000).

Administrative/APS Agencies

All states have adopted some form of adult protective services law that enables state agencies to offer remedies to victims of elder abuse (AARP, 2001) and each state generally has an APS agency designed to prevent and address problems the elderly may face (Dessin, 2000).[44] These agencies focus on maintaining a system for receiving reports of mistreatment, investigating cases, and providing protection or assistance to the elder person rather than punishing the perpetrator (Moskowitz, 1998b; Otto, 2000; Roby and Sullivan, 2000). They generally can take steps to protect the elder person from further abuse, including obtaining protective orders and the initiation of a guardianship to place the assets of the elder person in the hands of a guardian (Capezuti et al., 1997; Dessin, 2000).

Advocates for the elderly complain that the federal government has inappropriately reduced the financial assistance it gives the states to develop and maintain protective services for the elderly and should be more

---

[44]One exception is North Dakota, which has an APS law but does not have a functioning APS program (Stiegel, personal communication, October 2001).

actively involved (AARP, 2001; Moskowitz, 1998b; Otto, 2000). Also, concerns have been raised about state failures to designate an agency with primary responsibility for preventing, investigating, and responding to elder abuse and about the inadequate funding, staffing, and training of such agencies (Capezuti et al., 1997; Dessin, 2000; Macolini, 1995).

Victims Services Network

A number of commentators have noted the limited availability of the victim services network for elderly victims of financial abuse and the lack of resources made available to them. Because these services have historically been targeted for victims of violent crime, it has been asserted that victims of financial abuse are treated like "second class victims" in the victim services network (Deem, 2000). In some states, restitution, case status notification, and prison release information are available only to victims of violent crimes (Deem, 2000). Similarly, it has been asserted that state social service programs are generally underequipped to educate the elderly about financial abuse prevention, to provide prevention services, to address the emotional needs of financial abuse victims (e.g., by providing support groups and counseling), to provide restitution advocacy or to help victims recover their losses, to supply emergency funds, and to otherwise provide needed services (Deem, 2000; Nerenberg, 2000c). Furthermore, there is a lack of referral programs to assist victims to locate services designed to assist them (Deem, 2000). Some states have fiduciary abuse specialist teams (FASTs), which consist of an interdisciplinary group of representatives from law enforcement, adult protective services, the office of the public guardian, the prosecutor's office, health and mental health providers, and expert financial and legal consultants to help victims recover or to prevent further loss of their assets (Bernatz et al., 2001; Heisler, 2000).[45] Of those programs that have been established to assist victims of financial crimes, little systematic evaluation has been conducted of their availability, impact, or effectiveness.

Although Congress in 1984 created the Victims of Crime Act Fund (VOCA) to assist crime victims, victim compensation funds provided through state programs established under this legislation were until recently available only to victims of violent crimes. In 2001, the Office for Victims of Crime (OVC), United States Department of Justice, issued revised guidelines for implementation of the crime victim compensation grant program (OVC, 2001). Although OVC had been lobbied to specifically encourage

---

[45]For a brief summary of 12 programs designed to assist victims of financial crimes, see Deem (2000).

states to include economic crime as a compensable crime category and had initially included language to that effect, in its final guidelines the OVC instead noted in its preamble to the guidelines that economic crime (including financial fraud of the elderly) was one of four emerging trends and that states should consider covering the unmet needs of these crime victims. Although the text of the guidelines clarifies that VOCA does not prohibit coverage of nonviolent crimes, the guidelines also reiterate that the priority under VOCA continues to be coverage for victims of violent crime. In addition, although financial counseling services for victims of economic crime is an allowable compensable expense, the guidelines specify that compensation grants cannot generally be used to redress property damage and loss, a form of compensation particularly relevant to victims of financial abuse.

Furthermore, only as of 1997 could victim assistance programs funded under VOCA serve victims of financial crimes (Deem, 2000). The absence of a reference to financial victims in the proposed Victims' Rights Constitutional Amendment has been cited as symbolic of their second-class status (Deem, 2000).

Criminal Investigations and Prosecutions

Following a report of elder abuse, a local APS agency generally conducts an investigation and if criminal behavior is suspected refers the matter to a local prosecutor's office, which will typically undertake an investigation of its own. Alternatively, a law enforcement agency that has received a report of elder abuse may also conduct an investigation and subsequently refer the matter for prosecution. The successful prosecution of financial abuse of the elderly has been characterized as rare (Wilber and Reynolds, 1996), with few prosecutions extending beyond the investigatory phase and most cases being closed due to lack of evidence (Heisler, 2000; Hwang, 1996). It has been asserted that the criminal justice system provides little deterrence to the commission of financial abuse of the elderly (Hwang, 1996). The extreme difficulty in detecting and proving abusive transactions has been widely noted (Coker and Little, 1997; Dessin, 2000; Heisler and Tewksbury, 1992). A number of barriers have been identified as impeding these investigations and prosecutions.[46]

For example, the initial task of defining financial abuse has been characterized as "daunting" (Dessin, 2000). Evaluating whether financial abuse occurred often requires complex and subjective determinations to distin-

---

[46]For a description of some specialized law enforcement and prosecutor units established to address financial abuse and promising criminal justice practices, see Heisler (2000).

guish between acceptable transactions and exploitative conduct and to separate misconduct from mismanagement (Central California Legal Services, 2001).

Unlike physical abuse or neglect, the manifestations of financial abuse are generally not immediately evident and discoverable (Dessin, 2000). There is a general attitude that outsiders should not meddle in the financial affairs of another (Dessin, 2000). As discussed, the victim is frequently reluctant to report the abuse or may have been unaware of its occurrence (Deem, 2000; Dessin, 2000). Voluntarily or involuntarily, the management of the victim's financial affairs may have been entrusted to another. The perpetrator may have taken steps to hide the abuse from the victim, or the victim may lack the capacity to recognize that the acts taken constituted financial abuse (Dessin, 2000). Compounding the problem is that financial abuse generally occurs in a private setting, enhancing the difficulty of detection (Dessin, 2000).

Another barrier is that the victims' diminished mental capacity may make it unclear whether they understood and consented to the financial transaction (Central California Legal Services, 2001). Alternatively, it can be difficult to determine whether the elder person was the victim of unfair persuasion or coercion (Central California Legal Services, 2001). As one commentator has noted, "in a relationship in which one person is likely to want to give and the other is likely to feel an entitlement to receive, how can the law identify improper transactions?" (Dessin, 2000:213).

Officials responsible for investigating and prosecuting financial abuse must often review and evaluate complex records, frequently without the assistance of a witness capable of testifying or willing to testify (Dessin, 2000). Relevant documents may be in the hands of perpetrators or may have been destroyed (Nerenberg, 2000c). Bank officials may resist releasing records because of fear of breaching privacy or confidentiality laws (Nerenberg, 2000c).

Investigating and prosecuting financial abuse typically requires expertise across a range of subject areas, and most law enforcement personnel and many prosecutors lack this expertise, with training in these areas often not provided and rotation through assignments preventing the acquisition of needed knowledge (Coker and Little, 1997; Nerenberg, 2000c). As a result of a lack of expertise, responsible officials may fail to recognize financial abuse or to pursue it effectively (Nerenberg, 2000c). Alternatively, officers and prosecutors with expertise may be inundated with such cases and forced to prioritize and limit the scope of their efforts (Nerenberg, 2000c).

Also, officials often view financial crimes as strictly civil matters and discourage their prosecution (Nerenberg, 2000c). Alternatively, they may perceive them as less serious or important than violent crimes and give them low priority (Nerenberg, 2000c). Financial crimes may also be given a low priority because investigating and prosecuting financial abuse can be extremely labor-intensive and time consuming. In addition, most police and prosecutors' offices lack adequate resources for handling complex financial crimes. Advocates for the elderly argue that federal agencies should assist the states in prosecuting elder abuse (AARP, 2001).

Prosecutors may be unwilling to pursue such cases because the elderly may be poor witnesses, particularly if because of diminished mental capacity they are unable to recall details of the crime (Nerenberg, 2000c; Oh, 1999). Particularly frail victims are likely to decline, become incapacitated, or die during the course of what are often protracted proceedings (Nerenberg, 2000c). Elders may find the criminal justice system incomprehensible and inaccessible, particularly when the individual has a physical or mental disability (Nerenberg, 2000c). Calls have been made for improved communication with victims throughout the criminal justice process (Deem, 2000).

Even when a report has been received and an investigation is proceeding, the perpetrator may continue to deplete the elder person's assets because many states have inadequate laws to freeze the victim's assets or to limit the perpetrator's ability to access those assets during the investigation (Nerenberg, 2000c). Complaints have been lodged that victims are not permitted to provide input into how much restitution to impose and that such restitution is often not a priority of the criminal justice system (Deem, 2000). It has been claimed that many judges fail to order restitution, prosecutors seldom ask for it, the system fails to consider the full value of the victims' financial losses, there is an absence of a designated agency overseeing restitution, and victims are not provided help in recovering funds (Nerenberg, 2000c).

There may also be a lack of a clear definition of where jurisdiction lies in such a case, and if the activities crossed county, state, and federal boundaries, responsibility for investigation and prosecution may be unclear and resisted by various officials (Nerenberg, 2000c). Further complicating the assumption of responsibility is that financial abuse may occur in conjunction with other crimes, such as assault, neglect, or false imprisonment, which are handled by different police or prosecutorial units (Nerenberg, 2000c). Because securing needed evidence can take a long time and because the abuse may not be discovered until long after it occurred, the applicable statute of limitations may pose a significant barrier (Nerenberg, 2000c).

There are two general categories of criminal laws that the states use to punish individuals who financially abuse the elderly (Dessin, 2000). First, such abuse may be criminally prosecuted under the state's general theft, extortion, or fraud statutes (Dessin, 2000; Moskowitz, 1998b), with some states permitting the sentencing judge to treat the advanced age of the victim as an aggravating factor (Dessin, 2000; Moskowitz, 1998b; Nerenberg, 2000c). Alternatively, perpetrators may be prosecuted under a specific penal statute that addresses (1) abuse of vulnerable adults (which either by legislation or by judicial interpretation has been extended to include elder persons), (2) elder abuse in general, or (3) financial abuse of the elderly specifically (Dessin, 2000; Moskowitz, 1998b). It has been estimated, however, that fewer than half of the states provide criminal penalties that directly address elder abuse (AARP, 2001). Advocates for the elderly assert that the federal government should encourage all states to make financial exploitation of older people a specific criminal offense to promote its prosecution (AARP, 2001). Empirical evidence, however, has not been generated to establish that the availability of such specifically targeted penal statutes results in either increased prosecution rates or deterrence of such crimes.

Civil Remedies

Although there may be a tendency to turn first to the criminal justice system (Mixson et al., 1992),[47] a range of civil remedies is also available for responding to financial abuse of the elderly. For example, in 1991 the California legislature enacted the Elder and Dependent Adult Civil Protection Act (CAL. HtmlResAnchor Welf. and Inst. Code §5600 et seq.).[48] This legislation established civil remedies against individuals and entities that committed elder abuse and provided incentives for attorneys to pursue such cases. It has been asserted, however, that most litigators ignored this act until a relatively recent opinion by the California Supreme Court established that considerable financial exposure can result from elder abuse (*Delaney v Baker,* 971 P.2d 986 (Ca. 1999); Mehta, 2000).

In general, civil litigation for financial abuse of the elderly has been infrequent (Moskowitz, 1998a), although it has been suggested that there will be more such litigation as civil and criminal agencies work together more cooperatively (Heisler and Quinn, 1995). A number of difficulties have been identified in conjunction with pursuing a civil remedy for financial abuse of the elderly. They include that the standard of proof typically applied to abuse cases in the civil system is clear and convincing evidence that the abuse occurred. Some advocates believe that this standard is too

---

[47]But see Heisler (2000), "Because elder abuse was rarely viewed as criminal conduct, litigation historically has been brought in civil courts" (p. 52).

[48]Similarly, Illinois established that treble damages and attorney fees be available for a civil judgment deciding property has been converted or stolen from an elder person by threat or deception (Moskowitz, 1998b).

demanding considering the difficulties noted above in establishing that financial abuse occurred and that a preponderance of the evidence standard would be better (Nerenberg, 2000c).

Another barrier to the pursuit of a civil remedy is the frequent unwillingness of attorneys to handle these cases (Moskowitz, 1998a, 1998b; Nerenberg, 2000c). Factors attributed to this shortage are the lack of incentives for attorneys to take such cases, which can be financially risky for the attorneys who must typically invest considerable time in the case and risk not getting paid if the victim dies before the case is resolved (Moskowitz, 1998b; Nerenberg, 2000c). Also, attorneys' fees may be difficult to collect as the perpetrator may be judgment proof and judges may be unable or reluctant to award such fees (Nerenberg, 2000c). If attorneys' fees are not available from the perpetrator, the misappropriated property may represent the elder person's life savings but still represent a relatively small sum in comparison to the attorneys' fees and the costs of litigation (Moskowitz, 1998b). Publicly funded legal assistance programs could provide an alternative source of attorneys, but these programs have been significantly curtailed in recent years (Nerenberg, 2000c). Problems of proof have also been cited as a disincentive for attorneys considering whether to accept such a case as victims often suffer from diminished mental capacity, memory loss, or speech difficulties (Moskowitz, 1998b). In addition, such cases require multiskilled attorneys who possess both litigation and financial skills (Nerenberg, 2000c).

Another barrier is the lack of agreement over what level of decision-making capacity is needed for various contractual agreements. Although there is general agreement over the level of capacity necessary to make a will, there is less agreement, for example, over the level of capacity needed to give gifts or to get married (Nerenberg, 2000c). The following is a discussion of some specific civil remedies that may be available.

Fraud

Among the civil penalties for financial abuse are traditional tort remedies for conversion and fraud (Dessin, 2000). For the reasons discussed above, attorneys have been generally reluctant to pursue such civil remedies on behalf of elderly clients who have been the victims of financial abuse. One advantage, however, of these remedies is that punitive damages may be available against the perpetrator. For example, in 1998 the Alabama Supreme Court approved an award of punitive damages to a couple who were defrauded by an insurance agent into cashing in their paid-up policy and buying other coverage (Frolik, 2001). At the same time, curbs on punitive damages have been instituted in a number of states, and many judges are reluctant to allow them to be awarded.

Undue Influence

An alternative civil remedy that may be available is a claim that a transaction was the product of undue influence (Dessin, 2000). Although this remedy varies from state to state, the doctrine is generally available to set aside both *inter vivos* transfers and transfers at death (Dessin, 2000). Undue influence consists of the concerted, deliberate effort to assume control over another person's decision making (Nerenberg, 2000c). Just as transactions made by persons who lack mental capacity are not legal, transactions by persons who are victims of undue influence are also illegal (Nerenberg, 2000c). Undue influence occurs when individuals use their role and power to exploit the trust, dependency, and fear of others to deceptively gain control over the decision making of another (Bernatz et al., 2001; Quinn, 2000). Both mentally competent persons and persons with diminished mental capacity can be unduly influenced (Nerenberg, 2000c; Quinn, 2000). Elder persons have been identified as being vulnerable to undue influence when there is a close relationship in which the abuser is trusted and the elder person either suffers from cognitive impairments, is socially isolated, or is in a major life transition, such as widowhood (Quinn, 2000).

There have been complaints, however, that the standard used to establish undue influence is extremely vague and difficult to prove and that existing assessment mechanisms are inadequate (Nerenberg, 2000c). It has been noted that "[p]art of the difficulty in identifying and defining undue influence stems from the fact that it is a process as opposed to a discrete action, event, or condition" (Nerenberg, 2000c). It has also been noted that little is known about the close bonds that develop naturally between caregivers who provide personal care and companionship to elders in their own homes and what constitutes exploitation as opposed to gift giving under these circumstances (Quinn, 2000).

Protective Orders

A protective order is another type of civil remedy that may be available to redress or prevent financial abuse of the elderly. For example, an order could be obtained to prevent an individual from committing further financial abuse, to stay away from the victim, to provide a financial accounting, or to pay the costs the elder person incurred in seeking the protective order (Dessin, 2000; Moskowitz, 1998b). Such protective orders, however, do not appear to have been widely used in responding to the financial abuse of the elderly and have been asserted to be a relatively ineffective response (Brandl and Meuer, 2000).

Abuse of Power of Attorney[49]

A general power of attorney appoints one individual to act in place of, or on behalf of, another person. For example, a homebound elder person may grant a power of attorney to a family member to conduct transactions at the bank on his or her behalf. A durable power of attorney continues after the principal loses decision-making capacity. The power may become effective when signed or may be a "springing power of attorney" that takes effect at a specified future time or on the occurrence of a specified future event or contingency (e.g., the incapacity of the principal). States have enacted a range of statutes to punish those who abuse powers of attorney (Brandl and Meuer, 2000). The misuse of a power of attorney has been explicitly classified as a theft (Arizona), a violation of an elder adult abuse statute (Utah, Montana, Nevada), an embezzlement (California, Oklahoma), and an exploitation of an infirm individual (Louisiana) (Thilges, 2000).

A durable power of attorney provides a simple, easily implemented, inexpensive tool for providing financial assistance to the elderly, but it is also subject to abuse (Nerenberg, 2000c; Weiler, 1989). Indeed, abuse of the durable power of attorney has been called an "invisible epidemic," a "license to steal," and the crime of the 1990s by practitioners who work with the elderly, in part because of the ease with which people can obtain and misuse durable power of attorney authority (Coker and Little, 1997; Hwang, 1996; Weiler, 1989).[50]

Among the abuses of powers of attorney that have been identified are having a power of attorney signed by a person who has a cognitive impairment at the time, using the power after it has terminated (e.g., the principal becomes incapacitated and the power is not a durable power), or using the power for purposes beyond those for which it was intended (Nerenberg, 2000c). The law generally presumes that the agent has the principal's permission to transact whatever business the document authorizes and unless the victim is able to testify, which is often not possible, it is difficult to prove otherwise (Hwang, 1996). It has been noted that few states require any type of registration by an agent, there are no mechanisms to ensure the principal has mental capacity at the time of signing or has not been coerced into signing, elders may not realize the extent of the authority they are

---

[49]For a discussion of civil remedies available when a perpetrator has occupied a fiduciary status in general, see Moskowitz (1998b).

[50]A 1994 survey of attorneys and service providers for the elderly found that two-thirds of the 410 respondents reported cases of abuse of the durable power of attorney and 38 percent knew of five or more such cases (Sacks, 1996).

assigning, elder persons may be imbued with a false sense of security by the fact that a notary must witness the signing of a power of attorney,[51] there are no requirements that the principal be notified when the power of attorney has been exercised, and there are few means to ascertain if a power of attorney is no longer effective or has been revoked (Nerenberg, 2000c). Other identified limitations are that the agent does not have to post a bond guaranteeing adherence to his or her fiduciary responsibilities, notice of the assignment of such authority is not provided to other individuals, including relatives of the elder person, there is no third party monitoring of the actions taken, the agent is not required to maintain or present records, and there is no way to regain misappropriated or mishandled assets short of a civil law suit (Heisler and Quinn, 1995; Weiler, 1989).

In general, if abuses occur, they are difficult to prove or rectify (Nerenberg, 2000c). Not surprisingly, it has been reported that although financial abuse through the illegal use of a power of attorney is frequent, few legal actions alleging the abuse of this power have been filed and even fewer have been successful (Oh, 1999). Civil actions may be fruitless as agents may be relatively judgment proof having exhausted the assets obtained from the elder person and lacking assets of their own (Henningsen, 2000). Similarly, criminal actions may be precluded by broad grants of authority to the agent that make it difficult to prove beyond a reasonable doubt that the agents exceeded the scope of their authority (Henningsen, 2000). Although some states have explored ways to bring more accountability into the use of this mechanism, it has been reported that "[t]hese efforts have met with mixed success" (Nerenberg, 2000c).[52]

Appointment of Guardian/Conservator

Perhaps the most drastic step that can be taken in response to financial abuse of an elder person is the appointment of a guardian (alternatively referred to as a conservator or a committee in some states) to make financial decisions for an elder person. Such an appointment requires a showing that the elder person lacks decision-making capacity. Because of its relatively drastic nature, concerted efforts have been made to establish less restrictive alternatives such as limited or partial guardianships and temporary guardianships (Heisler and Quinn, 1995).

---

[51]The role of the notary is simply to attest that the person signing the document is who he or she claims to be.

[52]For an excellent description of how attorneys can better draft powers of attorney and advise clients to avoid financial abuse, see Henningsen (2000).

Although establishing a guardianship or a conservatorship can be a useful mechanism for conducting the financial affairs of elder persons who lack decision-making capacity and can help shield their assets from abuse or be used to recover lost assets (Heisler and Quinn, 1995), a number of difficulties have been associated with this mechanism, and it is a remedy that is dreaded by many elder persons. For example, the costs of establishing and administering a guardianship can pose a significant drain on an elder person's resources (Nerenberg, 2000c) and it can be relatively complex and intrusive.[53] Also, individuals seeking establishment of a guardianship for an elderly person may be acting in their own interests rather than attempting to assist an elderly person in need (Heisler and Quinn, 1995). In addition, although establishing a guardianship requires judicial involvement, the court may not be provided with critical information or conduct a neutral investigation that focuses on the capacity of a proposed guardian to provide needed services to the elder person (Heisler and Quinn, 1995).

In addition, it may be difficult to obtain a reliable and trustworthy candidate to serve as guardian (Nerenberg, 2000c). Family members and friends of the elder person may not be available or interested in assuming such a role. Also, adequate court monitoring of the guardian may not be available (Heisler and Quinn, 1995). Public guardianship programs were created to serve vulnerable individuals and are usually more accountable (Roby and Sullivan, 2000), but many communities do not have public guardians, and where they do exist, the demand often far exceeds the supply (Nerenberg, 2000c). As a supplement, some private nonprofit agencies have started guardianship programs. Another option that has emerged is the use of private professional guardians and fiduciaries, although there have been reports of professional criminals seeking to fill these roles. Each of these options may also provide a further drain on the elder person's assets.

In general, there is little screening of potential candidates and review of their qualifications, notwithstanding that they may be responsible for managing significant wealth and ensuring the financial health of the elder person (Nerenberg, 2000c). Ensuring subsequent accountability by appointed guardians can also be problematic (Nerenberg, 2000c). The powers as-

---

[53]As discussed, alternatives such as durable powers of attorney can also be subject to abuse. Research has not been conducted on which of these measures leaves an elderly person more vulnerable, is more likely to be misused, or has more egregious consequences for an elderly person when misused. However, the law pertaining to the establishment of guardianships generally expresses a preference for alternatives that have been established by the elderly person and that ostensibly are less comprehensive in their assigned powers than is typically true of a guardianship.

signed to a guardian can be abused to misappropriate the elder person's assets. Periodic exposés have found guardians stealing funds from their wards. Although courts are ostensibly charged with this responsibility, their resources are often not sufficient to provide adequate ongoing investigation and monitoring of guardianships.

Also, the negative stigma associated with the establishment of a guardianship has made it an unattractive alternative for many elder persons and their families. One commentator wrote, "[t]o some seniors, the threat of being placed under guardianship is as terrifying as the threat of nursing home placement" (Nerenberg, 2000c). Advocates for the elderly have argued that the federal government should encourage the states to create less restrictive alternatives to guardianship and to educate those who are acting as guardians (AARP, 2001).

Limitations of Legal Interventions in General

Beauchamp (2001) argues that legal interventions to redress financial abuse of the elderly will inevitably be flawed and that no set of laws can be made perfect. In particular, he asserts an inherent tension between competing priorities that, on the one hand, seek to protect elder persons from people who desire to financially abuse them and, on the other hand, seek to respect the wishes of elder persons, which often include a desire to retain their independence. Also, he notes that the greater the level and extent of protections established, the greater the cost. He concludes the problem may not be a need to reform the law or to create new laws, but a need to enforce existing law. Furthermore, he contends, any approach will necessitate reliance on the good faith and efforts of the people assisting elder persons with their financial affairs, whether it be a family member, a fiduciary, or a judge, and there is little that laws can do to make people more caring or diligent in their duties.

PREVENTIVE MEASURES

Because investigating and proving financial abuse is often difficult and because perpetrators often spend or dissipate assets before abuse is discovered, preventive measures are the preferred means for addressing financial abuse of the elderly (Central California Legal Services, 2001).[54] A number

---

[54]Addressing elder abuse in general, a report of the U.S. General Accounting Office concluded that creating a high level of public and professional awareness of elder abuse was the most effective means for redressing elder abuse, more so than either mandatory or voluntary reporting laws (U.S. General Accounting Office, 1991).

of factors have been identified as likely to prevent financial abuse of the elderly, although this identification is generally derived from personal experience rather than from empirical investigation. A variety of approaches for identifying or preventing financial abuse have also been proposed or implemented, although little systematic evaluation has been conducted of their effectiveness. These approaches can be organized according to the individuals charged with preventing this abuse.

Elder Persons or Family Members and Friends of the Elderly

The first set of preventive approaches addresses steps elder persons and family members and friends of the elderly should take. Many advocates argue that the best measure is to prevent isolation by helping the elder person to stay in close contact with multiple friends and relatives (Hoban, 2000; National Clearinghouse on Family Violence, 2001; Podnieks, 1992; Quinn, 2000; Wilber and Reynolds, 1996; Zimka, 1997). Although, as noted, family members have been identified as the most likely perpetrators of financial abuse of the elderly, anecdotal accounts suggest that such abuse is not the result of a conspiracy among a number of relatives, but rather represents the actions of a single family member who has isolated the elder person from other family members or friends. Greater involvement of family members and friends of the elderly person can help prevent or remedy this isolation. Such isolation, it has been argued, can also be avoided by encouraging or helping the elderly person to be active in community affairs, senior centers, or religious or charitable organizations (Hoban, 2000; National Clearinghouse on Family Violence, 2001; Zimka, 1997). Advocates also emphasize the importance of educating the elderly to recognize financial victimization (Coker and Little, 1997; Podnieks, 1992).

Another series of preventive steps addresses transactions conducted with financial institutions. Recommendations include that checks received on a regular basis be mailed directly to banks to reduce the risk of theft (Hoban, 2000; National Clearinghouse on Family Violence, 2001; Zimka, 1997). Similarly, it has been suggested that routine bills, such as utility bills, be paid automatically from checking or savings accounts (Zimka, 1997). Arrangements might also be made that any effort to expand the number of individuals with access to an elder person's bank account result in the notification or require the consent of a third party (National Clearinghouse on Family Violence, 2001).

Other steps identified to prevent financial abuse include arranging for the payment of bills by a trusted friend, family member, or bill paying service (Zimka, 1997) or asking a trusted friend or family member to review all papers before they are signed (Hoban, 2000; National Clearinghouse on Family Violence, 2001). A written plan for repayment should be signed before money is loaned (National Clearinghouse on Family Violence, 2001). References of people being hired to serve as caregivers should be carefully screened and attention given to a caregiver who tries to isolate an older person (Zimka, 1997).

A number of suggestions have been made to prevent abuse of a durable power of attorney. It has been suggested that the elder person carefully choose a trustworthy friend or relative to act as the agent, appoint two trustworthy persons to act jointly thereby creating a check on their individual actions, establish a "springing power of attorney" that does not take effect until a specific event occurs such as the loss of capacity, and specify that the power of attorney does not take effect until two doctors have certified that the individual is incapacitated (Hwang, 1996). Important legal actions, such as preparing or revising a will and establishing a power of attorney, should be done with a lawyer's assistance (Hoban, 2000; National Clearinghouse on Family Violence, 2001).

When financial abuse is suspected, a number of courses of action have been suggested for elder persons or for individuals who are concerned about the well-being of the elderly. They include contacting a bank and requesting that it flag and observe activity in the elder person's account, arranging for a review of account activity and associated signatures, transferring funds to a new account or closing an old account, and requesting a bank investigation (Central California Legal Services, 2001; National Clearinghouse on Family Violence, 2001). Similarly, steps can be taken to revoke a power of attorney and to request an accounting (Central California Legal Services, 2001; National Clearinghouse on Family Violence, 2001). The Social Security Administration, the Veteran's Administration, or a pension board can be notified of the possible theft of benefit or annuity checks, of a new representative payee, or of new arrangements for direct deposit or delivery of checks (Central California Legal Services, 2001). Finally, steps can be initiated to remove a perpetrator from the home of the elder person or to establish a guardianship to protect the assets of the elder person (National Clearinghouse on Family Violence, 2001).

Financial Institutions

A group of individuals frequently cited as being best positioned to provide early detection of possible financial abuse are employees of banks or other financial institutions who interact with the elderly person or process account activity (Choi et al., 1999; National Clearinghouse on Family Violence, 2001; Podnieks, 1992; Zimka, 1997). One commentator noted that "[b]ank employees, given their frequent contact with older clients who prefer personal bank visits to automatic teller machines, are often the first to spot suspicious banking activity that may be indicative of abuse" (Tom,

2001). The NEAIS report concluded that "banks are in a good position to observe financial abuse and concerted attention should be given to how to better involve them" (National Center on Elder Abuse, 1998).

Alternatively, some retirement communities provide financial advice and assistance to members of the community. For a description of one such service that provided assistance with daily money management, see Bassuk (2001). Many elderly individuals who are the most likely targets of financial abuse are not members of such communities. Nevertheless, it has been argued that such models should be expanded to be readily available to all elderly individuals who need such advice and assistance (Bassuk, 2001).

In general, a series of recommendations targeted at the financial industry and its employees have been generated to minimize financial abuse of the elderly (Commonwealth of Massachusetts, 2001).[55] Among the steps recommended are that financial institutions employ training programs to help employees identify and redress such abuse (Commonwealth of Massachusetts, 2001; National Clearinghouse on Family Violence, 2001). Such a program implemented in New York provides instruction on who commonly commits financial exploitation, typical scenarios that lead to financial exploitation, ways to detect financial abuse, a model protocol for action, and prevention training (New York State Department of Law, 2000). Similarly, bank employees in Massachusetts received special training in the identification of possible cases of abuse of older persons' bank accounts (Price and Fox, 1997).[56] This training led to the identification of a number of cases of financial abuse (Price and Fox, 1997). Also, employees can be encouraged to tell older customers about good financial practices and ways to prevent financial abuse (National Clearinghouse on Family Violence, 2001).

Along with the development of model programs, barriers limiting the banking industry's participation in efforts to curb financial abuse of the elderly have also been identified. For example, bank employees may be hesitant to report customer financial information and potential financial exploitation because of privacy laws and confidentiality requirements that prohibit the disclosure of a client relationship or account information (Jackson, 2000; Tom, 2001; U.S. Congress, 2000).[57] In response, advance

---

[55]For a compilation of warning signs and suggestions generated specifically for Certified Public Accountants, see Rush and Lank (2000).

[56]The Massachusetts program is also being employed in California, Maryland, New York, Oregon, Utah, and Virginia (Commonwealth of Massachusetts, 2001).

[57]The banking industry has been reported to believe that statutes encouraging the voluntary reporting of elder abuse do not adequately shield financial institutions from liability (Tom, 2001). However, others believe that exceptions within state and federal law allow

directives have been designed that specifically permit banks to notify account holders and other named parties of activity that is inconsistent with the account holders' usual banking patterns (Tom, 2001).[58] Alternatively, financial institutions could be included within the list of mandated reporters of elder abuse, as in Arizona, although the banking industry has been reported to resist such inclusion because of its fear of additional government control over and involvement in its operations (Choi et al., 1999; Tom, 2001). Some states have instituted laws that specifically provide immunity to employees of financial institutions who had reasonable suspicion that a consumer is a victim of financial abuse and reported this information to the proper authorities (Jackson, 2000).

Businesses Providing Services to the Elderly

Businesses that routinely provide services to the elderly can also help minimize the potential for financial abuse of the elderly. For example, it has been noted that many utility companies offer helpful services such as direct payment plans, warning programs to notify customers before services are turned off due to nonpayment, and payment averaging plans (Central California Legal Services, 2001).

Attorneys

Attorneys are another group of individuals who may be well positioned to identify and respond to the potential financial abuse of the elderly. It has been suggested that attorneys be sensitive to the potential for financial abuse when drawing up powers of attorney or other legal documents (Podnieks, 1992) and proactively advise clients to limit the authority granted when establishing a power of attorney (Zimka, 1997). In addition, it has been suggested that steps be implemented to monitor an agent's activity by requiring an annual reporting to an outside party of the financial transactions undertaken, including a listing of income and expenses (Zimka, 1997). Another avenue is to encourage attorneys to ensure that older persons who

---

financial institutions to contact government entities and disclose otherwise private customer records and information concerning suspected violations of the law and that this would encompass elder abuse reports (U.S. Congress, 2000).

[58]A similar approach has been implemented in Canada, where older persons have begun authorizing their banks to monitor their accounts for unusually large transactions or unusual patterns of transactions, to subsequently raise concerns with the account holder, and to warn of the possibility of fraud (Smith, 1999). Resistance to financial advance directives has reportedly come primarily from larger financial institutions that cite additional paperwork and exposure to large class-action lawsuits as their reasons for not endorsing this approach (Smith, 1999).

sign financial and legal documents are fully competent to do so (Moskowitz, 1998a; Smith, 1999) and have not been coerced by family members or others into inappropriately disposing of their assets (Smith, 1999). Also, it has been recommended that lawyers inform older clients of their fundamental right to asset control and personal decision making and explain to them the consequences of various legal actions (Moskowitz, 1998a).

Fiduciaries

A fiduciary appointed to act on behalf of an elder person by necessity exercises considerable control over the finances of the elder person. Although advance planning regarding financial affairs and the execution of a financial advance directive may be undertaken in an effort to avoid subsequent financial abuse, such efforts have been undercut when the elder person's designated agent engages in financial abuse (Kapp, 1995). A number of steps have been identified to minimize the likelihood of financial abuse by fiduciaries. For example, a need for greater numbers of specially trained fiduciaries has been asserted (Sampson, 1996). But most proposals call for improved tracking or accountability of the fiduciary (Nerenberg, 2000c).[59] It has been suggested that in appropriate cases individuals who act under a power of attorney be required to prepare an annual statement setting out details of the year's financial activities (Smith, 1999). Similarly, it has been suggested that guardians and conservators be subject to IRS-style audits that would be performed by a state agency that would randomly select a small percentage of guardianships or conservatorships to review their records and to investigate the wards' situations (Beauchamp, 2001). Another suggestion is to delegate some of the duties of judges who are ultimately responsible for supervising conservatorships and guardianships to other officials who specialize in these appointments and who may be better situated to investigate them (Beauchamp, 2001). It has also been argued that too many elders are not represented at their competency hearings, that assigned powers are overly broad and based on convenience rather than necessity, that statutorily required annual accountings often go unfiled, and that curtailed rights of the elderly are rarely reviewed and almost never restored, notwithstanding changes in the elder person's decision-making capacities (Sampson, 1996).

Some commentators suggest that the best solution is to avoid a conservatorship or guardianship altogether and to employ alternatives such as trusts, durable powers of attorney, representative payees, and joint tenancy

---

[59]For an annotated bibliography of materials addressing financial exploitation of the elderly by a conservator, see Sampson (1996).

that are more flexible, less costly, and avoid judicial scrutiny (Beauchamp, 2001; Weiler, 1989). At the same time, it has been recognized that these alternatives may also present problems, including a lack of oversight and means to ensure assets are devoted to the elder person's needs (Beauchamp, 2001; Heisler and Quinn, 1995; Weiler, 1989). At least one commentator has concluded no alternative is foolproof and "society may just have to rely on the person who takes care of the vulnerable and hope that that person does not take advantage of her position" (Beauchamp, 2001).

Health Care Providers

Finally, it has been suggested that health care providers are in a unique position to prevent financial abuse of the elderly (Bernatz et al., 2001; Lavrisha, 1997). Health care providers who see their elderly patients regularly may be in the best position to know if an older person's mental capabilities have declined to such an extent that the individual is subject to financial abuse (Smith, 1999).[60]

It has been suggested, for example, that nurses in the community and in clinics are likely to encounter elder persons at risk and can assess the level of social support available, provide education on how to avoid financial exploitation, and make appropriate referrals to volunteer companion programs and the like (Lavrisha, 1997). In addition, it has been argued that nurses have an ethical and often a legal responsibility to recognize and detect potential financial mistreatment and that gerontological nurses in particular can encourage the initiation of appropriate responses to financial abuse such as the establishment of a representative payee, a durable power of attorney, a trust, or a joint tenancy (Weiler, 1989). It has also been recommended that when a person is diagnosed with a disorder that diminishes mental capacity (e.g., Alzheimer's disease), health care providers should warn the patient and family members about the potential for financial abuse and provide practical suggestions on how to avoid such abuse (e.g., by having a cosigner on bank accounts) (Bernatz et al., 2001). One physician has suggested that clinicians working with older people should consider including questions about financial affairs in their routine history and be particularly concerned when socially isolated and frail older people talk of unpaid bills, new friends who are visiting regularly and borrowing money, ongoing home renovations, or frequent large purchases (Cohen, 1998).

---

[60]At the same time, an assessment of individuals 70 years of age or older who were presented for treatment at a hospital emergency room found that one of the three areas with which patients needed the most assistance was the management of finances (medications and ambulation were the other two areas) (Fulmer and Cahill, 1984).

Education regarding financial abuse of the elderly, warning signs, and steps that can be taken to minimize or remedy such abuse could be targeted at health care providers who regularly provide services to the elderly. In addition, protocols for detecting elder abuse that include questions pertaining to financial abuse have been developed for physicians (Kleinschmidt, 1997; Tueth, 2000), nurses (Fulmer and Cahill, 1984), and emergency department professionals (Fulmer et al., 1992) and could be made more readily available to them.

Social Services/Governmental Agencies

Social services agencies may already be responsible for providing services to elder persons who are vulnerable to financial abuse and they could be assigned a specific or enhanced role in preventing such abuse. Alternatively, they could be given responsibility for providing financial assistance to the elderly. For example, as noted, some states have fiduciary abuse specialist teams (FASTs), which include expert financial and legal consultants, to help victims recover or prevent further loss of their assets (Bernatz et al., 2001). Such teams could be made available to elder persons seeking advice on or assistance with financial decisions as a means to prevent financial abuse of the elderly.

Alternatively, assessment instruments for detecting elder abuse, which include signals of financial abuse, have been developed for caseworkers visiting elders in the community (Reis, 2000; Sengstock and Hwalek, 1986). However, one survey found little enthusiasm for involving social services agencies in these surveillance efforts, with caseworkers stressing that sorting out financial affairs was complex and time-consuming (Langan and Means, 1996). In addition, it has been noted that social service agencies have long recognized the need to provide financial assistance, including assistance with daily money management, but the scope and availability of such services vary greatly around the country and few free or low-cost programs provide a full range of such services (Bassuk, 2001). It is also likely that many elder persons would be reluctant to permit governmental agencies and personnel to become involved in their financial affairs. Moreover, it has been noted that elders and their relatives are often not aware of financial-management services offered by community-based agencies (Choi and Mayer, 2000).

FUTURE RESEARCH NEEDED

Two of the leading authorities on financial abuse of the elderly have identified what they consider to be the important research questions. Nerenberg writes:

> [L]ittle is known about the extent or nature of financial crime. Apart from a few studies on telemarketing fraud, very little is known about other types of financial crime, including fraud by family members. Even less is known about the impact of financial crime on its victims, victims' service needs, and promising approaches to meeting those needs. . . . Even less is known about victims' mental health or social service needs and effective approaches to addressing them (2000c:70).

In contrast, the NEAIS report (National Center on Elder Abuse, 1998) raised the following research questions:

> Are there characteristics of the caregiving relationships among younger family members who financially exploit their older relatives that could be affected by service interventions for the perpetrators? What are those interventions? Are there services or education for persons aged 60+ that would help them from becoming victims of financial abuse, particularly by younger family members? How can employees of banks be educated and encouraged to identify and report incidents of financial exploitation that may come to their attention while serving elderly customers?

The analysis provided in the course of this report has also identified a number of research questions. Although greater attention has been given to financial abuse of the elderly in recent years, most of the accompanying commentary relies on anecdotal evidence, personal experience, or commonly shared beliefs. There is a great need for a research foundation to be generated to inform the debate over how best to respond to this abuse. In addition to the many issues that have not been subject to systematic research, there is a need for existing studies that rely on small samples to be replicated at a national or regional level and for this research to be conducted in a methodologically rigorous manner. Conducting research on elder abuse in general has proven to be difficult (see Comijs et al., 2000; Thomas, 2000), and these same difficulties generally apply to research on financial abuse of the elderly.[61]

In addition, there are special challenges associated with conducting research on financial abuse of the elderly. These challenges include the absence of a consistent, objective operational definition of what constitutes financial abuse; ascertaining what impact, if any, cultural differences and subjective perceptions (especially those of the elderly person) should play; whether a minimal financial amount should be involved before financial abuse is considered to have occurred; particular difficulties associated with

---

[61]See Langan and Means (1996); Research on financial abuse is often quite limited, being based on very small samples or an investigation of case files of those elderly people defined by statutory agencies as victims of abuse.

detecting and establishing the occurrence of financial abuse; what role the intent of the alleged perpetrator should play; discerning the existence, relevance, and impact of the tacit acknowledgment and consent of the elder person; and whether, particularly for smaller financial amounts, a pattern of abuse is required or a single incident will suffice to establish abuse.

The following questions also need specific empirical examination. What is the prevalence of financial abuse of the elderly? Because it is underreported and difficult to detect, it is difficult to mobilize public interest in this issue without this baseline information. What is the impact of financial abuse on the elderly? For example, does it typically result in financial devastation and a loss of independence? What impact does it have on the health of the elder victims? What is its psychological impact, both short-term and long-term? In a world of limited resources, does financial abuse justify the same level of scrutiny or intervention as do other forms of elder abuse? What other forms of elder abuse co-occur with financial abuse and to what extent? Are reports of other types of elder abuse likely to address most instances of financial abuse? If financial abuse is a distinct phenomenon, it may need separate and distinct responses.

What types of financial abuse are most common? What are the characteristics of the victims? For example, are they socially isolated, where do they live, how old are they, what is their financial status, what is their cognitive state, what is their family history/status, and what is their ethnicity? Similarly, what are the characteristics of the perpetrators? For example, what are their motivations and how many are close family members, acquaintances, or caregivers of the elder person? What factors lead to financial abuse? For example, what is the nature of the interaction between victim and perpetrator and what risk factors associated with this interaction can be identified? What decreases the likelihood of abuse? For example, when do close family bonds buffer against financial abuse? What variations are associated with the cultural context in which the elderly person lives, and is it possible to develop objective standards that apply appropriately to all cultural groups? Such information is a prerequisite for developing and targeting interventions.

What are the barriers to detecting financial abuse of the elderly? What are indicators that family and professionals can watch for that suggest financial abuse may be occurring? What are the best ways to identify financial abuse? What are elder persons' perceptions of what constitutes financial abuse and how do they correspond with various professionals' perceptions? How effective are reporting requirements? Does mandatory reporting result in different rates of identification than voluntary reporting? Do the various means of responding to financial abuse serve as deterrents for future financial abuse? Do these various means adequately meet the needs of elder victims? Which venue is most effective in responding to the financial abuse of the elderly? Do adequate laws exist to address financial abuse, but the shortcoming lies with the enforcement of existing laws? What advantages would be associated with establishing a national standard/uniform law? Would such an approach fail to take into account local conditions and homogenize cultural variations?

Perhaps the most critical and pressing problem is how to prevent financial abuse of the elderly in the first place. A number of options have been identified, but information is lacking on which are the most effective. For example, can financial advice and assistance be provided to the elderly in such a way that their vulnerability to this abuse is decreased? What impact do public education programs, particularly those aimed at the elderly, have on the prevalence of financial abuse of the elderly?

Clearly, considerable information is needed regarding the occurrence of financial abuse of the elderly. In light of the nature of the problem and its impact, related research should be a high priority.

REFERENCES

AARP
  1993   *Abused Elders or Older Battered Women? Report on the AARP Forum.* Washington, DC: AARP Women's Initiative.
  2001   AARP on the Issues: Elder Abuse. Available: *http://www.aarp.org/ontheissues/issueelderab.html.*
Anetzberger, G.J.
  2000   Caregiving: Primary cause of elder abuse? *Generations* 24(2): 46–51.
Bassuk, K.
  2001   Financial abuse. In *The Encyclopedia of Elder Care,* M.D. Mezey, ed. New York: Springer Publishing Co.
Beauchamp, E.R.
  2001   Chapter 565: One more law to reform conservatorships and guardianships; but is it needed? *McGeorge Law Review* (Winter):647–669.
Beck, C.M., and L.R. Phillips
  1984   The unseen abuse: Why financial maltreatment of the elderly goes unrecognized. *Journal of Gerontological Nursing* 10(12):26–30.
Bernatz, S.I., S.J. Aziz, and L. Mosqueda
  2001   Financial abuse. In *The Encyclopedia of Elder Care,* M.D. Mezey, ed. New York: Springer Publishing Co.
Brandl, B.
  2000   Power and control: Understanding domestic abuse in later life. *Generations* 24(2):39–45.
Brandl, B., and T. Meuer
  2000   Domestic abuse in later life. *Elder Law Journal* 8:297–335.
Brown, A.S.
  1999   Patterns of abuse among Native American elderly. In *Understanding Elder Abuse in Minority Populations,* T. Tatara, ed. Philadelphia, PA: Brunner/Mazel.
Capezuti, E., B.L. Brush, and W.T. Lawson
  1997   Reporting elder mistreatment. *Journal of Gerontological Nursing* 23:24–32.

Carroll, J.
  2001   *Financial Abuse: Signs.* Colorado State University Cooperative Extension. Available: *http://www.colostate.edu/Depts/CoopExt/SEA/Jean/finabuse.html.*
Central California Legal Services (CCLS)
  2001   *Elder Financial Abuse.* Available: *http://www.las.org/abuse/elder financial.html.*
Choi, N.G., D.B. Kulick, and J. Mayer
  1999   Financial exploitation of elders: Analysis of risk factors based on county adult protective services data. *Journal of Elder Abuse and Neglect* 10(3/4):39–62.
Choi, N.G., and J. Mayer
  2000   Elder abuse, neglect, and exploitation: Risk factors and prevention strategies. *Journal of Gerontological Social Work* 33(2):5–25.
Cohen, C.A.
  1998   Conmen and confusion: Consumer fraud and vulnerable older people in the community. *Journal of the American Geriatrics Society* 46(1):118–119.
Coker, J., and B. Little
  1997   Investing in the future: Protecting the elderly from financial abuse. *FBI Law Enforcement Bulletin* (February):1–5.
Comijs, H.C., W. Dijkstra, L.M. Bouter, and J.H. Smit
  2000   The quality of data collection by an interview on the prevalence of elder mistreatment. *The Journal of Elder Abuse and Neglect* 12(1):57–72.
Commonwealth of Massachusetts
  2001   *The Bank Reporting Project: An Edge Against Elder Financial Exploitation–Employee Training Manual.* Boston, MA: Author.
Council on Ethical and Judicial Affairs, American Medical Association
  1992   Physicians and domestic violence: Ethical considerations. *The Journal of the American Medical Association* 267(23):3190–3193.
County Welfare Directors Association
  1988   *Protecting the Silent Population: Remedying Elder and Dependent Adult Abuse.* Sacramento, CA: Author.
Deem, D.L.
  2000   Notes from the field: Observations in working with the forgotten victims of personal financial crimes. *Journal of Elder Abuse and Neglect* 12(2):33–48.
Dessin, C.L.
  2000   Financial abuse of the elderly. *Idaho Law Review* 36:203–226.
Fielo, S.B.
  1987   How does crime affect the elderly? Most crimes against the elderly are sustained by the inner-city aged who live alone. *Geriatric Nursing* 1(March/April):80–83
Frolik, L.A.
  2001   Insurance fraud on the elderly. *Trial* (June):48–52.
Fulmer, T.T., and V.M. Cahill
  1984   Assessing elder abuse: A study. *Journal of Gerontological Nursing* 10(12):16–20.
Fulmer, T., D.J. McMahon, M. Baer-Hines, and B. Forget
  1992   Abuse, neglect, abandonment, violence, and exploitation: An analysis of all elderly patients seen in one emergency department during a six-month period. *Journal of Emergency Nursing* 18(6):505–510.
Gilbert, A.N.
  1986   The ethics of mandatory elder abuse reporting statutes. *Advances in Nursing Science* 8(2):51–62.
Giordano, J.A., B.L. Yegidis, and N.H. Giordano
  1992   Victimization of the elderly: Individual and family characteristics of financial abuse. *Arete* 17:26–37.

Gold D.T., and L.P. Gwyther
    1989   The prevention of elder abuse: An educational model. *Family Relations* 38(1):8–
            14.
Gordon, R.M.
    1986   Financial abuse of the elderly and state "Protective Services:" Changing strate-
            gies in the penal-welfare complex in the United States and Canada. *Crime and
            Social Justice* 26:116–134.
Griffin, L.W.
    1999   Elder maltreatment in the African-American community: You just don't hit your
            momma!!! In *Understanding Elder Abuse in Minority Populations,* T. Tatara,
            ed. Philadelphia, PA: Brunner/Mazel.
Hall, J.M.
    1999   Abuse of black elders in Rhode Island. In *Understanding Elder Abuse in Minor-
            ity Populations,* T. Tatara, ed. Philadelphia, PA: Brunner/Mazel.
Heisler, C.J.
    1991   The role of the criminal justice system in elder abuse cases. *Journal of Elder
            Abuse and Neglect* 3(1):5–33.
    2000   Elder abuse and the criminal justice system: New awareness, new responses.
            Generations 24(2):52–58.
Heisler, C.J., and M.J. Quinn
    1995   A legal perspective. In *Elder Mistreatment: Ethical Issues, Dilemmas, and Deci-
            sions,* T.F. Johnson, ed. Binghamton, NY: Haworth Press.
Heisler, C.J., and J.E. Tewksbury
    1992   Fiduciary abuse of the elderly: A prosecutor's perspective. *Journal of Elder
            Abuse and Neglect* 3(4):23–40.
Henningsen, E.
    2001   *Financial Abuse of the Elderly, Wisconsin Department of Health and Family
            Services—Programs and Services.* Available: *http://www.dhfs.state.wi.us/aging/
            Age_News/N0111/finabus.html.*
    2000   *Preventing Financial Abuse by Agents Under Powers of Attorney.* Available:
            http://www.wisbar.org/wislawmag/2000/09/henning.html (also *Wisconsin Law-
            yer* 73(9):2000).
Hoban, S.
    2000   Elder abuse and neglect: It takes many forms—if you're not looking, you may
            miss it. *American Journal of Nursing* 100(11):49–50.
Hudson, M.F., and J.R. Carlson
    1999   Elder abuse: Its meaning to Caucasians, African Americans, and Native Ameri-
            cans. In *Understanding Elder Abuse in Minority Populations,* T. Tatara, ed.
            Philadelphia, PA: Brunner/Mazel.
Hwang, M.H.
    1996   Durable power of attorney: Financial planning tool or license to steal? *Journal
            of Long-Term Home Health Care* 15(2):13–23.
Jackson, H.
    2000   Assemblymember Jackson's Bill to Combat Elder Financial Abuse Passes Assem-
            bly Floor with Bipartisan Support: Measure Will Allow Finacial Institutions to
            Report Financial Abuse More Quickly Available: *http://democrats.assembly.
            ca.gov/members/a35/press/p352000030.htm.*
Jecker, N.S.
    1993   Privacy beliefs and the violent family: Extending the ethical argument for physi-
            cal intervention. *The Journal of the American Medical Association* 269(6):776–
            780.

Kapp, M.A.
    1995   Elder mistreatment: Legal interventions and policy uncertainties. *Behavioral Sciences and the Law* 13:365–380.
Kleinschmidt, K.C.
    1997   Elder abuse: A review. *Annals of Emergency Medicine* 30:63–72.
Klingbeil, K.S., and V.D. Boyd
    1984   Emergency room intervention: Detection, assessment, and treatment. In *Battered Women and Their Families: Intervention Strategies and Treatment Programs*, A.R. Roberts, ed. New York: Springer Publishing Co.
Kosberg, J.I., and D. Nahmiash
    1996   Characteristics of victims and perpetrators and milieus of abuse and neglect. In *Abuse, Neglect, and Exploitation of Older Persons: Strategies for Assessment and Intervention*, L.A. Baumhover and S.C. Beall, eds. Baltimore, MD: Health Professions Press.
Lachs, M.S., and K. Pillemer
    1995   Current concepts: Abuse and neglect of elderly persons. *The New England Journal of Medicine* 332(7):437–443.
Langan, J., and R. Means
    1996   Financial management and elderly people with dementia in the UK: As much a question of confusion as abuse? *Ageing and Society* 16:287–314.
Lavrisha, M.
    1997   What can nurses do about financial exploitation of elders? *Journal of Gerontological Nursing* 23(7):49–50.
Macolini, R.M.
    1995   Elder abuse policy: Considerations in research and legislation. *Behavioral Sciences and the Law* 13:349–363.
Marshall, C.E., D. Benton, and J.M. Brazier
    2000   Elder abuse: Using clinical tools to identify clues of mistreatment. *Geriatrics* 55(2):42–53.
McGhee, J.L.
    1983   The vulnerability of elderly consumers. *International Journal of Aging and Human Development* 17(3):223–246.
Mehta, S.G.
    2000   Respecting our elders. *Los Angeles Lawyer* 23:35.
Menio, D., and B.H. Keller
    2000   CARIE: A multifaceted approach to abuse prevention in nursing homes. *Generations* 24(2):28–32.
Mixson, P., K. Chelucci, C. Heisler, W. Overman, P. Sripada, and P. Yates
    1992   The case of Mrs. M.: A multidisciplinary team staffing. *Journal of Elder Abuse and Neglect* 3 4):41–55.
Moon, A.
    1999   Elder abuse and neglect among the Korean elderly in the United States. In *Understanding Elder Abuse in Minority Populations*, T. Tatara, ed. Philadelphia, PA: Brunner/Mazel.
    2000   Perceptions of elder abuse among various cultural groups: Similarities and differences. *Generations* 24 (2):75–80.
Moskowitz, S.
    1998a   New remedies for elder abuse and neglect. *Probate and Property* 12:52–56.
    1998b   Saving granny from the wolf: Elder abuse and neglect—the legal framework. *Connecticut Law Review* 31:77–201.

National Center on Elder Abuse
1996   *Elder Abuse: Questions and Answers.* Washington, DC: National Center on Elder Abuse.
1998   *The National Elder Abuse Incidence Study: Final Report.* Washington, DC: National Aging Information Center.
2000   Summaries of the Statistical Data on Elder Abuse in Domestic Settings: An Exploratory Study of State Statistics for FY 93 and FY 94. Available: *http://www.aoa.gov/abuse/report/Cexecsum.html* [Accessed Feb. 28, 2000].
2001   The Basics: What Is Elder Abuse? What Are the Major Types of Elder Abuse? Available: *http://www.elderabusecenter.org/basic/.*

National Clearinghouse on Family Violence, Health Canada (NCFV)
2001   Financial Abuse of Older Adults. Available: *http://www.hc-sc.gc.ca/hppb/family violence/html/financialaben.html* .

National Committee for the Prevention of Elder Abuse (NCPEA)
2001   Elder Abuse: Financial Abuse. Available: *http://www.preventelder abuse.org/elderabuse/fin_abuse.html.*

Neale, A.V., M. Hwalek, C.S. Goodrich, and K.M. Quinn
1996   The Illinois elder abuse system: Program description and administrative findings. *The Gerontologist* 36(4):502–511.

Nerenberg, L.
1999   Culturally specific outreach in elder abuse. In *Understanding Elder Abuse in Minority Populations,* T. Tatara, ed. Philadelphia, PA: Brunner/Mazel.
2000a   Developing a service response to elder abuse. *Generations* 24(2):86–92.
2000b   Introduction. *Journal of Elder Abuse and Neglect* 12(2).
2000c   Forgotten victims of financial crime and abuse: Facing the challenge. *Journal of Elder Abuse and Neglect* 12(2):49–72.

New York State Department of Law
2000   Press Release, Financial Abuse of Elderly Targeted: Bank Employees to Receive Training to Combat Exploitation. Available: *http://www.oag.state.ny. us/press/2000/sep/sep21b_00.html.*

Office for Victims of Crime, United States Department of Justice (OVC)
2001   Victims of Crime Act Victim Compensation Grant Program. *Federal Register* 66(95):27158–27166.

Oh, S.
1999   The hidden horror: Many elderly are abused by the people they trust the most—their own kids. *Maclean's* 48.

Otto, J.M.
2000   The role of adult protective services in addressing abuse. *Generations* 24(2):33–38.

Paris, B.E.C., D.E. Meier, T. Goldstein, M. Weiss, and E.D. Fein
1995   Elder abuse and neglect: How to recognize warning signs and intervene. *Geriatrics* 50(4):47–51.

Paveza, G.J.
2001   Elder mistreatment: Overview. In *The Encyclopedia of Elder Care,* M.D. Mezey, ed. New York: Springer Publishing Co.

Pillemer, K., and D. Finkelhor
1988   The prevalence of elder abuse: A random sample survey. *The Gerontologist* 28(1):51–57.

Podnieks, E.
1992   National survey on abuse of the elderly in Canada. *Journal of Elder Abuse and Neglect* 4(1/2):5–58.

Price, G., and C. Fox
    1997   The Massachusetts bank reporting project: An edge against elder financial exploitation. *Journal of Elder Abuse and Neglect* 8(4):59–71.
Quinn, M.J.
    2000   Undoing undue influence. *Journal of Elder Abuse and Neglect* 12(2):9–16.
Ramsey-Klawsnik, H.
    2000   Elder-abuse offenders: A typology. *Generations* 24(2):17–22.
Reis, M.
    2000   The IOA Screen: An abuse-alert measure that dispels myths. *Generations* 24(2): 13–16.
Roby, J.L., and R. Sullivan
    2000   Adult protection service laws: A comparison of state statutes from definition to case closure. *Journal of Elder Abuse and Neglect* 12(3/4):17–51.
Rosenblatt, D.E., K.H. Cho, and P.W. Durance
    1996   Reporting mistreatment of older adults: The role of physicians. *Journal of the American Geriatrics Society* 44(1):65–70.
Rush, R.L., and R.J. Lank
    2000   How to Thwart Financial Fraud of Elderly Clients. Available: *http://www. elderweb.com/default.php3?PageID=2206.*
Sacks, D.
    1996   Prevention of financial abuse focus of New Institute at the Brookdale Center on Aging. *Aging Magazine* 367:86–89.
Sampson, D.
    1996   Annotated Bibliography: Elder Abuse—Financial Exploitation by a Conservator. Available: *http://www.keln.org/bibs/sampson.html.*
Sanchez, Y.M.
    1996   Distinguishing cultural expectations in assessment of financial exploitation. *Journal of Elder Abuse and Neglect* 8(2):49–59.
Schiamberg, L.B., and D. Gans
    2000   Elder abuse by adult children: An applied ecological framework for understanding contextual risk factors and the intergenerational character of quality of life. *International Journal of Aging and Human Development* 50(4):329–359.
Sengstock, M.C., and M.A. Hwalek
    1986   *Sengstock-Hwalek Comprehensive Index of Elder Abuse.* Detroit, MI: Social Program Evaluators and Consultants, Inc.
Shiferaw, B., M.B. Mittelmark, J.L. Wofford, R.T. Anderson, P. Walls, and B. Rohrer
    1994   The investigation and outcome of reported cases of elder abuse: The Forsyth County Aging Study. *The Gerontologist* 34(1):123–125.
Sklar, J.B.
    2000   Elder and dependent adult fraud: A sample of actual cases to profile the offenders and the crimes they perpetrate. *Journal of Elder Abuse and Neglect* 12(2):19–32.
Smith, R.S.
    1999   Fraud and Financial Abuse of Older Persons. No. 132 Australian Institute of Criminology. Canberra, Australia.
Stark, E., Flitcraft, A., and W. Frazier
    1979   Medicine and patriarchal violence. *International Journal of Health* 9:461–493.
Stiegel, L.
    2000   The changing role of the courts in elder-abuse cases. *Generations,* 24(2):59–64.
Sugg, N.K., and T. Inui
    1992   Primary care physicians' response to domestic violence: Opening Pandora's Box. *The Journal of the American Medical Association* 267(23):3157–3160.

Tatara, T., ed.
  1999 *Understanding Elder Abuse in Minority Populations.* Philadelphia, PA: Brunner/ Mazel.
Thilges, A.A.
  2000 Comment, Abuse of a power of attorney: Who is more likely to be punished, the elder or the abuser? *Journal of the American Academy of Matrimonial Lawyers* 16:579–592.
Thomas, C.
  2000 The first national study of elder abuse and neglect: Contrast with results from other studies. *Journal of Elder Abuse and Neglect* 12(1):1–14.
Tom, C.
  2001 Model advance directive combats financial abuse Available: *http://www.asaging. org/at/at-201/model.html.*
Tueth, M.J.
  2000 Exposing financial exploitation of impaired elderly persons. *American Journal of Geriatric Psychiatry* 8(2):104–111.
U.S. Congress, House Select Committee on Aging
  1981 *A Report: Elder Abuse (An Examination of a Hidden Problem).* Washington, DC: U.S. Government Printing Office.
  1991 *Elder Abuse: What Can Be Done?* Washington, DC: U.S. Government Printing Office.
U.S. Congress, Senate Special Committee on Aging
  2000 *Elder Fraud and Abuse: New Challenges in the Digital Economy.* Washington, DC: U.S. Government Printing Office.
U.S. General Accounting Office
  1991 *Elder Abuse: Effectiveness of Reporting Laws and Other Factors.* Washington, DC: U.S. Government Printing Office.
Vinton, L.
  1991 Abused older women: Battered women or abused elders? *Journal of Women and Aging* 3(3):5–19.
  1999 Working with abused older women from a feminist perspective. *Journal of Women and Aging* 11(2/3):85–100.
Vinton, L., J.A. Altholz, and S.T. Lobell-Boesch
  1997 A five-year follow up study of domestic violence programming for older battered women. *Journal of Women and Aging* 9(1/2):3–15.
Weiler, K.
  1989 Financial abuse of the elderly: Recognizing and acting on it. *Journal of Gerontological Nursing* 15(8):10–15.
Wilber, K.H., and S.L. Reynolds
  1996 Introducing a framework for defining financial abuse of the elderly. *Journal of Elder Abuse and Neglect* 8(2):61–80.
Wolf, R.S.
  2000 Introduction: The nature and scope of elder abuse. *Generations* 24(2):6–12.
Wolf, R.S., and K.A. Pillemer
  1989 *Helping Elderly Victims: The Reality of Elder Abuse.* New York: Columbia University Press.
Zimka, K.
  1997 Financial Exploitation of the Elderly. Colorado State University Cooperative Extension, Jefferson County. Available: *http://www.ext.colostate.edu/pubs/ columncc/cc970710.htm.*

14
Elder Abuse in Residential Long-Term Care Settings: What Is Known and What Information Is Needed?

Catherine Hawes *

There has been very limited research on elder abuse, although there is some evidence that suggests it may be nearly as widespread in the community as child abuse (Bourland, 1990; Fulmer, 1989; Kleinschmidt et al., 1997; National Center on Elder Abuse, 1998; Pillemer and Finkelhor, 1988; U.S. House of Representatives, 1990). Although attention has increased somewhat in recent years, most research on elder abuse and neglect has focused on incidence, causes, and risk factors in the community. Elderly who live in settings other than their own homes or apartments or those of relatives have received relatively little attention from either the research or policy communities. However, elderly who live in residential settings that offer long-term supportive services are at particular risk for abuse and neglect.[1] They are particularly vulnerable because most suffer from several chronic diseases that lead to limitations in physical and cognitive functioning and are dependent on others (Spector et al., 2001). In addition, many are either unable to report abuse or neglect or fearful that

---

*Catherine Hawes, Ph.D., is a professor in the Department of Health Policy and Management, School of Rural Public Health, at Texas A&M University System Health Science Center.

[1]Marshall and his colleagues assert that elder abuse is more common in homes than in institutional or residential facility settings but offer no evidence to support this assertion (Marshall et al., 2000). What they ignore is that although there may be more cases of community-dwelling elderly, proportionally, there may be more cases in residential/institutional long-term care settings.

such reporting may lead to retaliation or otherwise negatively affect their lives (Hayley et al., 1996). Thus, as Shapira (2000) noted, "The elderly in skilled nursing facilities are among the most vulnerable members of our society. They are dependent on the . . . nursing facility operator for their food, medicine, medical care, dental care, and a bed; a roof over their heads; for assistance with virtually every daily activity."

On any given day, approximately 1.6 million people live in approximately 17,000 licensed nursing homes, and another estimated 900,000 to 1 million live in an estimated 45,000 residential care facilities, variously known as personal care homes, adult congregate living facilities, domiciliary care homes, adult care homes, homes for the aged, and assisted living facilities (Strahan, 1997; Hawes, et al., 1999, 1995a). Research suggests that the 2.5 million vulnerable individuals in these settings are at much higher risk for abuse and neglect than older persons who live at home, as discussed below. Moreover, these figures may underestimate the number of persons who are actually at risk for abuse or neglect in a nursing home. Based on data from the National Mortality Followback Survey, researchers estimate that more than two-fifths (43 percent) of all persons who turned 65 in 1990 or later will enter a nursing home at some time before they die (Kemper and Murtaugh, 1991; Murtaugh et al., 1990). Moreover, of those who enter a nursing home, more than half (55 percent) will have a total lifetime use of at least one year. The probability of use increases dramatically with age, rising from 17 percent for those aged 65 to 74 to 60 percent for persons aged 85 to 94. Because women live longer than men, their relative risk of lifetime use of a nursing home is higher (i.e., 52 percent versus 33 percent). In addition, because the most rapidly growing segment of the population is those aged 85 and older, the proportion of persons estimated at risk for nursing home use at some time in their lives is expected to increase over time. Thus, while only 2.5 million elders living in a residential long-term care facility on any given day may be at risk for abuse, over their lives many elderly may be at risk during a period of long-term care facility use.

The general goals of this paper are to present the available evidence about the nature and scope of abuse and neglect in nursing homes and other residential care facilities and the causes, as well as to suggest a research agenda. To accomplish these goals, the paper is organized as follows:

- Section 2 presents definitions of abuse and neglect;
- Section 3 provides the available evidence about the nature and scope of abuse and neglect in nursing homes;
- Section 4 presents the available evidence about the nature and scope of abuse and neglect in residential care facilities;
- Section 5 explains the limitations of these estimates;

• Section 6 discusses the sample design and data collection issues associated with studies to determine the prevalence of abuse and neglect in nursing homes and residential care facilities;

• Section 7 discusses what is known about the causes of abuse and neglect and presents the author's recommendations for additional research.

DEFINITIONS OF ABUSE AND NEGLECT

The definition of *physical abuse* is the area about which there is the greatest agreement, both in terms of being "wrong" and in terms of what constitutes physical abuse; it involves injury or harm to a person carried out with the intention of causing suffering, pain, or impairment (Clarke and Pierson, 1999; Lachs et al., 1994; Lachs and Pillemer, 1995; Tatara and Kuzmeskus, 1996–1997). The Administration on Aging, in its instructions to long-term care ombudsmen, defines abuse as "the willful infliction of injury, unreasonable confinement, intimidation or cruel punishment with resulting physical harm, pain, or mental anguish or deprivation by a person, including a caregiver, of goods or services that are necessary to avoid physical harm, mental anguish, or mental illness" (1998:13). This is consistent with the definition used by the Centers for Medicare and Medicaid Services (CMS, formerly the Health Care Financing Administration) in its guidelines to the states on reporting of abuse and neglect in nursing homes, as reported below.

Physical abuse is generally thought to include hitting, slapping, pushing, or striking with objects. In nursing homes, other types of actions have been included, such as improper use of physical or chemical restraints. Physical abuse also typically includes *sexual abuse* or nonconsensual sexual involvement of any kind, from rape to unwanted touching or indecent exposure.[2]

There is somewhat less agreement about whether *verbal* or *psychosocial abuse* should be included in the general category of abuse when applied to older persons. This is generally thought of as "intentional infliction of anguish, pain, or distress through verbal or nonverbal acts" and includes threats, harassment, and attempts to humiliate or intimidate the older person (Clarke and Pierson, 1999:632).

In focus group interviews conducted in 2000 (Hawes et al., 2001),

---

[2]Clarke and Pierson (1999:635) argue that examples (or possibly indicators of potential abuse and neglect) of abuse are "falls and fracture, physical or chemical restraints, malnutrition, dehydration, bed sores, defective equipment, lack of supervision, weight gain or loss, theft of money and personal property, unexpected or wrongful death, unsanitary conditions, untrained or insufficient staff, over-sedation, substandard medical care, and poor personal hygiene."

certified nursing assistants (CNAs) defined abusive actions that included both physical and verbal or psychological abuse, such as:

- aggressiveness with a resident;
- rough handling;
- pulling too hard on a resident;
- yelling in anger;
- threats;
- punching, slapping, kicking, hitting; and
- speaking in a harsh tone, cursing at a resident, or saying harsh or mean things to a resident.

Neglect of older persons is another area that has received increased attention in recent years. As Clarke and Pierson noted, "Definitions of neglect are probably the most disputed of any category" of maltreatment of elderly persons (Clarke and Pierson, 1999:632). However, in general, neglect is thought of as including "the refusal or failure of a caregiver to fulfill his or her obligations or duties to an older person, including . . . providing any food, clothing, medicine, shelter, supervision, and medical care and services that a prudent person would deem essential for the well-being of another" (Clarke and Pierson, 1999).

CNAs who participated in focus groups also had very clear and specific ideas about what constituted neglect in nursing homes (Hawes et al., 2001). They mentioned a number of examples:

- no oral/dental care;
- not doing range of motion exercises;
- not changing residents each time they are wet after an episode of incontinence;
- ignoring residents who are bedfast, particularly not offering activities to them;
- not doing prescribed wound care;
- not giving residents regular baths;
- doing a one-person transfer when the resident requires a two-person transfer;
- not providing cuing or task segmentation to residents who need that kind of assistance to maximize their independence;
- not doing scheduled toileting or helping residents when they ask;
- not keeping residents hydrated; and
- turning off a call light and taking no action on the resident's request.

The federal government also has formal definitions of abuse and neglect in nursing homes. The nursing home reforms contained in the Omnibus Budget Reconciliation Act of 1987 (OBRA 1987. Pub L. No. 100-203) specified that nursing home residents had the "right to be free from verbal, sexual, physical, and mental abuse, corporal punishment, and involuntary seclusion" (42 CFR Ch. IV (10-1-98 Edition) §483.13 (b)). HCFA issued regulations and guidelines implementing these provisions of the OBRA 1987 legislation. These regulations specified the following definitions:

> *Abuse* means the willful infliction of injury, unreasonable confinements, intimidation, or punishment with resulting physical harm, pain, or mental anguish.
> *Neglect* means failure to provide goods and services necessary to avoid physical harm, mental anguish, or mental illness.

The federal regulations implementing OBRA 1987 also specified long-term care facilities' responsibility to "develop and implement written policies and procedures that prohibit mistreatment, neglect, and abuse of residents and misappropriation of resident property" (42 CFR Ch. IV (10-1-98 Edition) §483.13 (c)). Furthermore, the law required that the facility "must not employ individuals who have been found guilty of abusing, neglecting, or mistreating residents by a court of law or have had a finding entered into the state nurse aide registry concerning abuse, neglect, mistreatment of residents, or misappropriation of their property" (42 CFR Ch. IV (10-1-98 Edition) §483.13 (c)(1) (ii) (A) (B)).[3]

EVIDENCE ABOUT THE NATURE AND PREVALENCE OF ABUSE AND NEGLECT IN NURSING HOMES

For decades, nursing homes have been plagued with reports suggesting widespread and serious maltreatment of residents, including abuse, neglect, and theft of personal property (Douglass et al., 1980; Fontana, 1978; Institute of Medicine, 1986; Mendelson, 1974; Moss and Halamandaris, 1977; New York State Moreland Act Commission, 1975, 1976; Ohio General Assembly Nursing Home Commission, 1978; Stannard, 1973; U.S. Senate, 1970; U.S. Senate, 1971; U.S. Senate Special Committee on Aging, 1974–1975; Vladeck, 1980). In addition, a number of case studies, participant-observation studies, interviews with nursing home staff, and interviews with residents and ombudsmen provided evidence of abuse (Doty and

---

[3]This lifetime ban was modified in certain cases under provisions of the 1997 Balanced Budged Act. Balanced Budget Act of 1997, Conference Report to Accompany H.R. 2015. 105th Congress, 1st Session. House of Representatives, Report 105-217 (July 30, 1997).

Sullivan, 1983; Douglass et al., 1980; Fontana, 1978; Gubrium, 1975; Jacobs, 1969; Kayser-Jones, 1990; Monk et al., 1984; Stannard, 1973; U.S. House of Representatives, Select Committee on Aging, 1990). Such conditions were major factors in the passage of the nursing home reforms contained in the Omnibus Budget Reconciliation Act (OBRA) of 1987 (OBRA, 1987).[4] The OBRA 1987 reforms, the most sweeping set of legislative changes to the way nursing homes were regulated since the passage of Medicaid and Medicare, addressed multiple areas of resident care and quality of life. They also specified that residents had the right to be free from verbal, sexual, physical, and mental abuse, including corporal punishment and involuntary seclusion, and limited the use of physical restraints and inappropriate use of psychotropic medications (Hawes, 1990; Elon and Pawlson, 1992).

Despite this federal law and reports over the preceding decades that raised the possibility of widespread and serious abuse, there has never been a systematic study of the prevalence of abuse in nursing homes. Indeed, it is important to note that none of the studies discussed below involving interviews with residents or with facility staff were designed with the intention of producing generalizable estimates to the nation as a whole. Nevertheless, the disparate evidence that is available and discussed below suggests the existence of a serious problem that warrants further study.

Resident Risk Factors

Several studies have examined the characteristics of individuals living in community settings (e.g., their own home or that of others) in an attempt to identify factors that place an older person at greater risk for being abused or neglected. Such studies found that persons suffering abuse or neglect were more likely to be old and nonwhite and to have greater limitations in physical and cognitive functioning, although there has been some disagreement about whether functional impairment in the activities of daily living (ADL) is a risk factor for abuse (Bristowe and Collins, 1989; Johnson, 1991; Lachs et al., 1994; Lachs et al., 1996, 1997; Pillemer and Finkelhor, 1988; Podnieks, 1992). However, there is strong evidence that the presence of cognitive impairment or dementia is associated with higher risk for being abused (Coyne et al., 1993; Dyer et al., 2000; Homer and Gilleard, 1990; O'Malley et al., 1983; Paveza et al., 1992; Pillemer and Finkelhor, 1988; Pillemer and Suitor, 1992; Wolf and Pillemer, 1989).

Studies of individual risk factors for elderly living in residential long-term care facilities are more limited but generally suggest the existence of

---

[4]The Omnibus Budget Reconciliation Act of 1987 ~ PL 100-203.

TABLE 14-1 Characteristics of Nursing Home Residents

Characteristic	Percent
Aged ≥ 85 years	49
Nonwhite	9
Receives assistance with ≥3 ADLs	83
Mild to moderate cognitive impairment	71
Exhibits physically aggressive behaviors	9
Exhibits any behaviors (e.g., verbally or physically aggressive, resists nursing care, socially inappropriate)	30

SOURCE: Krauss and Altman (1998).

similar risk factors for individual residents. For example, Burgess and her colleagues argued, "The risk for abuse increases simply as a function of their dependence on staff for safety, protection, and care" (Burgess et al., 2000). They found that a diagnosis of Alzheimer's or other dementia or some type of memory loss or confusion was present at a somewhat higher rate among nursing home residents who had been sexually abused than among the average nursing home population, although those data were from a small case study (Burgess et al., 2000). Similarly, the findings from another study suggest that residents with behavioral symptoms, such as physical aggressiveness, appear to be at higher risk for abuse by staff (Pillemer and Bachman-Prehn, 1991), a finding supported by focus group interviews with CNAs (Hawes et al., 2001) and studies of precipitating factors among community-dwelling elders who have been abused (Pillemer and Suitor, 1992; Ehrlich, 1993).

Unfortunately, dependence on others for help with physical functioning and impairment in cognitive functioning are common among the vast majority of nursing home residents, and difficult or challenging behaviors are not uncommon, as displayed in Table 14-1. These behaviors are often a product of neurological changes, memory loss, and communication deficits associated with diseases such as Alzheimer's. However, many staff members often view aggressive resident behaviors or attempts to resist care as intentional attempts by the resident to be difficult or to hurt staff, a belief that makes such residents more likely to be handled roughly or abused by staff (Hawes et al., 2001).

Reports of Abuse from Residents and Families

I saw a nurse hit and yell at the lady across the hall because the nurse told the lady she didn't have all day to wait on her. The lady made some remark. The nurse hit the lady and said, "Shut up."

Georgia Nursing Home Resident
(Atlanta Long-Term Care Ombudsman Program, 2000)

A few studies have interviewed residents and family members about their experiences in nursing homes and asked specific questions about abuse. The Atlanta Long Term Care (LTC) Ombudsman Program (Atlanta Long-Term Care Ombudsman Program, 2000) conducted the most recent study under a grant funded by the National Ombudsman Resource Center. In this study, ombudsmen interviewed 80 residents in 23 nursing homes in Georgia.[5] This survey found that 44 percent of the residents reported that they had been abused, while 48 percent reported that they had been treated roughly. For example, one resident noted:

They throw me like a sack of feed . . . [and] that leaves marks on my breast.

Georgia Nursing Home Resident
(Atlanta Long-Term Care Ombudsman Program, 2000)

In addition, 38 percent of the residents reported that they had seen other residents being abused, and 44 percent said they had seen other residents being treated roughly. For example, as one resident reported:

My roommate—they throw him in the bed. They handle him any kind of way. He can't take up for himself.

Georgia Nursing Home Resident
(Atlanta Long-Term Care Ombudsman Program, 2000)

---

[5]The ombudsmen initially identified what they considered 10 problem facilities and recruited residents from those nursing homes. The process was subsequently expanded to a total of 23 facilities, based on local ombudsman identification of residents willing to speak with the interviewers about issues of abuse and neglect. The authors reported, "Almost all those approached agreed to be interviewed." Those who declined cited fear of retaliation. Finally, the ombudsmen used CMS Survey protocols to identify "interviewable" residents in long-term care facilities (Atlanta Long-Term Care Ombudsman Program, 2000).

Focus groups and individual interviews with residents and family members for a study of the nursing home complaint-investigation process also produced reports of abuse and severe neglect. Families reported finding residents with bruises and abrasions, unexplained falls, some of which caused fractures, and residents left for days with broken bones before the family or resident's physician were notified, such as the case reported below.

> *Have I seen abuse? No, not directly. But I've come in and found my mom battered and bruised. I mean, her whole face was bruised and swollen, the backs of her hands and arms were bruised, as if she tried to protect herself.*
>
>   Daughter of a Texas Resident, 1999 (Hawes et al., 2000)

Reports of Abuse from Facility Staff

> *Oh, yeah. I've seen abuse. Things like rough handling, pinching, pulling too hard on a resident to make them do what you want. Slapping, that too. People get so tired, working mandatory overtime, short-staffed. It's not an excuse, but it makes it so hard for them to respond right.*
>
>   CNA from South Carolina (Hawes et al., 2000)

A 1987 survey of 577 nursing home staff members from 31 facilities found that more than one-third (36 percent) had witnessed at least one incident of physical abuse during the preceding 12 months (Pillemer and Moore, 1989).[6] As displayed in Table 14-2, such incidents included excessive use of physical restraints (21 percent); pushing, shoving, grabbing, or pinching a resident (17 percent); slapping or hitting (13 percent); throwing something at a resident (3 percent); kicking or hitting with a fist or object (2 percent). Ten percent of the staff members surveyed reported they had committed such acts themselves.

A total of 81 percent of the staff reported that they had observed and 40 percent had committed at least one incident of psychological abuse during the same 12-month period. Psychological abuse included yelling in anger, insulting or swearing at a resident, inappropriate isolation, threatening to hit or throw an object, or denying food or privileges. Yelling at a resident in anger and insulting or swearing at a resident were the most common acts observed, with 70 percent having observed yelling and 50 percent having observed a staff member insulting or swearing at a resident

---

[6]Thirty-one of a potential sample of 77 facilities in one state met the facility size criteria, agreed to participate in the study, and provided complete lists of staff.

TABLE 14-2 Results of Surveys of CNAs about Committing or Witnessing Abuse and Neglect of Residents

Abusive Behaviors	Rates of Self-Reported Behaviors[a]	
	Pillemer and Moore (percentage)	Pillemer and Hudson (percentage)
Yelled at a resident in anger	23	51
Insulted or swore at a resident	10	23
Threatened to hit or throw something at a resident	2	8
Pushed, grabbed, or shoved	3	17
Slapped or hit a resident	3	2
Thrown something at a resident	1	1
Excessive use of physical restraints	4	Not reported
	Rates of Behaviors Witnessed by CNAs Not Asked	
Yelling at a resident	70	
Insulting or swearing at a resident	50	
Excessive use of physical restraints	21	
Pushing, grabbing, shoving, or pinching	17	
Slapping or hitting a resident	13	
Throwing something at a resident	3	
Kicking or hitting a resident	2	

[a]Pillemer and Moore (1989) surveyed 577 staff (nurses and CNAs) about incidents over a 12-month period. Pillemer and Hudson (1993) interviewed 211 staff about incidents during the preceding 1-month period.

(Pillemer and Moore, 1989). Interviews with more than 200 staff members who subsequently participated in an abuse-prevention training program also indicated substantial levels of abusive behaviors by staff caregivers in nursing homes.

Focus groups with CNAs also provided quantitative and qualitative data that supported the findings reported by Pillemer and Moore. For example, North Shore Elder Services in Danvers, Massachusetts, conducted a recent project on reducing abuse and neglect in nursing homes (MacDonald, 2000). In this project, 77 CNAs from 31 nursing facilities received training. As part of this project, CNAs were surveyed about whether they had witnessed any incidents of abuse or neglect. Verbal abuse was reported as fairly common: 58 percent of the CNAs said they had seen a staff member yell at a resident in anger; 36 percent had seen staff insult or swear at a resident; 11 percent had witnessed staff threatening to hit or throw something at a resident (MacDonald, 2000).

These CNAs also reported that they had witnessed incidents of rough treatment and physical abuse of residents by other staff. Twenty-five percent of the CNAs witnessed staff isolating a resident beyond what was needed to manage his/her behavior; 21 percent witnessed restraint of a resident beyond what was needed; 11 percent saw a resident being denied food as punishment.

In addition, the staff reported witnessing more explicit instances of abuse. Twenty-one percent saw a resident pushed, grabbed, shoved, or pinched in anger; 12 percent witnessed staff slapping a resident; 7 percent saw a resident being kicked or hit with a fist; 3 percent saw staff throw something at a resident; and 1 percent saw a resident being hit with an object.

Reports of Abuse from Health Care Professionals

There are relatively few studies of health care professionals and issues of abuse of nursing home residents, and most that exist focus on underreporting and reasons for that phenomenon. However, one study did suggest that abuse might be widespread. Emergency department physicians conducted retrospective chart review of 328 nursing home residents admitted to the emergency room. In nearly 1 in 5 (19 percent) of 253 cases with adequate documentation of when the injury occurred, there was an unexplained delay in seeking medical treatment of 24 hours or more (Barlow et al., 1998).

Reports of Abuse from Ombudsmen and Adult Protective Services Agencies

Another source of information on abuse and neglect in nursing homes is data from the Long-Term Care Ombudsman program. The ombudsman program was established in the early 1970s to "identify, investigate, and resolve individual and systems level complaints" that affect residents in nursing homes and residential care facilities (Huber et al., 2001:1). Federal funds for the program are through the Older Americans Act, and some programs also receive state funding (Huber et al., 1996).

For some years, ombudsmen have reported incidents of abuse and neglect in nursing homes (Monk et al., 1984). For example, one study that surveyed agencies in 22 states reported 15,612 cases involving allegations of abuse of nursing home residents received by such agencies as Adult Protective Services, ombudsmen, and state Medicaid fraud units, which are responsible for prosecuting abuse cases involving nursing homes (Tatara, 1990).

Reports of abuse and neglect from ombudsmen are thought to have become more reliable in recent years, even as their data suggest increasing incidence. As part of their responsibilities, the ombudsman program established a National Ombudsman Reporting System (NORS), using standardized definitions of complaint types and resolutions (Administration on Aging, 1998). The 1998 compilation of complaints received by the state Long-Term Care Ombudsman program and its parent agency, the Administration on Aging, using the NORS system, found that, nationwide, physical abuse was one of the five most frequent complaints to ombudsmen about nursing homes (Administration on Aging, 2000). Ten percent, or about 20,000, of the complaints received by ombudsmen during FY 1998 involved allegations of abuse, gross neglect, or exploitation, while another 5 percent related to financial abuse and misappropriation of property. In addition, ombudsmen reported more than 1,700 allegations of sexual abuse of nursing home residents during a two-year period (Burgess, personal communication,[7] November 2000; see also Burgess et al., 2000).

Deficiency Citations for Abuse

Ninety-six percent of all facilities nationwide participate in the Medicare or Medicaid programs or both (Strahan, 1997). These facilities are subject to annual surveys and to complaint investigations under federal law and regulation governing participation in these programs. These surveys also provide evidence of abuse and neglect in nursing homes.

Office of the DHHS Inspector General

The Office of the Inspector General (OIG) in the U.S. Department of Health and Human Services reviewed data from the Health Care Financing Administration's (HCFA) Online Survey Certification and Reporting System (OSCAR) for one full survey cycle (1997–1998) in 10 states. The OIG found 4,707 abuse complaints, involving nearly one-third of the facilities certified to participate in the Medicare or Medicaid programs.[8]

Centers for Medicare and Medicaid Services

The Centers for Medicare and Medicaid Services (CMS, formerly HCFA) has reported even more current data on abuse in nursing homes. In

---

[7]Personal communication and presentation at the Forensic Conference on Elder Abuse and briefing for Attorney General Reno, sponsored by the U.S. Department of Justice, Washington, DC, November 2000.

[8]The vast majority of complaints (e.g., about two-thirds) were not substantiated, an issue discussed at greater length in the body of this report.

its Quarterly Report on the Progress of the Nursing Home Initiative for January 2001, CMS reported the rate of citations for various types of deficiencies, including abuse (U.S. Department of Health and Human Services, Center for Medicare and Medicaid Services, 2001). These citations do not represent prevalence measures (e.g., the proportion of residents who were abused); however, they do suggest the potential severity of the problem. The CMS/HCFA data indicated an increase in citations for deficiencies related to abuse between 1988 and 2000. Although the data show an increase in citations for abuse, the increase has been seen in deficiencies related to facility processes rather than to actual, documented abuse of residents. Four deficiencies, listed below, are related to abuse. Only one (F223) is cited when there is a substantiated incident of abuse.

  •   F223 is cited when a facility fails to protect its residents from abuse;
  •   F224 is cited when a facility fails to write and use policies that forbid mistreatment, neglect, abuse, and theft of resident's property;
  •   F225 is cited when a facility fails to hire employees without histories of abusive behaviors or fails to report and investigate allegations of abuse;
  •   F226 is cited when a facility fails to implement the policies it writes to forbid mistreatment, neglect, abuse, and misappropriation.

Changes in the rates of these deficiencies across the first quarters of 1998, 1999, and 2000 are displayed in Figure 14-1. These rates represent the proportion of facilities that were cited for resident abuse. In 1999, for example, 326 facilities were cited for F223, the deficiency representing substantiated cases of abuse. However, it is important to note that these probably represent minimal estimates of abuse because, as discussed below, very few allegations are substantiated. Furthermore, even among substantiated cases of abuse and neglect, relatively few result in a deficiency citation (Hawes et al., 2001).

In addition to increases in substantiated cases of abuse for which deficiencies are cited, there have been significant increases in citations for failure to hire persons without a history of abusive behaviors or to adequately investigate and report allegations of abuse.

These reported increases are more serious than the data suggest for two main reasons. First, as discussed later, most cases are not substantiated, often for reasons having little to do with the likely truth of the allegation. Second, as also discussed later, even when abuse allegations are substantiated, there is rarely a deficiency citation against the facility that would be recorded as an "F-Tag." Third, in most states the agencies responsible for investigating abuse and neglect in nursing homes acknowledge their depen-

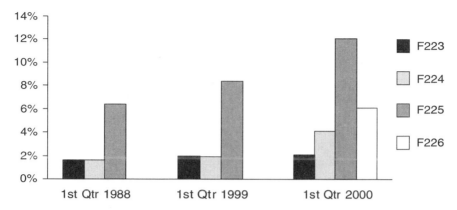

FIGURE 14-1   Rates of deficiency citations for abuse, 1988–2000.

dence on such reports from facilities, as illustrated by the following quote from a state official responsible for state investigations of abuse and neglect:

> We are struggling with [the] responsibility to do our investigations and how reliant we are on facility investigations. . . . [W]e would need more staff to do all investigations. To do an on-site investigation to verify a facility's investigation takes us a day. To do an investigation from scratch would take us three days.
>
> Nurse Aide Registry Director (Hawes et al., 2001)

Indeed, the bulk of the allegations of abuse in most states start with reports filed by facilities (Hawes et al., 2001). Some agencies reported concern that facilities may fail to report cases, simply discharging the CNA in question. If this view is correct and some facilities are failing to report allegations or to investigate them adequately, there may be large numbers of unreported cases of resident abuse or neglect.

U.S. House of Representatives, Committee on Government Reform

Recently, the Minority Staff of the Special Investigations Division of the House Committee on Government Reform issued a report asserting that abuse of residents "is a major problem in U.S. nursing homes" (U.S. House of Representatives, 2001). This report analyzed data from the OSCAR system and the nursing home complaint database covering all surveys and complaint investigations during a 2-year period (i.e., January 1999 through

January 2000) and included all four of the deficiency codes related to abuse (F223, 224, 225, and 226). The report concluded:

• During the 2-year period, nearly one-third of all certified facilities had been cited for some type of abuse violation that had the potential to cause harm or had actually caused harm to a nursing home resident.

• Ten percent of the nursing homes in the United States were cited for abuse violations that caused actual harm to residents or placed them in immediate jeopardy of death or serious injury.

• The percentage of homes with abuse violations has been increasing, probably as a result, at least in part, of more stringent reporting requirements and increased vulnerability among residents.

• The cases involving abuse included physical and sexual abuse as well as verbal abuse involving threats and humiliation.

Reports from the Nurse Aide Registries

One potential source of data on abuse in nursing homes is the nurse aide registries. Under federal law, states were required to establish a nurse aide registry and investigate any complaints of abuse, neglect, and misappropriation of resident property by any nurse aide in a nursing home that participates in the Medicare or Medicaid program.[9] The law provided that "if a state found that a nurse aide had neglected or abused a nursing facility resident or misappropriated property of a resident, then the state must have such information included in the state's nurse aide registry" and the aide would be barred from nursing home employment.[10] In addition, under federal regulations, states were obligated to determine whether facility practices or policies caused or contributed to the substantiated abuse, neglect, or misappropriation.

In a recent study for CMS (formerly HCFA), researchers surveyed the state agencies administering the nurse aide registries (Hawes et al., 2001). Forty of the 51 agencies responded, but those agencies varied widely in their ability to provide data and in the operation of their systems, from intake to investigation and resolution. Nevertheless, some of the results were instructive about the prevalence of abuse and neglect. For example, only 14 states provided a detailed breakdown of the types of complaints or allegations they received. However, for the vast majority (79 percent) of those states that provided a breakdown of cases by type, more than 70

---

[9]Sections 1819 (e) (2) (A) and 1919 (e) (2) (A) of the Social Security Act.

[10]42 CFR Ch. IV (10-1-98 Edition) §483.156 (a) (5) (c) (iv) (D). The lifetime ban was modified in certain cases under provisions of the 1997 Balanced Budged Act.

TABLE 14-3 Rates of Allegations per 1,000
Nursing Facility Beds

Rate	Number of States
1 to 6.99 per 1,000 beds	4
7 to 9.99 per 1,000 beds	3
10 to 19.99 per 1,000 beds	5
20 to 29.99 per 1,000 beds	3
>30 per 1,000 beds	5

Total states reporting = 20 of 41 surveyed.
SOURCE: Hawes et al. (2001).

percent of the cases involved allegations of abuse. Fewer than 20 percent of the cases involved neglect, and less than 10 percent of the reported allegations involved misappropriation.

States also varied in the rate of complaints they received. Because of very limited data systems, only about half of the participating states could provide statistics on the total number of allegations broken out by category—abuse, neglect, or misappropriation. As displayed in Table 14-3, there was tremendous variation in the rate of reported complaints across the states. The reported number of complaints or allegations of abuse, neglect, and misappropriation that were logged into the nurse aide registry system varied from 1 per 1,000 nursing home beds to 174 per 1,000 beds across the states that reported these statistics. It is important to note that this finding is very similar to that reported by the U.S. Department of Health and Human Services, OIG (1998), which also found widespread variability between states in reported rates. The OIG found that in the states it examined, the rates of abuse complaints varied from less than 1 percent to more than 17 percent of the state's nursing home population.

Because of this variability and because most states were unable to break out complaints by type, it is difficult to estimate the underlying prevalence of complaints about abuse. The modal rate of complaints is between 10 and 20 complaints per 1000 beds. If this rate were applied to the 1.8 million beds nationwide, that would suggest a nationwide average of 18,000 to 36,000 complaints per year. If 70 percent of these were about abuse, then the estimate would be 12,600 to 25,200 abuse complaints annually. Of course, there is no way to discern what the underlying rate would be if all states had effective outreach and reporting systems and inclusive definitions of abuse and neglect. For example, in a state with a model education and outreach program, the rate was 54 complaints per 1,000 beds.[11,12]   If that state's rate were applied nationwide, there would be 97,200 complaints, with more than 54,000 complaints about abuse.

Prevalence of Neglect in Nursing Homes

I have seen my roommate left lying in the bed for more than one hour with her behind exposed. I feel sorry for my roommate. They treat her so bad. She can't talk or walk.

Georgia Nursing Home Resident
(Atlanta Long-Term Care Ombudsman Program, 2000)

Neglect is more difficult than abuse to identify and thus to quantify. Neglect is typically thought of as "the failure by the responsible caretaker to provide services to maintain [the elder's] physical and mental health" (Lachs et al., 1997).   The federal definition, as applied to the nurse aide registry, is "failure to provide goods and services necessary to avoid physical harm, mental anguish, or mental illness."   The Washington state survey agency branch that manages the nurse aide registry distinguishes between two types of neglect.   One type is represented by the failure to provide needed assistance and services.   A second type occurs when a CNA performs a task inappropriately, such as doing a one-person transfer when a resident actually requires a two-person transfer for safety or when a CNA does a task for which he or she is not qualified and not supervised (e.g., performing a procedure that should be done by a licensed nurse).   While the second type of neglect is distinct, the first is difficult to separate from a more general quality of care problem rooted in broader facility practices and policies rather than in the circumscribed action of one individual staff member.

Sadly, there is considerable evidence of the "failure to provide goods and services necessary to avoid physical harm, mental anguish, or mental illness" in the nation's nursing homes.

---

[11]In this state with a model program, a much higher proportion of complaints addressed issues related to neglect (e.g., 56 percent were about abuse in this state, versus a national average of 70 percent; 38 percent were about neglect).   In addition, most of the complaints in this model state were about verbal or psychological abuse rather than physical abuse, unlike other states.

[12]One state with a relatively low rate noted that it had instituted fingerprinting as part of the criminal background check for applicants for the CNA position.   The state agency reported that the number of people rejected had quadrupled as a result of the greater accuracy of the background checks and that this might account for the drop in complaints the state experienced recently.

Resident and Family Reports of Neglect

Ninety-five percent of the residents who were interviewed as part of the Atlanta Long-Term Care Ombudsman study reported that they had experienced neglect or witnessed other residents being neglected (Atlanta Long-Term Care Ombudsman Program, 2000). The kinds of things they reported included residents being left wet or soiled with feces; not being turned and positioned, which can lead to pressure ulcers; shutting off call lights without helping the resident seeking assistance; not receiving enough help at mealtimes; and residents who needed help with eating and drinking or not getting enough to eat or drink. In focus group interviews, families also discussed instances of neglect, including residents who needed help with eating not receiving it and dying of malnutrition and dehydration, residents being put in tubs of water that were too hot and being scalded, and residents being left for hours or even days in wet and soiled clothing and bedding. They also reported incidents in which pressure ulcers were improperly treated, leading to sepsis and death.

CNA Reports of Neglect

In focus group interviews, CNAs reported that neglect was not unusual. They reported that in times of shortstaffing, neglect of range of motion exercises to prevent contractures, failure to turn and reposition to prevent development of pressure ulcers, neglect of residents' hydration needs (e.g., not taking them fresh water or not reminding cognitively impaired residents to drink), and giving residents too little help with eating were the most common areas of neglect (Hawes et al., 2001). In a survey of CNAs preparing to go through a special training session aimed at preventing abuse and neglect, 37 percent of the CNAs reported they had seen neglect of a resident's care needs (MacDonald, 2000).

Ombudsman Reports

The 1998 compilation of complaints received by the state Long-Term Care Ombudsman program reported that 27 percent of the complaints ombudsmen received had to do with the types of inadequate care that are typically thought of as neglect (e.g., improper handling, accidents, neglected personal hygiene, and unheeded requests for assistance) (Administration on Aging, 2000). Further, the U.S. Department of Health and Human Services, OIG (1999a) found that ombudsman complaints about quality of care have also been increasing in recent years.

Survey Deficiencies

The U.S. Department of Health and Human Services, OIG (1999a) found an increase in the frequency with which deficiencies were cited for neglect and poor quality-of-care. In recent years, deficiency citations increased in 13 of 25 quality of care areas, including such problems as improper care for pressure ulcers, inadequate care to maximize physical functioning in activities of daily living (ADL), and lack of adequate supervision to prevent accidents.

Research Studies

Other studies have raised similar concerns. For example, in a detailed review of records of a sample of residents who died in California nursing homes, U.S. General Accounting Office (1999a) found that more than half had received unacceptable care, including lack of appropriate attention to dramatic, unplanned weight loss, failure to properly treat pressure ulcers, and failure to manage pain. This was a follow-up to a review of deaths from 1986 to 1993 in California nursing homes by an attorney who argued that 7 percent of all residents died as a result of severe neglect (Thompson, 1997). A review of records and care practices in 14 facilities in 11 states, conducted with protocols similar to the GAO's, documented inadequate treatment in one-third of the facilities in the areas of nutritional support, pressure ulcer care, prevention of contractures, pain management, and personal assistance (Johnson and Kramer, 1998). Other studies and hearings by the U.S. Senate Special Committee on Aging have documented similar problems (Bernabei et al., 1998; Blaum et al., 1995; Fries et al., 1997; Hawes et al., 1997; Hawes, 1997; Kayser-Jones, 1997; Phillips et al., 1997). For example, Blaum and her colleagues (1995) found that a major predictor of unintended weight loss and low body-mass index among nursing home residents was that a resident needed help with eating. Similarly, Kayser-Jones and Schell (1997) found that many facilities were so understaffed that even though trays were taken into rooms, residents were not fed.

EVIDENCE ABOUT THE NATURE AND PREVALENCE OF ABUSE AND NEGLECT IN RESIDENTIAL CARE FACILITIES

There are no federal standards that govern residential care facilities, which are known by more than 30 different names across the country.[13]

---

[13]Those names include personal care homes, adult care homes, adult congregate living facilities, residential care homes for the elderly, shelter care homes, homes for the aged, domiciliary care homes, board and care homes, and assisted living facilities.

As a result, there are no national databases containing information on deficiencies. Thus, it is even more difficult than with nursing homes to generate anything approaching estimates of the prevalence or nature of abuse of neglect. This section of the paper briefly reviews what is known about these types of facilities and issues related to abuse and neglect.

What Are Residential Care Facilities?

Other than nursing homes, the most common form of residential settings with services for people with disabilities are generically known as board and care homes, or residential care facilities (RCFs). These terms describe a variety of settings; however, in general they refer to nonmedical community-based residential settings that house two or more unrelated adults and provide some services such as meals, medication supervision or reminders, organized activities, transportation, and help with bathing, dressing, and other activities of daily living (ADL). RCFs are known by more than 30 different names, including adult congregate care, personal care homes, homes for the aged, adult care homes, and group homes. In addition, many states have expanded the category of RCFs to include a specific classification known as assisted living (Mollica, 1998).

There are three basic types of RCFs: (1) group homes serving a clientele with mental retardation or developmental disabilities (MR/DD); (2) homes serving persons with mental illness; and (3) homes serving a mixed population of physically frail elderly, cognitively impaired elderly, and persons with mental health problems. All but 7,000 facilities are in the last category and are the focus of our initiative. They serve a mainly elderly population, although many house a mixed population of frail elderly and residents who have some type of psychiatric condition. In the early 1990s, there were an estimated 46,000 licensed and unlicensed RCFs with more than 700,000 beds (Clark et al., 1994; Hawes et al., 1993; Hawes et al., 1995a). The rapid growth since then of assisted living facilities has probably increased the total number of all types of residential care facilities to more than 50,000 facilities with more than 1 million beds (Hawes, et al., 1999; Assisted Living Federation of America, 1998; American Seniors Housing Association, 1998). As a point of comparison, there are an estimated 16,700 licensed nursing homes with approximately 1.8 million beds serving more than 1.5 million residents (Strahan, 1997). Thus, RCFs are a significant care setting for persons with chronic illness and disability.

Risk Factors: Vulnerability of Consumers

Consumers in RCFs face a number of daunting challenges to protecting their interests and securing adequate health care. Indeed, many RCF resi-

TABLE 14-4   RCF Resident Characteristics

RCF Resident Characteristic	ASPE, 1993[a]	NC, 1994[b]	Maine, 1999[c]
Female	66%	66%	67%
White	91%	71%	98%
Black/African American	7%	29%	—
Aged 85+	34%	24%	33%
Average age	75	—	77
Currently married	13%	8%	8%
Mental retardation/DD	11%	23%	11%
Self-report mental, emotional or nervous condition	33%	51%	42% (with diagnosis)
Moderate to severe cognitive impairment	40%	64%	44%
Received help with 1 to 2 ADLs	21%	21%	32%
Received help with 3+ ADLs	10%	20%	19%
Urinary incontinence	23%	39%	37%
Any behavioral symptom (e.g., wandering, physical aggression)	—	29%	31%
Received any psychotropic medication	41%	—	40%
Medicaid or SSI eligible	34%	71%	18%

[a]The Office of the Assistant Secretary for Planning and Evalaution (ASPE) 1993 study is based on a random sample of residents in 10 states (Hawes et al., 1995a and b).

[b]The 1994 North Carolina study is based on a probability sample of residents statewide (Hawes et al., 1995c).

[c]The Maine data are from the resident universe (Fralich et al., 1997).

dents exhibit the characteristics that place elders at risk of abuse and neglect in other settings. First, RCFs house a population with chronic disease and significant disabilities, as shown in Table 14-4 (Fralich et al., 1997; Hawes et al., 1995a, 1995b, 1995c, 2000). In particular, residents exhibit relatively high levels of cognitive impairment or another mental health condition, with the exception of residents in relatively high-level assisted living facilities (Phillips et al., 2000). Moreover, the average age of residents and their level of functional and cognitive impairment have increased significantly over the last decade (Hawes et al., 1995a). Several studies confirm these findings of significant chronic disease and disability, including significant levels of cognitive impairment and behavioral symptoms, which place them at high risk for abuse and neglect (Fralich et al., 1997; Hawes et al., 1995a, b, c; Hodlewsky, 1998; Kane et al., 1991; National Investment Center Conference, 1998).

A second factor that places RCF residents at risk for abuse and neglect is that they experience considerable social isolation. Several studies found that 83 to 85 percent were unmarried, and one-quarter of the residents had no living children (Fralich et al., 1997; Hawes et al., 1995a, b, c; Phillips et al., 2000). In one study conducted in the mid-1990s, the research found that one-third of 3,200 residents in 10 states reported they had not left the facility in the preceding 14 days; 19 percent reported no visits with family or friends in the preceding 30 days; and 24 percent had visited with friends or family only one or two times in the preceding 30 days (Hawes et al., 1995b). Similarly, in a 1998 survey of a national probability sample of residents in assisted living facilities that offered high services or high privacy, 9 percent reported no visit with family or friends in last 30 days, and 27 percent had visited with friends or family only once or twice in the last 30 days (Hawes et al., 2000). Thus, many residents lacked close family or friends who could be their advocates. In addition, ombudsmen programs that help fill this gap in nursing homes are largely absent in RCF settings, their activities mainly limited to complaint investigation (Phillips et al., 1994). Also, one study interviewed staff and residents and found that most residents and staff were ignorant of the ombudsman program (Hawes et al., 1995a).

Third, many RCF residents have additional characteristics that have been associated with disparities between services and unmet health care needs. Many of these have been identified as risk factors for abuse or neglect in other settings. Although estimates vary across states and types of residential care facilities, an estimated one-third of residents are poor— their care paid for by a combination of Supplemental Security Income (SSI), state supplemental payments, and Medicaid (Hawes et al., 1995a, b, c; Fralich et al., 1997). The majority of residents in traditional RCFs (outside of higher-priced assisted living facilities) would be classified as poor or near-poor (i.e., income less than 200 percent of poverty). Furthermore, about one-third of all residents have mental retardation, developmental disabilities, or persistent, severe mental illness (Fralich et al., 1997; Hawes et al., 1995a, b, c; Mor et al., 1986). As an example of disparities associated with these characteristics, one 10-state study[14] that included a random sample of residents found that residents with SSI as a payor were twice as likely as other residents to have unmet need for assistive devices (Hawes et al., 1995c).

---

[14]The 10 states were selected based on whether they had extensive or limited regulatory systems. Facilities were selected on a stratified, random basis, and residents were randomly selected within the study facilities.

Evidence of Abuse in Residential Care Facilities

Unfortunately, there are no published quantitative studies of abuse in residential care facilities, and there have not even been published qualitative studies, such as focus groups, that addressed issues of abuse. The 10-state study described above interviewed staff members in RCFs using the items developed by Pillemer and Moore (1989); however, rather than interviewing staff by telephone, these were in-person interviews. Fifteen percent of the staff reported witnessing other staff engage in verbal abuse (e.g., threats, cursing, yelling) or forms of punishment, such as withholding food, excessive use of physical restraints, or isolating difficult residents (Hawes et al., 1995b).

The only other available estimates of abuse or neglect in RCFs are from the LTC ombudsman program and the NORS data. However, the ombudsman presence in residential care facilities is much more limited than in nursing homes (Phillips et al., 1994). For example, ombudsmen handled 121,686 cases in FY 1998, but 82 percent of those cases were in nursing home settings; only 17 percent were residents in residential care facilities. However, of the cases handled by ombudsmen in residential care facilities and reported in NORS, physical abuse was one of the top five complaints registered with the ombudsman program (Administration on Aging, 2000).

Neglect and Quality Concerns

The vulnerability of consumers is particularly troubling because of long-standing concerns about quality in RCFs and residents' access to needed health care services. As noted above in the section on defining neglect, it is difficult to define neglect and separate it from poor quality, in general. Moreover, relatively few studies have focused on quality in residential care, and most of those concentrated on medication errors and overuse of psychotropics. Thus, there is only relatively limited evidence available about neglect in residential care facilities.

Several studies throughout the 1980s suggested that RCF residents were not receiving adequate care or were being neglected. Such findings included unsafe and unsanitary conditions, widespread use of psychotropic drugs suggesting some level of chemical restraints, lack of staff knowledge about medication administration, and other problems (Avorn et al., 1989; Budden, 1985; Hartzema et al., 1986; Mor et al., 1986; U.S. General Accounting Office, 1992a, b; U.S. House of Representatives, Select Committee on Aging, 1989).

These concerns were heightened in the 1990s because of the increasingly complex health care needs of residents and continued reports of quality problems (Hawes et al., 1995a). These problems included medication

TABLE 14-5 Resident Reports of Unmet Care
Needs in RCFs Known as Assisted Living

Unmet Need	Percent	Standard Error
Dressing	12	2.89
Locomotion	12	3.29
Toileting	26	12.07
Eating	0.0	0.0

Data for only those residents who received some help with
that ADL.
SOURCE: Phillips et al. (2000).

errors, high rates of psychotropic drug use, poor management of behavioral
symptoms among residents with Alzheimer's disease or other dementias,
including inappropriate use of physical restraints, and poorer functional
outcomes for RCF residents compared to nursing home residents, which
suggested neglect of care needs (Baldwin, 1992; Bates, 1997; Spore et al.,
1995, 1996, 1997a, b; Stark et al., 1995; U.S. General Accounting Office,
1992a). In addition one study asked a national probability sample of
assisted living residents who could respond about whether they had unmet
care needs (Phillips et al., 2000).[15] As shown in Table 14-5, among those
residents who needed assistance with various ADLs, some residents did
report needing more help than they received (e.g., had to wait so long for
help with toileting that they wet or soiled themselves).

These findings are troubling, because state policymakers wish to expand the role of RCFs (Mollica, 1998). States have been permitting higher
levels of acuity (e.g., admission or retention of residents who are bedfast,
chairfast, or use wheelchairs), and many have begun allowing provision of
daily or intermittent nursing care, skilled home care, and hospice care in
RCFs (Hawes et al., 1993; Kane and Wilson, 1993; Manard, et al., 1992;
Mollica, 1998).

LIMITATIONS OF ESTIMATES OF PREVALENCE OF ABUSE AND NEGLECT IN LONG-TERM CARE SETTINGS

The results of these studies suggest that abuse and neglect are widespread across residential long-term care settings. However, there is no

---

[15]This was a national probability sample of residents in ALFs that, relative to the general
population of places calling themselves "assisted living," provided either high services or high
privacy.

definitive evidence about prevalence. There are several reasons for this. First, existing estimates are based on reports to a multiplicity of agencies, each of which uses different definitions, investigative protocols, and standards of proof. Second, research and well-established protocols are needed to distinguish incidents involving abuse and neglect from the natural consequences of multiple chronic diseases and disabilities experienced by long-term care residents. Third, there is significant underreporting by health care professionals, residents and families, and the official mechanisms for receiving formal complaints of abuse and neglect are deeply flawed.

Multiple Reporting Agencies and Differing Definitions

The chief impediment to rigorous epidemiologic research has been widely differing definitions of abuse.

Lachs and Pillemer (1995:437)

There are multiple agencies with some responsibility for investigating cases of abuse or neglect (U.S. Department of Health and Human Services, OIG, 1998, 1999b; Tatara, 1990; Hawes et al., 2001). For residents in nursing homes and residential care facilities, those agencies differ across states but typically include ombudsmen, adult protective services, the state survey agency responsible for licensing nursing homes, the state agency responsible for the operation of the nurse aide registry, Medicaid fraud units in the attorney general's office, and professional licensing boards, such as the Board of Nursing or Boards of Nursing Home Administrators.

As a result, the data from one agency, such as the ombudsmen, should not be taken as an indicator of the amount of abuse, because "many abuse complaints are reported to other state agencies, not to the ombudsman program" (Administration on Aging, 2000). In addition, the existence of multiple reporting agencies means that data on the prevalence of abuse are often incomplete, generated using different definitions and methods of data collection (Baron and Wellty, 1996). In practice, reporting individuals and agencies use different definitions and have different standards and practices for the timing and nature of investigations and for classifying an allegation as substantiated (Hawes et al., 2001; Huber et al., 2001; U.S. Department of Health and Human Services, OIG, 1999b). For example, some of the reporting agencies, such as the Boards of Nursing, use different definitions of abuse, excluding anything that would be classified as verbal or psychological abuse, such as threats or yelling at a resident in anger (Hawes et al., 2001). Similarly, in general, ombudsmen are not held to a standard of beyond a reasonable doubt (Huber et al., 2001). However, in most states, the investigations of abuse by the nurse aide registries do adhere to the standard of beyond a reasonable doubt (Hawes et al., 2001).

Finally, even within the two systems that maintain a national database on abuse and neglect in nursing homes—the NORS used by ombudsmen and the Online Survey Certification and Reporting System (OSCAR) used by state survey agencies—there are variations across states in the definitions, standards of proof, and rates of substantiation they use, despite having uniform requirements (Administration on Aging, 2000; Hawes et al., 2001; Huber et al., 2001; U.S. Department of Health and Human Services, OIG, 1991, 1999b).

Difficulty Detecting and Distinguishing Abuse and Neglect from Effects of Chronic Disease Among the Aging

One of the factors that complicates the task of generating accurate estimates of the prevalence of abuse and neglect is that it is often difficult to distinguish abuse from the effects of the chronic diseases found among many elderly, particularly those at risk for abuse and neglect because of their functional limitations. Signs that may indicate abuse or neglect tend to be attributed to either the normal processes of aging or to the chronic diseases and disabilities experienced by many frail elders (Wolf, 1988). The fact that some injuries thought of as potential markers for abuse may be a product of medical conditions (e.g., spontaneous fractures of the long bones among nursing home residents who were non-weight-bearing) makes the issue singularly complex (Kane and Goodwin, 1991). This problem is accentuated by the lack of care some physicians take when examining elderly residents admitted to hospitals or emergency rooms from nursing homes or residential care facilities and investigating and documenting their injuries. For example, one study examined charts of all elderly nursing home residents admitted to a Level I trauma center for an injury during 1997. The study found that 17 percent of cases reviewed had inadequate documentation to differentiate accidental trauma from abuse or neglect (Barlow et al., 1998).

Widespread Underreporting

As noted earlier, reporting of suspected cases of elder abuse is required in most states under mandatory elder abuse reporting laws; moreover, it is required in all states if it occurs in nursing homes under the provisions governing the Nurse Aide Registry (Hawes et al., 2001; Morris, 1998; Steigel, 1995). Despite this, there is general agreement that there is significant underreporting of cases of suspected elder abuse (Administration on Aging, 2000; American Medical Association, 1992; Atlanta Long-Term Care Ombudsman Program, 2000; Bowers et al., 2001; Pillemer and Finkelhor, 1988). Indeed, most authorities acknowledge that incidents of abuse are underreported, both by mandated "reporters," such as physicians and nurses, and by residents and families (Kleinschmidt et al., 1997; U.S. Department of Health and Human Services, OIG, 1990a; Pettee, 1997; Pillemer and Finkelhor, 1988;Tatara, 1990).[16]

Underreporting by Health Care Professionals

There have been relatively few studies of elder abuse, compared to child abuse (Kleinschmidt et al., 1997; Lachs and Pillemer, 1995). However, there is some evidence that physicians rarely or never report suspected cases of elder abuse involving nursing home residents (U.S. Department of Health and Human Services, OIG, 1990b). Other studies have had similar findings with regard to staff in hospitals. Several studies have found that hospital and emergency department (ED) personnel, such as physicians and nurses, were often unfamiliar with mandatory elder abuse reporting laws (Blakely and Dolon, 1991; Clark-Daniels et al., 1990; Wolf, 1988). In addition, one study found that only 27 percent of emergency physicians had established protocols for identifying and addressing suspected cases of elder abuse (MacNamara et al., 1992). Furthermore, relatively few cases of elder abuse are reported to authorities (Pillemer and Finkelhor, 1988). The same is true for other health care professionals who are in a position to detect abuse and neglect.

A study of emergency department (ED) nurses in Florida found that 83 percent reported seeing what they thought was evidence of abuse of older persons admitted to an emergency room for treatment, but only 36 percent had reported abuse (Reynolds and Stanton, 1983). Two more recent studies demonstrated similar findings, as displayed in Table 14-6. The studies reported on interviews with ED nurses, home health agency nurses, and nurses who worked in acute care (i.e., medical or surgical units) or a long-term psychiatric facility. As shown, most nurses reported observing abuse, including instances of severe injuries, such as skull fractures, sexual assault, bites, and severe bruising (Pettee, 1997). Yet in both studies, there was a significant discrepancy between the proportion of nurses who had observed suspected abuse and those who had reported it (e.g., 73 percent reportedly observed abuse but only 36 percent had reported it). In addition, both

---

[16]One report, however, suggested that aside from nursing home employees, hospital staff were the most likely to report abuse to an ombudsman program (Watson et al., 1993). On the other hand, as noted earlier in this paper, another study found that documentation of injuries occurring among elderly nursing home residents was inadequate to differentiate accidental trauma from abuse or neglect in 47 percent of the 328 cases reviewed (Barlow et al., 1998).

TABLE 14-6 Nurse Observation and Reporting

Topic	Indiana Nurses (percent)[a]	Michigan Nurses (percent)[b]
Abuse Observed	73	60
Type of Abuse Observed		
Physical	22	32
Psychological	10	29
Neglect	39	37
Abuse Reported	36	34
Nurse Knowledge Of...		
Laws on elder abuse	41	34
Mandatory reporting law	57	85
APS	72	50
Immunity	33	23

[a] Nurses (n = 83) in ED and home health agencies.
[b] Nurses (n = 90) in acute care (medical and surgical units) and long-term psychiatric facility.
SOURCE: Adapted from Pettee (1997).

studies found that the majority of nurses (59 percent and 66 percent, respectively) were unaware of laws on elder abuse, and a surprising number of nurses (43 percent) working in EDs or home health were unaware of state mandatory reporting requirements.

Underreporting by Residents and Family Members

There is also evidence from surveys and focus group interviews of underreporting by residents and family members (Atlanta Long-Term Care Ombudsman Program, 2000; Bowers et al., 2001; Hawes et al., 2001; Pettee, 1997). In focus group interviews, surveys, and individual interviews, some residents and family members expressed a general reluctance to complain, evidently feeling that there were other mechanisms for resolving problems, such as working through the resident and family councils or speaking with the administrator. Others feared that a formal complaint might generate retaliation by the facility against the resident. For example, in a recent survey by the Atlanta ombudsman program, 44 percent of the residents who had seen abuse of other residents did not report it. Half (50 percent) did not tell because they feared retaliation (Atlanta Long-Term Care Ombudsman Program, 2000). Other residents and family members did not file formal complaints because they felt the process was futile. For example, in the study by the Atlanta ombudsmen, 38 percent of the residents said reporting "wouldn't do any good" (Atlanta Long-Term Care Ombudsman Program, 2000). Finally, some families reported that they did not file formal complaints in some cases because all their energy was directed at getting adequate medical care for their loved one who had been abused, moving them to the hospital, and then finding a new nursing home for the resident following acute care discharge (Bowers et al., 2001).

Underreporting by Ombudsmen

There is also some underreporting of complaints by ombudsmen (Administration on Aging, 2000; Tatara, 1990). For example, some residents and family members do not consent to having a formal complaint filed. In addition, in a recent survey, one-third of the ombudsmen (36 percent) reported that they viewed their role as resolving complaints with the facility and filing a complaint only if unable to resolve the complaint. Another four percent reported that they would resolve problems between the resident or family and facility without ever filing a complaint (Hawes and Blevins, 2001).

Unreliable Reporting by the Nurse Aide Registries

There is considerable disagreement among the directors of the state nurse aide registries about whether there is overreporting or underreporting of complaints about abuse and neglect, as displayed in Figure 14-2. The situation is complicated by at least two factors. First, facilities are obligated by federal regulation to investigate and report incidents alleged to involve abuse, neglect, or misappropriation. Some respondents felt this encouraged some facilities to report even incidents that were not abuse or neglect just to ensure that they were in compliance with federal regulations. Other respondents felt that some facilities simply discharged CNAs involved in incidents or allowed them to resign, thus terminating any investigation or reporting process. Only 39 percent of the state nurse aide registry directors felt that facilities reported allegations of abuse or neglect "all of the time" (Hawes et al., 2001). Second, it was clear that differing concepts of the nature of abuse led some respondents to label reports of verbal or psychological abuse as overreporting, as illustrated by the following quote from on agency's director/program manager.

> Oh, there is just tremendous overreporting. You know, things like yelling at or threatening a resident. That's not really abuse, and we don't count it.

Aide Registry Director (Hawes et al., 2001)

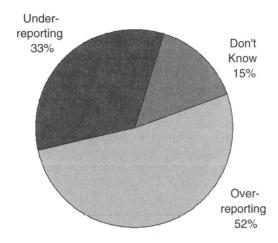

FIGURE 14-2 Agencies' views on the rate of allegations.
SOURCE: Hawes et al. (2001).

There is also reason to believe that data from the nurse aide registries represent an underestimate based on the historically low rates at which these agencies substantiate allegations of abuse and neglect. As reported by the nurse aide registries, the substantiation rates for allegations of abuse and neglect ranged from a low of zero (i.e., no allegations substantiated) to a reported high of 98 percent, although the norm appeared to be a substantiation rate of about one-third for all allegations of abuse or neglect. Fewer than one in five of the state agencies (18 percent) had substantiation rates above 60 percent. About half of the state agencies (47 percent) reported substantiation rates of 20 to 39 percent, while slightly more than one-third of the agencies (35 percent) had rates between zero and 19 percent (Hawes et al., 2001).

There are several reasons for such low substantiation rates. First, in some states considerable time elapsed between the time the alleged incident occurred and the formal investigation by the state nurse aide registry. Second, if the only witnesses were the alleged perpetrator and the victim, most state registries closed the case, classifying it as either insufficient evidence or unsubstantiated. Many nurse aide registry respondents reported being uncomfortable with this decision to essentially drop cases that were based only on the word of a resident. They attributed this decision to the fact that the penalty for a CNA found to have committed abuse was being barred for life from nursing home employment. Thus, the states felt they were held to such a high burden of proof in these cases (e.g., beyond a reasonable doubt)—or would be held to such a standard if the case were appealed to an administrative law judge—that they would not accept cases they viewed as being essentially "he said/she said." Third, if the facility were unable (or unwilling) to identify the alleged perpetrator of abuse, some states would close the case, classifying the injury as "an incident of unknown origin" and the case as unsubstantiated, as illustrated below in a case reported by the adult child of a resident.

> *The DON called me and said my mother had waked up with a bump, a red bump, on her forehead. When I got to the facility that morning, I found her horribly bruised on her face and [the backs of her] forearms, as you can see in the photograph. She looked as if someone had gone seven rounds with her, except she has advanced Parkinson's. The only movement she can make is to raise her arms like this [indicating she could raise them defensively in front of her face]. The facility said she must have gotten them [the bruises and contusions] falling against her bedrails, but she can't move independently in bed. . . . So then they said they didn't know how it happened. When I called the state's toll-free number [for the abuse hotline], I was told they couldn't do anything if the facility couldn't identify the perpetrator. . . . Did anyone suggest I call the police? No, no one.*
>
>   Daughter of a resident, speaking in a focus group with
>   other family members (Hawes et al., 2001)

Finally, there is some evidence to suggest that if the nursing home terminated the employment of the alleged perpetrator or if the CNA in question quit after an alleged incident, the case was closed. However, it appears that some such cases never appear as substantiated nor is the CNA in question ever listed on the registry as barred from nursing home employment (Hawes et al., 2001).

As a result of these factors, the actual number of abuse and neglect cases reported by the nurse aide registries as substantiated is quite small relative to the number of allegations received. In focus group interviews, the directors of the state survey agencies that had overall administrative authority for the nurse aide registries expressed concern about the relatively low rates of substantiation, particularly because most tended to believe that residents and families complained only when something significant had occurred.

Underreporting in the OSCAR Database

The surveys of the state nurse aide registries also suggest that the deficiency data on abuse in OSCAR represent an underestimate of the prevalence of abuse cases. Even when cases of abuse or neglect were substantiated, most states did not cite the facility for a sanction. Indeed, four-fifths of the states (63 percent) that could provide data on deficiency citations reported that they cited a deficiency in fewer than 10 percent of the substantiated cases (Hawes et al., 2001).

RESEARCH CHALLENGES ASSOCIATED WITH DETERMINING THE PREVALENCE OF ABUSE AND NEGLECT IN NURSING HOMES AND RESIDENTIAL CARE FACILITIES

The preceding sections were intended to show that abuse and neglect are apparently widespread and serious problems in long term care settings. Millions of elderly are at risk over the course of their lives, and this population at risk will increase, given current demographic trends. Despite this, there is no conclusive evidence about the prevalence of abuse and neglect. Determining the nature and prevalence of abuse and neglect is important for several reasons. First, policymakers need to know how serious and extensive the problem is in order to determine the priority that should be accorded to remedying the problem. Second, information about prevalence is often an important determinant of funding for research.

This section discusses issues related to research on prevalence of abuse and neglect in long-term care settings. First, we discuss nursing homes and then residential care facilities, if there are different issues. In addition to deciding on how to define abuse and neglect for purposes of research, several additional critical decisions and challenges must be addressed.

Prevalence of Abuse or Neglect

The available evidence has been based on extremely diverse units of analysis and resident, facility, and staff samples. Determining what the focus should be in future research is challenging. One challenge involves defining the nature of the phenomenon. Abuse is probably more easily defined operationally than neglect, because neglect and general issues of substandard quality are difficult to separate. Given that, the following are the types of questions that might reasonably be asked, but each involves a different sample design and data collection strategy.

- How many residents in a given period experience abuse or neglect?
- How many incidents of abuse and neglect occur in nursing homes or residential care facilities (e.g., one resident might experience multiple episodes of abuse over a period of time)?
- How many staff members have abused or neglected one or more residents?
- How many staff members have witnessed abuse or neglect?
- In what proportion of facilities does abuse or neglect occur?

Sampling Issues

There are a number of challenging issues to be decided relative to the sample design for studies of the nature and prevalence of abuse and neglect in long-term care settings. For example, most studies seeking to establish prevalence will involve a multistage sample design. For example, a study that proposed in-person interviews with residents or staff would probably select geographic areas at the first stage, facilities at the second stage, and residents or staff at the third stage.[17]

Sampling Facilities

For nursing homes, a sampling list exists at the national level from the OSCAR database listing all facilities that participate in Medicare or Medicaid. This covers nearly all licensed nursing homes (i.e., more than 95 percent) (Strahan, 1997).

For residential care facilities, there is no national list of facilities. Indeed, securing a list will be a challenging task. First, the list must be constructed at the state level. Second, there are multiple licensing agencies in many states. Thus, a decision must be made about what types of facilities to include and what types to exclude. In general, there are two types of residential care facilities. One group includes facilities specifically licensed for special populations, such as for persons with substance abuse, mental illness, or developmental disabilities. They represent a small proportion of all residential care facilities (e.g., about 7,000 of more than 40,000 facilities) and an even smaller proportion of beds (Clark et al., 1994; Hawes et al., 1995a). Moreover, they tend to receive special funding for programmatic services and to have higher staffing levels than traditional residential care facilities. A second group of facilities, the most common, is licensed for general populations and includes frail elderly and persons with psychiatric conditions. These facilities are generally licensed by state health departments, departments of aging, and departments of community services. In some states, there is a separate licensure category for very small homes (e.g., two to six beds). Moreover, as noted, in a few states, even for the general, mixed population facilities, there are multiple licensing agencies, or some that license while others offer registration (e.g., for Medicaid waiver programs) or certification. Thus, securing a comprehensive, unduplicated list is a challenge.

Another critical sampling issue is whether to oversample among larger facilities. An estimated two-thirds of all residential care facilities have 2 to

---

[17]This will also mean that researchers will need to use analytic software, such as SUDAAN.

10 beds. However, an estimated two-thirds or more of all residents are found in larger facilities (e.g., 11 beds or more).

Sampling Residents

Decisions about sampling residents are intertwined with decisions about data collection, and they too are challenging. As noted above, research suggests that residents at highest risk for abuse and neglect are those with cognitive impairment and behavioral symptoms. Research is more mixed about whether greater levels of impairment in ADLs represent a risk factor. In nursing homes, the majority of residents receive assistance in three or more ADLs, so a random sample would produce adequate numbers of residents with significant physical impairment. Most residents also have moderate to severe cognitive impairment. Many (though not necessarily all) of those will not be candidates for interviews. So, one key issue is how one can collect valid information about the experience of these residents. However, it will not be difficult in even a random sample to secure an adequate number of residents with this risk factor.

Other potential risk factors for abuse or neglect are less common among nursing home residents. For example, the most recent data suggest that fewer than 10 percent of residents are African American and only 9 percent exhibit physically aggressive behaviors. Similarly, if one wished to have results that were generalizable to short-stay residents, one would need to oversample such residents.

Fortunately, there are two sources of data that can inform sampling decisions in nursing homes. The Medical Expenditure Panel Survey (MEPS) Institutional Component provides estimates of the prevalence of various conditions and risk factors among a national probability sample of residents (Krauss and Altman, 1998). Even more immediate data are available through the national database CMS maintains on all nursing home residents in every nursing home certified to participate in the Medicare or Medicaid programs. These data, taken from the Minimum Data Set (MDS), provide information on hundreds of characteristics for the universe of residents.

In residential care facilities, there is less current information available with which to make sampling decisions about residents. The most recent multistate study of residential care facilities is the 10-state study conducted for the U.S. Department of Health and Human Services, Office of the Assistant Secretary for Planning and Evaluation (Hawes et al., 1995a,b). These data are from interviews conducted during 1993, and the states were selected on the basis of their regulatory environment. Within those states, facilities were selected on a random, stratified basis (i.e., size and licensure status), and residents were randomly selected, as were staff members. However, the estimates these data produce are somewhat dated, particularly because there is some expectation that acuity levels have been increasing in RCFs in most states. A more recent ASPE study has produced data on a national probability sample of assisted living facilities, residents, and staff (Hawes et al., 1999, 2000). Rough estimates of resident acuity levels in physical functioning (i.e., ADL) and cognitive status are available for all facilities (Hawes et al., 1999), while more detailed data (e.g., behaviors, falls) are available for residents in assisted living facilities that offer either high services or high privacy (Hawes et al., 2000).

Sampling decisions in residential care are complicated by the fact that there appears to be significant variation across states. Some, like North Carolina, have made aggressive use of RCFs to limit use of nursing homes. In these states, the resident mix is considerably more impaired physically and cognitively than in other states that have not pursued an aggressive expansion in the number of RCFs and in the level of care that may be provided in those facilities. In addition, there appear to be important differences in resident characteristics among different types of residential care facilities. For example, small homes are more likely to have residents with primary psychiatric diagnoses. Similarly, the assisted living sector of residential care is largely populated by persons who have higher incomes and are more racially homogeneous than residents in traditional RCFs. If these factors are expected to have an effect on the prevalence of abuse or neglect, this must be considered in designing the sampling plan of any study aimed at examining prevalence.

Sampling Staff

There does not appear to be sufficient information about staff risk factors from prior studies that would facilitate decisions about whether to oversample certain types of staff. For example, one study suggests that the belief that nursing home residents are childlike makes a staff member somewhat more likely to abuse residents, but there is no obvious way to initially select a sample based on this characteristic. However, the MEPS study provides general demographic data on nursing home staff, and the two ASPE studies also provide such data on staff demographics, training and education, and other characteristics.

My strong recommendation would be to depart from prior studies that interviewed only staff working during the shifts that field interviewers were on site. In practice, when in-person interviews have been used to collect data, this has meant that staff members who work during the morning and evening shifts during the week were overrepresented in staff samples. Night shifts and weekends, however, have a tendency to be short-staffed and to have the fewest supervisors available. Thus, staff working on these shifts may be in situations when abuse and neglect are more likely to occur.

Other decisions involve the type of staff to be studied. Although CNAs provide more than 80 percent of hands-on care, other staff members—from nurses to maintenance staff—are potential perpetrators as well as sources of information about the prevalence and nature of abuse and neglect.

Data Collection Issues

Data collection issues are extremely complex. Interviews with staff members could be conducted by telephone or in person, with some research suggesting that respondents are more willing to self-report illegal or questionable behavior when they are not being interviewed in person. In addition, this would facilitate interviewing staff who work night and weekend shifts.

Interviews with residents are more problematic on several fronts. Most experts agree that in-person interviews are most likely to produce valid and complete information about such sensitive information as their experiences in nursing homes or RCFs. In interviews with residents about whether they had ever had complaints about the care they received and how they handled it, Barbara Bowers and I had great difficulty getting residents to discuss this difficult topic. The Atlanta Ombudsman program, however, had substantial success in its resident interviews, and it is probably worth speaking with Karen Boyles, the Ombudsman Coordinator, about the methods they used.[18]

There is somewhat less agreement about what proportion of residents can be interviewed. Many researchers use a set cutoff point on a scale that measures cognitive function (e.g., Simmons and Schnelle, 2001). Others argue for less reliance on set cut-points, opting to base decisions on initial attempts to interview residents who are able to communicate and have some remaining skills for daily decision making (e.g., Gwen Uman, personal communication, 1999; Morris, personal communication, 2000). Moreover, researchers may wish to apply techniques used in the field of research on persons with developmental disabilities to improve their ability to secure information directly from residents with cognitive impairment.

Whatever the decision about how many residents can be interviewed and how to interview them more effectively, the fact remains that many residents who are presumably at highest risk for abuse and neglect will not be good subjects for interviews. There are at least four basic options for proxy respondents for residents unable to respond verbally:

---

[18]Karen Boyles, Atlanta Long-Term Care Ombudsman Coordinator, (404) 371-3800.

- Use family members who regularly visit the cognitively impaired resident as a proxy respondent. They can be interviewed in person or by telephone. However, some studies suggest that family members report levels of satisfaction with care higher than expressed by residents.
- Use family members who are regularly present in the facility at different times of the day. They may be good observers and reporters about life in the facility or a good supplement to the reports of cognitively intact residents.
- Use cognitively intact residents as proxies. They may know more about the day-to-day life of residents in the facility than family members, who visit only at certain times of the day or week. On the other hand, in facilities with special care units for persons with dementia or even those that locate residents on different units by the type and level of acuity of the resident, intact residents may not be in a position to observe directly the care of residents who cannot respond for themselves.
- Use multiple sources of information for residents who are unable to respond for themselves, including medical records, interviews with family members, interviews with roommates who are cognitively intact, observation of the resident, and interviews with direct care staff. This technique demands highly trained and well-educated interviewers (e.g., RNs) but has been effective in producing reliable information about residents' health and functional status, activities, mood, and preferences (Hawes et al., 1995d).

Another challenging data collection issue is related to protection of human subjects. Staff may be asked to report behavior by themselves or others that is illegal, so confidentiality protections will be crucial. For residents the issue is more complex. Residents and family members fear retaliation if they complain about the care they receive. This is a particularly problematic issue with respect to interviewing residents, because it is difficult to find a place in which they can be interviewed in privacy, completely outside the hearing of others. Most residents in nursing homes and RCFs (except assisted living facilities) have a roommate. In addition, CNAs, housekeeping staff, laundry staff, and maintenance staff may be in and out of a resident's room as a normal course of business. Data collection efforts must take this into account.

It will also be difficult to provide reasonable information about the nature of the study to the facility administrators while still protecting residents. It will be important to stress that the data collection is not aimed at producing any report on individual facilities but rather at producing national estimates. In addition, it will be important to ensure that residents who are selected for interviews are not placed at heightened risk for retaliation.

Furthermore, any data collection efforts must consider what the responsibility is of the field interviewers in terms of mandatory abuse reporting laws. Most state laws require reporting only if the individual witnesses abuse, but some may be broader. In any event, some interviewers will be told about incidents that involve illegal behavior—from rape to assault. Such incidents will represent ethical, legal, and moral challenges for the field interviewers and for the data collection firm.

Finally, the National Institute on Aging (NIA) and other potential funding agencies should work closely with the IRB(s) of any grantees who are selected to study abuse and neglect in nursing homes. In their attempts to protect subjects, some IRBs place such severe restrictions on researchers that meaningful and important research cannot be accomplished.

CAUSES OF ABUSE AND NEGLECT AND IMPLICATIONS FOR RESEARCH

Research on the causes of abuse and neglect may be more important even than prevalence, because it should provide clues to prevention. Such research may address resident and staff risk factors, as well as institutional and environmental factors.

Research on Causes

A male nurse grabbed me, slung me on the floor, and threw me into the bed. He was in a bad mood because we were short-staffed, and he had to work two floors.

Georgia nursing home resident
(Atlanta Long-Term Care Ombudsman Program, 2000)

Facilities place CNAs in situations where abuse is bound to happen.

Aide registry director (Hawes et al., 2001)

Individuals come in who are not adequately trained, and then they have a heavy workload, frustrated, under-oriented, under-supervised, under-paid, under-trained.

Aide registry director (Hawes et al., 2001)

Although there has been only minimal research on the causes of abuse and neglect in residential long-term care settings, there is remarkable consensus among diverse studies and surveys of stakeholders. Three factors about which there is widespread agreement are largely situational and include:

- stressful working situations, particularly staffing shortages;
- staff burnout, often a product of staffing shortages and mandatory overtime; and
- combination of resident aggression and poor staff training on how to handle such challenging behaviors (Hawes et al., 2001; Pillemer and Bachman-Prehn, 1991; Pillemer and Moore, 1989).

Staff Shortages

As shown in Table 14-7, the directors and managers of the nurse aide registries felt strongly that issues related to nursing home staffing levels, training, and turnover were major factors causing or contributing to abuse and neglect. Indeed, nearly all the responses, including the role of low wages, emphasized the role of staffing shortages and poor staff to resident ratios as major causes of abuse and neglect in nursing homes (Hawes et al., 2001). This was consistent with prior studies. A recent study (U.S. Department of Health and Human Services, Health Care Financing Administration, 2000) found major staffing shortages in many nursing homes. Similarly, hearings before the U.S. Senate Special Committee on Aging (1998) and reports by the U.S. General Accounting Office and the U.S. Office of the Inspector General for the U.S. Department of Health and Human Services identified staffing problems as major impediments to quality of care in nursing homes. For example, in 10 states surveyed by the Office of the Inspector General (U.S. Department of Health and Human Services, Office of the Inspector General, 1999a), survey and certification

TABLE 14-7 Nurse Aide Registry Agency Views on Main Causes of Abuse and Neglect

Cited Cause	Percent[a]
Staffing shortages, too few staff, bad staff to resident ratios	85
Staffing shortages and difficulty hiring qualified staff	71
Poor training	61
Poor supervision, management	51
Staff turnover	63
Low wages	78
Combative residents	56
Vulnerable consumers/residents	29

[a]Multiple responses were allowed.
SOURCE: Hawes et al. (2001).

staff, state and local ombudsmen, and directors of state units on aging identified inadequate staffing levels as one of the major problems in nursing homes. The OIG report concluded that the type of deficiencies commonly cited "suggest that nursing home staffing levels are inadequate" (U.S. Department of Health and Human Services, Office of the Inspector General, 1999a). Too few staff, low staff-to-patient ratios, and overworked employees result in increased stress levels, and in focus group interviews, CNAs identified short-staffing as the major cause of abuse and neglect (Hawes et al., 2001).

Staff Training and Aggressive Residents

Staff in many of the state aide registry agencies believed that inadequate training for CNAs was a major factor causing or contributing to abuse and neglect. In part, they suggested, some CNAs might lack an understanding of what constituted abuse. In addition, they argued that cultural factors might play a role. For example, in some families slapping is not considered abusive but an appropriate response to certain behaviors. A prior study that surveyed nursing home staff who acknowledged abusing a resident found that such CNAs were more likely to view the elderly "as children" (Pillemer and Moore, 1989).

> There is this aphasic man from stroke. He's a messy eater but likes to feed himself. He can be aggressive if I try to wipe his mouth. One day, he grabbed me, tried to bite me. If I grab him and sit him down, or even shove him into his chair to keep him from biting me [that] is not abuse. . . . Or some resident will come up behind you and pinch your bottom. I mean, if our spouses treated us like this, they'd be in jail . . . for domestic abuse. This man [the resident who had a stroke and tried to bite her] is cognitively alert. He knows what he is doing; I know he does, because all the time he was grabbing my hand and trying to bite me, he was grinning. And I don't want my fingers in his mouth. I've seen what he puts in there. He puts BM [fecal matter] in his mouth and eats it. If I'm rough with him, I'm just protecting myself from injury.
>
> CNA (Hawes et al., 2001)

Several nurse side registry directors felt that many staff had difficulty in handling residents with behavioral symptoms, particularly combative or aggressive behaviors. Focus group interviews with CNAs demonstrated that, in fact, many CNAs believed that combative behaviors, even among residents with psychiatric illnesses or Alzheimer's disease, were purposive and that some "rough handling" by staff in response or to protect themselves was justified and not abusive (Hawes et al., 2001).

It's OK to be a little rough with a resident if it's defense from attack by a resident. But you know, if the nurse sees fingerprints [bruises] on the resident, she will charge you with abuse. CNA #3

We hear, if they have Alzheimer's, they don't know what they're doing. But I mean it, if our husbands hit us like some residents do, he would be in jail. CNA #12

If someone hits you on the head, surprises you, it's sort of a body mechanism. You raise your arm. You might hit, but it's reflex, not intentional. CNA #3

I had a co-worker [who] had gotten a hepatitis B shot, and it was sore. A resident hit her. Her [the CNA's] arm went up [she demonstrates raising her arm in a threatening way, as if to hit someone]. Automatic reflex. She lost her job. CNA #7

Somebody sneaks up and hits you or pinches. You jump; you might hit someone. It's automatic. CNA #12

That's not abusive. I agree. [That] resident should be brought up on disciplinary procedures. CNA #11

(Hawes et al., 2001)

Indeed, one troubling finding from the CNA focus groups was that there was disagreement among the CNAs about behaviors that were a reaction to something a resident did. In particular, some of the CNAs felt that rough handling of a resident who was physically aggressive with them was justified and not abusive, especially if they perceived the behavior as intentional. Some felt those reflexive actions—or what they termed a startle response—were acceptable. In part, these CNAs felt they had a right to defend and protect themselves from injury. In part, they believed the residents' aggressive behaviors were intentional, that is, that the resident was aware of what he or she was doing. This belief often persisted even when the examples given by the CNAs indicated that the residents had some level of cognitive impairment.

I have a somewhat different opinion on the reflex issue [of hitting back if startled by a resident]. You might get startled, but you know where you are. You're in a nursing home. I tell my staff, who is the resident? The residents, they are who we're here to care for. CNA #9

But you know, it's from physical reaction, not a thought process. CNA #3

Well, you can't let your physical reaction [control]. CNA #8

I agree with . . . [CNA #9]. I think the startle reaction is a result of being overly stressed and overworked. I worked on a [Alzheimer's] Special Care Unit, and I was having a really rough day. It was near the end of my shift, and we had been short-staffed all day. And this one resident who was really confused all the time just kept asking me the same question, over and over and over. She wouldn't let me finish changing her, because she kept going on at me. I was so frustrated. And I just took her by the shoulders and kind of shouted [at her] "Why are you doing this?" And she looked at me, and with perfect clarity, said, "I don't know." And then . . . [she] cried. She cried, and I cried. CNA #8

You never ever had a startle reflex? CNA #12

Not on the job. You remember where you are; remember they are the residents. If you can't control that startle thing without raising your hand to a resident, you shouldn't work in a nursing home. CNA #9

(Hawes et al., 2001)

In the focus groups, other CNAs argued that they had a right to protect themselves from injury but spoke of multiple ways of achieving that without resorting to rough handling of a resident. For example, two staff members noted that their facility had a behavior committee that was specially trained to deal with residents who engaged in challenging or physically aggressive behaviors. This team could be called on if a CNA was having difficulty. Other CNAs said that the policy in their facility was to have a team of CNAs work with a physically difficult or aggressive resident, for protection of both the resident and staff.

In addition, there was disagreement about whether staff members were justified in reflexive hitting, shoving, or yelling at a resident. Some CNAs noted that these reactions and actions were more likely to occur when staff members were tired and overworked, conditions more likely to arise when the facility was short-staffed.

Finally, it is worth noting that some research suggests that some attitudes and experiences intrinsic to the staff member may play a role. Such characteristics included staff having the view that residents were children who needed discipline, staff who reported high levels of arguments or conflict with residents, and those who reported having stressful personal lives (Pillemer and Hudson, 1993; Pillemer and Moore, 1989).

Implications for Research Topics

The following are a few suggestions about the types of research topics that might generate better estimates of prevalence and inform efforts to prevent abuse and neglect in nursing homes and residential care facilities.

Are There Ways to Improve Detection?

• Autopsies might reveal more about prevalence if more deaths in nursing homes and RCFs were examined (Collins et al., 2000).

• Most nurses in two studies reported that the topic of elder abuse and reporting requirements were not part of their nursing education (Pettee, 1997). It would be useful to determine whether curricula in schools of nursing and continuing education programs include information on how to recognize abuse and the responsibility of nurses to report suspected cases of abuse, as recommended by Pettee (1997) and Weiler and Buckwalter (1992). The same is true about neglect. It would be even more useful to determine the effectiveness of different approaches to informing licensed nurses of their responsibilities.

• Do any EDs have protocols in place for identifying suspected cases of abuse and neglect among residents of nursing homes and residential care facilities, for documenting adequately to differentiate between accidental trauma and abuse or neglect, and for reporting such cases to appropriate authorities? Are these protocols followed? Are there any differences in prevalence of reports and substantiated cases among EDs that have such protocols and those that do not?

• What has been the role of medical directors in facilities and resident physicians in detecting, reporting, and preventing abuse and neglect? What might increase their ability to recognize abuse and neglect and their willingness to report it when it occurs? What role can physician licensing boards play?

• What is the effect of ombudsman programs? Prior studies suggested that the existence of the ombudsman program and presence of ombudsmen visiting nursing homes on a regular basis did not influence abuse reporting or even resulted in fewer survey deficiencies (Cherry, 1991; Litwin and Monk, 1987). However, a more recent study analyzed the program after legislation that enhanced its authority and found that the presence of ombudsmen was associated with increased abuse reporting, higher substantiation rates, higher rates of survey deficiencies, and increased use by state survey agencies of enforcement sanctions (Nelson et al., 1995). In addition to conflicting study findings, a current study surveyed state ombudsmen and found differing views among them of their role in addressing complaints about abuse from residents and families (Hawes and Blevins, 2001). This study found many ombudsmen did not routinely file large numbers of complaints with the state survey agencies (e.g., 38 percent of the ombudsmen reported filing fewer than 10 complaints during the preceding year, while 17 percent filed more than 100 complaints in the past 12 months). In addition, they had differing views of the proper role of ombudsmen. Only 24 percent of the ombudsmen reported that they made follow-up calls to the state survey agency when a complaint of abuse or neglect had been filed. Similarly, about one-third of the ombudsmen (36 percent) reported that they filed a complaint only if they were unable to resolve the individual case (Hawes and Blevins, 2001).

These diverse findings suggest the need for:

• Studies that identify different models of ombudsman programs and examine their effect on the prevalence of reports, substantiation rates, deficiency citations, and the use of enforcement sanctions.
• An examination of the effect of various ombudsman interventions on the prevalence and nature of abuse, including an analysis of the conditions under which such interventions will be adopted, fully implemented, and maintained over time in various types of facilities. Examples include programs developed by CARIE (1991) (advocates in Philadelphia), the Atlanta Long-Term Care Ombudsman program, and the North Shore Legal Services Program.
• An examination of the effects of different types of training for nursing facility and RCF staff, resident and family education and empowerment interventions provided by ombudsmen programs (effects on both detection and reporting as well as on prevention).

Causes

• What is the relationship between abuse of residents and the work conditions experienced by direct care staff (e.g., management style, staff satisfaction with working conditions and management support, staff satisfaction with wages and benefits)?
• What is the relationship between aggressive or difficult behaviors by residents and abusive behaviors by staff and whether aggressive staff responses are moderated by staff training, staffing levels, or specific interventions (e.g., use of behavior management teams for residents with challenging behaviors)?
• What staff characteristics are associated with a greater propensity for abuse or neglect, including such factors as gender, reason for choosing work in residential long-term care, attitudes about the elderly, and others?
• What are risk factors for individual staff members—both situational, having to do with their work environment, and intrinsic?

Prevention

• Evaluate different facility management styles (e.g., administrator, director of nursing, unit charge nurses) associated with variations in rates and types of abuse and neglect. In particular, one might follow up on Vince Mor's "good nursing home study" (Mor et al., 1986) and Bowers and Becker's work (1992) to determine whether certain management styles are associated with less abuse and neglect.

- Examine the effect of environmental factors (e.g., that make work in nursing homes more or less difficult or burdensome for staff) and more or less confusing (or in the case of bathrooms, unfamiliar and disturbing) for residents with cognitive impairment.

- Identify and evaluate any model employee screening and hiring practices.

- Evaluate the effects of different staffing models, particularly use of permanent staff assignment to a group of residents (e.g., the primary care model versus the floating CNA model).

- Evaluate the effect of different staffing patterns, particularly in terms of staff-to-resident ratios, on the prevalence and severity of abuse and neglect.

- Identify and evaluate interventions aimed at CNAs that are intended to improve quality or explicitly to prevent abuse. The one most highly regarded by ombudsmen is a training program developed by an advocacy group, the Coalition of Advocates for the Rights of the Infirm Elderly (CARIE), and researcher Karl Pillemer. This program has been evaluated and found to be effective in changing both staff attitudes and behaviors (Pillemer and Hudson, 1993). It would be useful to examine the extent to which the effects persist and whether effects vary across different facility types (e.g., different management styles, different staffing patterns and staffing levels). Another training program worth evaluation might be the one developed by North Shore Legal Services Program (MacDonald, 2000); however, they found difficulties in maintaining and expanding the intervention in facilities.

- Evaluate staff empowerment models, such as Wellspring. Such research should include an analysis of the conditions under which such interventions will be adopted, fully implemented, and maintained over time in various types of facilities.

- Evaluate models of culture change, such as the Eden Alternative, to determine whether they reduce the prevalence or severity of abuse and neglect. Such research should include an analysis of the conditions under which such interventions will be adopted, fully implemented, and maintained over time in various types of facilities.

- Evaluate the effect of different regulatory systems. For example, Washington state has been identified as having a model program for quality assurance and for detection and prevention of abuse and neglect, and ombudsmen, facility administrators, and state agency nurse aide registry staff report that incidents of physical abuse are much less common than the rates reported in other states (Hawes et al., 2001; Hawes, based on site visit interviews in 2001).

REFERENCES

Administration on Aging
1998 *Instructions for Completing the State Long-term Care Ombudsman Program Reporting Form for the National Ombudsman Reporting System (NORS)*. Washington, DC: Department of Health and Human Services, Office of the Secretary of the Administration on Aging.
2000 *FY 1998 Long-Term Care Ombudsman Report with Comparisons of National Data for FY 1996-1998*. Washington, DC: Administration on Aging, Department of Health and Human Services. Available at: *http://www.aoa.gov/ltcombudsman/98report/98finalreport.html*.
American Medical Association
1992 *Diagnostic and Treatment Guidelines on Elder Abuse and Neglect*. Chicago, IL: American Medical Association.
American Seniors Housing Association
1998 *Seniors Housing Construction Report—1998*. Washington, DC: American Seniors Housing Association.
Assisted Living Federation of America (ALFA)
1998 *The Assisted Living Industry: An Overview—1998*. Fairfax, VA: Price Waterhouse for ALFA.
Atlanta Long-Term Care Ombudsman Program
2000 *The Silenced Voice Speaks Out: A Study of Abuse and Neglect of Nursing Home Residents*. Atlanta, GA: Atlanta Legal Aid Society and Washington, DC: National Citizens Coalition for Nursing Home Reform.
Avorn, J., P. Dreyer, K. Connely, and S.B. Soumerai
1989 Use of psychoactive medication and the quality of care in rest homes. *New England Journal of Medicine* 320(4):227–232.
Baldwin, V.R.
1992 *An Analysis of Subjective and Objective Indicators of Quality of Care in North Carolina Homes for the Aged*. Dissertation, University of North Carolina at Chapel Hill, School of Public Health, Department of Health Policy and Administration.
Barlow, B., C. Puetz, J.S. Jones, and D.J. Ray
1998 Institutional 'accidents': Is emergency department documentation adequate for assessment of elder abuse? *Annals of Emergency Medicine* 32(3)(Supplement, Part 2):S60.
Baron, S., and A. Wellty
1996 Elder abuse. *Journal of Gerontological Social Work* 25(1/2):33–57.
Bates, E.
1997 Mining the golden years: Homes for the elderly dig deep into tar heel politics— and hit pay dirt. *The Independent*. A series that ran from April 30 to May 6, 1997.
Bernabei, R., G. Giovanni, K. Lapane, F. Landi, C. Gatsonis, R. Dunlop, L. Lipsitz, K. Steel, and V. Mor
1998 Management of pain in elderly patients with cancer. *Journal of the American Medical Association* 279(23):1877–1882.

Blakely, B.E., and R. Dolon
    1991   The relative contributions of occupation groups in the discovery and treatment of
            elder abuse and neglect. *Journal of Gerontological Social Work* 1(17):183–199.
Blaum, C.S., B.E. Fries, and M.A. Fiatarone
    1995   Factors associated with low body mass index and weight loss in nursing home
            residents. *Journal of Gerontology: Medical Sciences* 50A(3):M162–M168.
Bourland, M.D.
    1990   Elder abuse: From definition to prevention. *Postgraduate Medicine* 87(2):139–
            144.
Bowers, B., C. Hawes, S. Burger
    2001   Focus group interviews with family members of nursing home residents and indi-
            vidual interviews with residents about the complaint process. Conducted for the
            Complaint Investigation Improvement Project (CIP). Working papers at the
            School of Nursing, University of Wisconsin at Madison (Bowers) and the School
            of Rural Public Health, Texas A&M University System Health Science Center,
            College Station, TX (Hawes).
Bowers, B., and M. Becker
    1992   Nurse's aides in nursing homes: The relationship between organization and qual-
            ity. *The Gerontologist* 32(3):360–366.
Bristowe, E., and J.B. Collins
    1989   Family mediated abuse of non-institutionalized frail elderly men and women liv-
            ing in British Columbia. *Journal of Elder Abuse and Neglect* 1:45–64.
Budden, F.
    1985   Adverse drug reactions in long-term care facility residents. *Journal of the Ameri-
            can Geriatrics Society* 33:449–450.
Burgess, A.W., E. Dowdell, and R. Prentky
    2000   Sexual abuse of nursing home residents. *Journal of Psychosocial Nursing* 38:11–
            18.
California Advocates for Nursing Home Reform
    1998   *Status Report on California's Nursing Home Industry.* San Francisco, CA: Cali-
            fornia Advocates for Nursing Home Reform.
Cherry, R.L.
    1991   Agents of nursing home quality of care: Ombudsmen and staff ratios revisited.
            The Gerontologist 31:302-308.
Clark, R., J. Turek-Brezina, C. Hawes, and C. Chu
    1994   *The Supply of Board and Care Homes: Results from the 1990 National Health
            Provider Inventory.* Presentation at the Gerontological Society of America, At-
            lanta, Georgia, November, 1994.
Clark-Daniels, C.L., R.S. Daniels, and L.A. Baumhover
    1990   Abuse and neglect of the elderly: Are emergency department personnel aware of
            mandatory reporting laws? *Annals of Emergency Medicine* 19:970–977.
Clarke, M.E., and W. Pierson
    1999   Management of elder abuse in the emergency department. *Emergency Medical
            Clinics of North America* 17(3):631-644.
The Coalition of Advocates for the Rights of the Infirm Elderly (CARIE)
    1991   *Ensuring an Abuse-Free Environment: A Learning Program for Nursing Home
            Staff.* Philadelphia, PA: CARIE.
Collins, K.A., A.T. Bennet, R. Hanzlick, and the Autopsy Committee of the College of Ameri-
can Pathologists
    2000   Elder abuse and neglect. *Archives of Internal Medicine* 160(11):1567–1569.

Coyne, A.C., W.E. Reichman, and L.J. Berbig
1993   The relationship between dementia and elder abuse. *American Journal of Psychiatry* 150:643–646.

Doty, P., and E.W. Sullivan
1983   Community involvement in combating abuse, neglect, and maltreatment in nursing homes. *Milbank Memorial Fund Quarterly Health and Society* 61:2.

Douglass, R.L., T. Hickey, and C. Noel
1980   *A Study of Maltreatment of the Elderly and Other Vulnerable Adults.* Ann Arbor, MI: University of Michigan, Institute of Gerontology, unpublished manuscript.

Dyer, C.B., V. Pavlik, K.P. Murphy, and D.J. Hyman
2000   The high prevalence of depression and dementia in elder abuse or neglect. *Journal of the American Geriatrics Society* 48(2):205–208.

Ehrlich, F.
1993   Patterns of elder abuse. *Medical Journal of Australia* 158(4):292.

Elon, R., and L.G. Pawlson
1992   The impact of OBRA on medical practice within nursing facilities. *Journal of the American Geriatric Society* 40:958-963.

Fontana, A.
1978   Ripping off the elderly inside nursing homes. In: *Crime at the Top: Deviance in Business and the Professions*, J.M. Johnson and J.M. Douglass, eds. Philadelphia, PA: Lippincott.

Fralich, J.T., C.A. McGuire, and J. DiMillo
1997   *Developing a Case Mix System for Residential Care Facilities in Maine: Options and Issues.* Prepared for the Maine-Net Demonstration Project (HCFA Grant #11-C904731/1-0) by the Edmund S. Muskie School of Public Service, University of Southern Maine, Portland, ME.

Fries, B., C. Hawes, J. Morris, C. Phillips, V. Mor, and P. Park
1997   Effect of the national resident assessment instrument on selected health conditions and problems. *Journal of the American Geriatrics Society* 45(8):994-1001.

Fulmer, T.T.
1989   Mistreatment of elders: Assessment, diagnosis, and intervention. *Nursing Clinics of North America* 24:707–716.

Gubrium, J.F.
1975   *Living and Dying at Murray Manor.* New York: St. Martin's.

Hartzema, A.G., N.P. Godbout, S.D. Lee, T.R. Konrad, and F.M. Eckel
1986   Evaluation of an educational intervention to reduce medication administration errors in domiciliary care facilities. Unpublished manuscript. Chapel Hill, N.C.: University of North Carolina, School of Pharmacy.

Hawes, C., M. Rose, and C. Phillips
1999   *A National Study of Assisted Living: Results of a National Survey of Facilities.* Washington, DC: U.S. Department of Health and Human Services, Office of the Assistant Secretary for Planning and Evaluation.

Hawes, C.
1997   *The Prevalence of Undernutrition Among Nursing Home Residents.* Testimony before the U.S. Senate Special Committee on Aging–Forum on the Risk of Malnutrition in Nursing Homes. Washington, DC, October 22, 1997.

Hawes, C., V. Mor, C.D. Phillips, B.E. Fries, J.N. Morris, E. Steele-Friedlob, A. Greene, and M. Nennstiel
    1997   The OBRA-87 nursing home regulations and implementation of the resident assessment instrument: Effect on process quality. *Journal of the American Geriatrics Society* 45(8):977–985.

Hawes, C., and D. Blevins
    2001   *The Role of the Ombudsman in Nursing Home Complaint Investigations.* Presentation prepared for the annual meeting of the National Citizens Coalition for Nursing Home Reform, Arlington, DC (September 30 to October 3, 2001, postponed). College Station, TX: Texas A&M University System Health Science Center School of Rural Public Health.

Hawes, C., D. Blevins, and L. Shanley
    2001   *Preventing Abuse and Neglect in Nursing Homes: The Role of the Nurse Aide Registries.* Report to the Centers for Medicare and Medicaid Services (formerly HCFA) from the School of Rural Public Health, Texas A&M University System Health Science Center, College Station, TX.

Hawes, C., M. Rose, and C. Phillips
    1999   *A National Study of Assisted Living for the Frail Elderly: Results of a National Telephone Survey of Facilities.* Washington, DC: U.S. Department of Health and Human Services, Office of the Assistant Secretary for Planning and Long-Term Car. Available at: *http://aspe.hhs.gov/daltcp/home.htm.*

Hawes, C., V. Mor, J. Wildfire, L. Lux, R. Green, V. Iannacchione, and C. Phillips
    1995a   *Executive Summary: Analysis of the Effects of Regulation on the Quality of Care in Board and Care Homes.* Report to the U.S. Department of Health and Human Services, Office of the Assistant Secretary for Planning and Evaluation, Washington, DC. Research Triangle Park, NC: Research Triangle Institute.

Hawes, C., J. Wildfire, V. Mor, V. Wilcox, D. Spore, V. Iannacchione, L. Lux, R. Green, A. Greene, and C. Phillips, C.
    1995b   *A Description of Board and Care Facilities, Operators and Residents: Analysis of the Effect Of Regulation on the Quality of Care in Board and Care.* Report to the U.S. Department of Health and Human Services, Office of the Assistant Secretary for Planning and Evaluation, Washington, DC. Research Triangle Park, NC: Research Triangle Institute.

Hawes, C., L. Lux, J. Wildfire, R. Green, L. Packer, V. Iannacchione, and C. Phillips
    1995c   *Study of North Carolina Domiciliary Care Home Residents.* Research Triangle Park, NC: Research Triangle Institute.

Hawes, C., J. Morris, C.D. Phillips, V. Mor, and B. Fries
    1995d   Reliability estimates for the minimum data set for nursing facility resident assessment and care screening (MDS). *The Gerontologist* 35(2):172–178.

Hawes, C., J. Wildfire, and L. Lux
    1993   *The Regulation of Board and Care Homes, Results of a 50-State Survey: National Summary.* Washington, DC: American Association of Retired Persons.

Hawes, C.
    1990   The Institute of Medicine study: Improving quality of care in nursing homes. In: *Advances in Long-Term Care,* P. Katz, R.L. Kane, and M. Mezey, eds. New York: Springer.

Hayley, D.C., C.K. Cassel, L. Snyder, and M.A. Rudberg
    1996   Ethical and legal issues in nursing home care. *Archives of Internal Medicine* 156(3):249–256.

Hodlewsky, R.T.
1998   *Facts and Trends: 1998—The Assisted Living Sourcebook.* Washington, DC: National Center for Assisted Living, American Health Care Association.

Homer, A.C., and C. Gilleard
1990   Abuse of elderly people by their caregivers. *British Medical Journal* 301:1359–1362.

Huber, R., K. Borders, F.E. Netting, and H.W. Nelson
2001   Data from long-term care ombudsman programs in six states—The implications of collecting resident demographics. *The Gerontologist* 41:61–68.

Huber, R., F.E. Netting, and J.R. Kautz
1996   Differences in types of complaints and how they are resolved by local ombudsmen operating in/not in Area Agencies on Aging. *Journal of Applied Gerontology* 15(1):87–101.

Institute of Medicine
1986   *Improving the Quality of Care in Nursing Homes.* Committee on Nursing Home Regulation. Washington, DC: National Academy Press.

Jacobs, R.H.
1969   One-way street: An intimate view of adjustment to a home for the aged. *The Gerontologist* 9:268–275.

Johnson, M.F., and A. Kramer
1998   *Quality of Care Problems Persist in Nursing Homes Despite Improvements since the Nursing Home Reform Act.* Paper prepared for the Committee on Quality on Long-Term Care, Institute of Medicine. Denver, CO: University of Colorado Health Sciences Center.

Johnson, T., ed.
1991   *Elder Mistreatment: Deciding Who Is at Risk.* Westport, CT: Greenwood Press.

Kane, R.A., R.L. Kane, L.H. Illston, J.A. Nyman, and M.D. Finch
1991   Adult foster care for the elderly in Oregon: A mainstream alternative to nursing homes? *American Journal of Public Health* 81(9):1113–1120.

Kane, R.A., and K.B. Wilson
1993   *Assisted Living in the United States: A New Paradigm for Residential Care for Frail Older Persons?* Washington, DC: American Association of Retired Persons.

Kane, R.S., and J.S. Goodwin
1991   Spontaneous fractures of the long bones in nursing home patients. *American Journal of Medicine* 90:263–266.

Kayser-Jones, J.
1990   *Old, Alone, and Neglected: Care of the Aged in Scotland and the United States.* Berkeley, CA: University of California Press.

Kayser-Jones, J., and E. Schell
1997   The effect of staffing on the quality of care at mealtime. *Nursing Outlook* 45(2):64–72.

Kemper, P., and C. Murtaugh
1991   Lifetime use of nursing home care. *New England Journal of Medicine* 324(9):595–600.

Kleinschmidt, K.C., P. Krueger, and C. Patterson
1997   Elder abuse: A review. *Annals of Emergency Medicine* 30(4):463–472.

Krauss, N.A., and B.M. Altman
1998   *Characteristics of Nursing Home Residents—1996 (AHCPR Pub. No. 99-0006).* Rockville, MD: Agency for Health Care Policy and Research. MEPS Research Findings No. 5.

Kyle, D.
    1998   *Management and Oversight of Long-term Care in Louisiana.* Legislative Audi-
            tor, Performance Audit Division. Baton Rouge, LA.
Lachs, M.S., L. Berkman, T. Fulmer, and R.I. Horowitz
    1994   A prospective community-based pilot study of risk factors for the investigation of
            elder mistreatment. *Journal of the American Geriatrics Society* 42:169–173.
Lachs, M.S., and K. Pillemer
    1995   Abuse and neglect of elderly persons. *New England Journal of Medicine*
            333(7):437.
Lachs M.S., C. Williams, S. O'Brien, L. Hurst, and R. Horwitz
    1996   Older adults: An 11-year longitudinal study of adult protective service use. *Ar-
            chives of Internal Medicine* 156:449–453.
    1997   Risk factors for reported elder abuse and neglect: A nine-year observational
            cohort study. *The Gerontologist* 37:469–474.
Litwin, H., and A. Monk
    1987   Do nursing home patient ombudsmen make a difference? *Journal of
            Gerontological Social Work* 2:95–104.
MacDonald, P.
    2000   *Make a Difference: Abuse/neglect Pilot Project.* Danvers, MA: North Shore
            Elder Services. Project report to the National Citizens' Coalition for Nursing
            Home Reform, Washington, DC.
Manard, B., N.B. Altmn, L. Kane, and A. Zeuschner
    1992   *Policy Synthesis on Assisted Living for the Frail Elderly.* Report to the U.S.
            Department of Health and Human Services, Office of the Assistant Secretary for
            Planning and Evaluation. Fairfax, VA: Lewin-VHI, Inc.
Marshall, C.E., D. Benton, and J.M. Brazier
    2000   Elder abuse: Using clinical tools to identify clues of mistreatment. *Geriatrics*
            (Feb):55:42–53.
McNamara, R.M., E. Rousseau, and A.B. Sanders
    1992   Geriatric emergency medicine: A survey of practicing emergency physicians.
            Annals of Emergency Medicine 21:796–801.
Mendelson, M.A.
    1974   *Tender Loving Greed.* New York: Knopf.
Mollica, R.
    1998   *State Assisted Living Policy–1998.* Portland, ME: National Academy for State
            Health Policy.
Monk, A., L.W. Kaye, and H. Litwin
    1984   *Resolving Grievances in the Nursing Home: A Study of the Ombudsmen Pro-
            gram.* New York: Columbia University Press.
Mor, V., S. Sherwood, and C. Gutkin
    1986   A national study of residential care for the aged. *The Gerontologist* 26(4):405–
            417.
Morris, R.M.
    1998   Elder abuse: What the law requires. Available at: *www.rnweb.com.*
Moss, F., and V. Halamandaris
    1977   *Too Old, Too Sick, Too Poor, Too Bad.* Germantown, MD: Aspen Systems
            Corporation.
Murtaugh, C.M., P. Kemper, and B.C. Spillman
    1990   The risk of nursing home use in later life. *Medical Care* 28:952–962.

National Center on Elder Abuse
  1998 *The National Elder Abuse Incidence Study.* Report prepared for the Administration on Aging and Administration for Children and Families in collaboration with Westat, Inc. Washington, DC: Author.
National Investment Center Conference
  1998 *National Survey of Assisted Living Residents: Who Is the Customer?* Annapolis, MD: National Investment Center.
Nelson, H.W., R. Huber, and K.L. Walter
  1995 The relationship between volunteer long-term care ombudsmen and regulatory nursing home actions. *The Gerontologist* 35:509–514.
New York Nursing Home Community Coalition
  1992 *The Nursing Home Complaint System in New York State—Does It Work?* New York: Nursing Home Community Coalition.
New York State Moreland Act Commission
  1975 *Regulating Nursing Home Care: The Paper Tigers.* Albany, NY: New York State Moreland Act Commission.
  1976 *Long-term Care Regulation: Past Lapses, Future Prospects.* Albany, NY: New York State Moreland Act Commission.
Ohio General Assembly Nursing Home Commission
  1978 *A Program in Crisis: An Interim Report.* Columbus, OH: Ohio General Assembly Nursing Home Commission.
O'Malley, T.A., D.E. Everitt, H.C. O'Malley, and E.W. Campion
  1983 Identifying and preventing family-mediated abuse and neglect of elderly persons. *Annals of Internal Medicine* 99:998–1005.
Paveza, G.J., C. Cohen, C. Eisdorfer, S. Freels, T. Semla, J.W. Ashford, P. Gorelick, R. Hirschman, D. Luchins, and P. Levy
  1992 Severe family violence and Alzheimer's disease: Prevalence and risk factors. *The Gerontologist* 32:493–497.
Pettee, E.J.
  1997 Elder abuse: Implications for staff development. *Journal of Nursing Staff Development* 13(1):7–12.
Phillips, C., C. Hawes, and M. Rose
  2000 *A National Study of Assisted Living for the Frail Elderly: High Service or High Privacy Assisted Living Facilities, Their Residents and Staff: Results from a National Survey.* Washington, DC: U.S. Department of Health and Human Services, Office of the Assistant Secretary for Planning and Long-Term Care. Available at: *http://aspe.hhs.gov/daltcp/home.htm.*
Phillips, C., L. Lux, J. Wildfire, and C. Hawes
  1994 *Long-term Care Ombudsman Activities in Board and Care Facilities.* Paper commissioned by the Institute of Medicine, Committee on Long-Term Care Ombudsmen. Research Triangle Park, NC: Research Triangle Institute.
Phillips, C.D., J.N. Morris, C. Hawes, B.E. Fries, V. Mor, M. Nennstiel, and V. Iannacchione
  1997 Association of the resident assessment instrument (RAI) with changes in function, cognition, and psychosocial status. *Journal of the American Geriatrics Society* 45(8):986–993.
Pillemer, K., and R. Bachman-Prehn
  1991 Helping and hurting: Predictors of maltreatment of patients in nursing homes. *Research on Aging* 13:74–95.
Pillemer, K., and D. Finkelhor
  1988 The prevalence of elder abuse: A random sample survey. *The Gerontologist* 28(10):51.

Pillemer, K., and B. Hudson
    1993   A model abuse prevention program for nursing assistants. *The Gerontologist*
            33:128–131.
Pillemer, K., and D.W. Moore
    1989   Abuse of patients in nursing homes: Findings from a survey of staff. *The Geron-
            tologist* 29:314–320.
Pillemer, K., and J.J. Suitor
    1992   Violence and violent feelings: What causes them among family caregivers? *Jour-
            nal of Gerontology* 47:S165–S172.
Podnieks, E.
    1992   National survey on abuse of the elderly in Canada. *Journal of Elder Abuse and
            Neglect* 4:5–58.
Reynolds, E., and S. Stanton
    1983   Elder abuse: A nursing perspective. In: *Abuse and Maltreatment of the Elderly:
            Causes and Interventions*, J.I. Kosberg, ed. Boston: John Wright.
Shapira, E.Z.
    2000   Elder abuse: Society's forgotten issue. *General Dentistry* (Sept./Oct.) 48(5): 490,
            492.
Simmons, S.F., and J.F. Schnelle
    2001   The identification of residents capable of accurately describing daily care: Impli-
            cations for evaluating nursing home care quality. *Gerontologist* (Oct.) 41(5):
            605–611.
Spector, W.D., J.A. Fleishman, L.E. Pezzin, and B.C. Spillman
    2001   *Characteristics of Long-Term Care Users.* Paper commissioned by the Institute
            of Medicine, Committee on Improving Quality in Long-Term Care. Publication
            No. 00-0049. Rockville, MD: Agency for Healthcare Research and Quality.
Spore, D., V. Mor, J. Hiris, E.P. Larrat, and C. Hawes
    1995   Psychotropic use among older residents of board and care facilities. *Journal of
            the American Geriatrics Society* 43(12):1403–1409.
    1996   Regulatory environment and psychotropic use in board and care facilities: Re-
            sults of a 10-state study. *Journal of Gerontology: Medical Sciences* 51A(3):
            M131–M141.
    1997a   Inappropriate drug prescriptions for elderly residents of board and care facilities.
            American Journal of Public Health 87(3):404–409.
    1997b   Suboptimal drug prescriptions for elderly residents of board and care facilities.
            Journal of Gerontology: Medical Sciences 87(3):404–409.
Stannard, C.
    1973   Old folks and dirty work: The social conditions for patient abuse in a nursing
            home. *Social Problems* 20:329–342.
Stark, A.J., R.L. Kane, R.A. Kane, and M. Finch
    1995   Effects on physical functioning of care in adult foster homes and nursing homes.
            Gerontologist 35(5):648–655.
Steigel, L.A.
    1995   *Recommended Guidelines for State Courts Handling Cases Involving Elder Abuse.*
            Washington, DC: American Bar Association.
Strahan, G.W.
    1997   *An Overview of Nursing Homes and Their Current Residents: Data from the
            1995 National Nursing Home Survey, Advance Data from Vital and Health Sta-
            tistics (No. 280).* Hyattsville, MD: National Center for Health Statistics.
Tatara, T.
    1990   *Elder Abuse in the United States: An Issue Paper.* Washington, DC: National
            Aging Resource Center.

Tatara, T., and L. Kuzmeskus
  1996-   *Elder Abuse in Domestic Settings.* Elder Abuse Information Series, No 1. Wash-
  1997   ington, DC: National Center on Elder Abuse.
Thompson, M.
  1997   Fatal neglect: In possibly thousands of cases, nursing home residents are dying
            from a lack of food and water and the most basic level of hygiene. *Time*
            150(17):34–38 (October 27).
U.S. Department of Health and Human Services, Center for Medicare and Medicaid Services
  2001   *Quarterly Report on the Progress of the Nursing Home Initiative* (January). Bal-
            timore, MD: Center for Medicare and Medicaid Services, U.S. Department of
            Health and Human Services.
U.S. Department of Health and Human Services, Health Care Financing Administration
  2000   *Appropriateness of Minimum Nurse Staffing Ratios in Nursing Homes: Phase 1
            Report.* Baltimore, MD: Health Care Financing Administration.
U.S. Department of Health and Human Services, Office of the Inspector General
  1990a   *Resident Abuse in Nursing Homes: Resolving Physical Abuse Complaints.* Wash-
            ington, DC: U.S. Government Printing Office.
  1990b   *Resident Abuse in Nursing Homes: Understanding and Preventing Abuse.* Wash-
            ington, DC: U.S. Government Printing Office.
  1997   *State of Maryland's Ombudsman Program for Processing of Elder Abuse and
            Neglect Complaints and Accuracy of Geriatric Nurse Aide Registry.* Washing-
            ton, DC: U.S. Government Printing Office.
  1998   *Safeguarding Long-term Care Residents.* Washington, DC: U.S. Government
            Printing Office.
  1999a   *Quality of Care in Nursing Homes: An Overview.* Washington, DC: U.S.
            Government Printing Office.
  1999b   *Abuse Complaints of Nursing Home Residents* (OEI-06-98-00340). Washing-
            ton, DC: U.S. Government Printing Office.
U.S. General Accounting Office
  1989   *Insufficient Assurances That Residents' Needs are Identified and Met.* Report to
            Congressional Requesters. Washington, DC: U.S. Government Printing Office.
  1992a   *Board and Care Homes: Elderly at Risk from Mishandled Medications.* Report
            to House Subcommittee on Health and Long-Term Care. Washington, DC: U.S.
            Government Printing Office.
  1992b   *Drug Use and Misuse in America's Board and Care Homes: Failure in Public
            Policy.* Report to House Select Committee on Aging. Washington, DC: U.S.
            Government Printing Office.
  1999a   *California Nursing Homes: Care Problems Persist Despite Federal and State
            Oversight* (GAO/HEHS-98-202). Washington, DC: U.S. Government Printing
            Office.
  1999b   *Nursing Homes: Complaint Investigation Processes Often Inadequate to Protect
            Residents* (GAO/HEHS-99-80). Washington, DC: U.S. Government Printing
            Office.
  1999c   *Nursing Homes: Additional Steps Needed to Strengthen Enforcement of Federal
            Quality Standards* (GAO/HEHS-99-46). Washington, DC: U.S. Government
            Printing Office.
U.S. House of Representatives
  2001   *Abuse of Residents Is a Major Problem in U.S. Nursing Homes.* Committee on
            Government Reform, Special Investigations Division, Minority Staff report pre-
            pared for Representative Henry A. Waxman. Washington, DC: U.S. Govern-
            ment Printing Office.

U.S. House of Representatives, Select Committee on Aging
    1989   *Board and Care Homes in America: A National Tragedy* (Comm. Pub. No. 101-711). A report by the Chairman of the Subcommittee on Health and Long-Term Care, House of Representatives.
    1990   *Elder Abuse: A Decade of Shame and Inaction.* Hearing by the Subcommittee on Health and Long-Term Care.

U.S. Senate
    1970   *Medicare and Medicaid: Problems, Issues and Alternatives.* Report of the Staff to the Committee on Finance. Committee Print, 91st Congress, 1st Session. Washington, DC: U.S. Government Printing Office.
    1971   *Trends in Long-Term Care—Part 18.* Subcommittee on Long-Term Care, Senate Special Committee on Aging. Washington, DC: U.S. Government Printing Office.

U.S. Senate Special Committee on Aging
    1974-   *Nursing Home Care in the United States: Failure in Public Policy.* An Introduc-
    1975   tory Report; (1975—a series of additional reports). Senate Report No. 73-1420, 93rd Congress, 2nd Session. Subcommittee on Long-Term Care, Special Committee on Aging. Washington, DC: U.S. Government Printing Office.
    1998   *Hearing on Crooks Caring for Seniors: The Case for Criminal Background Checks* (Print 105-33). Washington, DC: U.S. Government Printing Office.

Vladeck, B.C.
    1980   *Unloving Care: The Nursing Home Tragedy.* New York: Basic Books.

Watson, M.M., T.C. Cesario, S. Ziemba, and P. McGovern
    1993   Elder abuse in long-term care environments: A pilot study using information from long-term care ombudsmen reports in one California County. *Journal of Elder Abuse and Neglect* 5:95–111.

Weiler, K., and K.C. Buckwalter
    1992   Geriatric mental health: Abuse among rural mentally ill. *Journal of Gerontological Nursing* 30(9):32–36.

Wolf, R.S.
    1988   Elder abuse: Ten years later. *Journal of the American Geriatrics Society* 36:758–762.

Wolf, R.S., and K. Pillemer
    1989   *Helping Elderly Victims: The Reality of Elder Abuse.* New York: Columbia University Press.

15

Elder Abuse Intervention: Lessons from Child Abuse and Domestic Violence Initiatives

*David A. Wolfe**

Despite being in the public eye for many years, progress in all areas of research, causes, consequences, and interventions of elder abuse has been very slow. Consequently, there is a noticeable lack of intervention initiatives or evaluations in this field. A recent review of interventions in child abuse, elder abuse, and domestic violence identified 144 controlled evaluations, yet only 2 dealt with the topic of elder abuse (Chalk and King, 1998). This is not surprising, however, when one considers how intervention in related areas of domestic violence developed slowly at first, hampered by a lack of research findings on causes and limited funding directives. Almost in stages, the related fields of child abuse and domestic violence grew from the voices of concerned practitioners as well as survivors, gaining the attention of the public and the recognition of researchers and professionals. Efforts to understand and deal with abuse of the elderly by family members or other caregivers are reminiscent of where the study of child abuse and woman abuse was 20 years ago. Although there is still much to be done in terms of detection and investigation in these two related fields, knowledge gained from past and recent efforts may benefit current intervention planning in elder abuse.

The current chapter is intended to offer insights into intervention and

---

*David A. Wolfe, Ph.D., is a professor in the Department of Psychology at the Social Science Center, University of Western Ontario.

prevention possibilities with elder abuse on the basis of findings in related, but somewhat more advanced, areas of child abuse and domestic violence. Importantly, this chapter does not address the full extent of the problem of elder abuse or the full range of interventions available to address it; rather, it examines intervention possibilities involving some form of elder abuse based on other forms of family violence. The common denominator for this discussion is that all three populations involve close, interdependent relationships with others, which form the potential circumstances and context for abuse. At the same time, there are many important differences between the contexts and consequences of elder abuse when compared to other abused populations, and these differences have important implications for how one might intervene with the elderly. Nonetheless, lessons derived from progress in child abuse and domestic violence initiatives provide a valid starting point for drawing more attention to elder abuse.

Cynically, one could argue that little progress has been made in addressing the fundamental causes and consequences of the many forms of domestic violence, as well as their effects on children, over the past three decades. These problems seem as serious as ever and major underlying causes, such as abuse of power, inequality, and modeling of violence in the home, remain largely unchanged. Unfortunately, society's response to these difficult problems has been largely one of detection and management, in which services are given on an individual basis only when it becomes absolutely necessary. Although crisis management makes sense when the intervention is critically needed and highly effective at a particular point in time, it is poorly suited to address fully the dynamics of woman, child, and elder abuse (Wolfe and Jaffe, 2001). Unless additional resources and strategies are brought to bear, the task far exceeds the capabilities of most crisis intervention approaches, which are a necessary but insufficient part of our response to domestic violence.

From a more optimistic perspective, in less than two decades scientific, professional, and activist groups have played a prominent role in recognizing the links between various forms of domestic violence and serious mental health and other issues (Peled et al., 1995). Shelters for battered women and their children have increased dramatically, there are more laws on the books, and there is consensus that family members who are maltreated by other family members must be protected (Family Violence Prevention Fund, 1998). Increased interest and understanding by researchers and clinicians in the field of domestic violence make it possible to establish a scientific foundation for implementing prevention and treatment initiatives and public policy to end elder abuse and related forms of violence.

Society's responses to woman abuse and child abuse, in particular, took more than two decades to turn from preliminary recognition and acknowledgment to more uniform opposition and action. While legal changes created an impetus for change, an initiative for change is also emerging from various professions to recognize the signs of domestic violence and to conduct proper inquiries and referrals when such cases come to their attention. Despite their pivotal role, however, the training and education of health care professionals about family violence remain inadequate for proper intervention (Institute of Medicine, 2001).

Mental health professions have adopted standards, procedures, and practices for dealing with many forms of domestic violence, which have been implemented sporadically at community, state, and national levels. Social service professionals have supported and often been responsible for the development of new treatment orientations and options for both victims and perpetrators of domestic violence. At a preventative level, many communities have recognized their responsibility in dealing with woman and child abuse issues through training programs, education, and the allocation of resources to relevant individuals and families. Finally, the general public's level of consciousness has been raised by the widespread use of hot lines, abuse registries, and public education campaigns.[1] This chapter considers how these developments in related areas of domestic violence can inform the field of elder abuse intervention.

ASSESSMENT AND INTERVENTION ISSUES

Screening and Detection

There have been numerous attempts in the last decade to develop screening instruments to identify persons at risk for elder abuse or neglect, following the lead of child welfare authorities. However, detection of abuse and neglect of the elderly is complicated by a number of factors, such as the recognition that older adults are often unwilling to report abuse due to feelings of shame, fear of retaliation, or fear of being placed in an institution (Mulligan, 1990). By and large, elder abuse investigators have developed screening instruments much like those aimed at detecting child or woman abuse, which are designed and put into place by persons in hospitals and other front-line community-based settings.

The goals of risk assessments are to guide and structure decision-making, to predict future harm and classify cases, to aid in resource manage-

---

[1] Although these changes have had a dramatic impact on the problem of domestic violence, especially considering the relatively short period of time in which a social change of this magnitude has been accomplished, they have been far from universal and consistent across North America

ment by identifying service needs for children and families, and to facilitate communication within the agency and other community stakeholders (Hollinshead and Fluke, 2000). Evidence suggests that risk and safety assessments have benefited children and families in the child welfare system. Implementation of an immediate safety assessment protocol for children in Illinois, for example, resulted in a 23 percent decrease of recurrence in a six-month period; three years after the implementation of this tool the recurrence rates were down by over 28 percent (Fluke et al., 1999).

The problem of woman abuse has also been approached through improved screening and detection, especially in relation to suspicious injury. Like elder abuse, the problem is complicated by the fact that most battered women are reluctant to volunteer the circumstances related to their injuries. However, when they are directly asked if this is the case, most women disclose the relevant information (Hotch, 1994). The conventional wisdom that women in abusive relationships are reluctant to disclose such information or that they resist efforts to change the nature of their relationship is not supported—more often than not, battered women will share their experiences with medical personnel when provided with a nonconfrontational and nonjudgmental atmosphere. Consequently, many hospitals now have protocols for screening woman abuse and other forms of domestic violence, which typically include a list of warning signs and symptoms that should prompt specific questions during the history-taking procedure. Such protocols may also serve as training instruments to ensure ongoing awareness and sensitivity to potential domestic violence victims. The Vancouver General Hospital, for example, reported that their rate of correctly detecting domestic violence cases increased 2.5 times as the result of introducing such a protocol (Jaffe et al., 1996).

The assessment of elderly persons who may be at risk for maltreatment by a family member is currently less formalized than is true of the other types of domestic violence. Whereas the medical system plays a prominent role in elder abuse, there are important insights that the mental health and social service systems can add to the overall assessment of persons at risk for family abuse, especially concerning victim and family characteristics.

Several elder abuse-screening instruments are currently available, which direct attention toward characteristics of the person, the caregiver, or the family system (e.g., Kozma and Stones, 1995; McDonald, 1996; Reis and Nahmiash, 1995, 1998). These measures are used as brief screening tools to identify persons who may be at risk for further follow-up and assessment, based on known indicators of elder abuse. The 29-item Indicators of Abuse (IOA) screening measure, for example, is based on an abuse-indicator model comprised of three main types of abuse signals: (a) caregiver personal problems/issues; (b) caregiver interpersonal problems/issues; (c) care receiver social support shortages and past abuse. Although practical, screening methods are limited by the few studies in this area. Some measures overly focus on adult children as potential perpetrators of elder abuse or fail to recognize some of the contextual aspects of abuse, such as chronic stress resulting from long-term responsibilities of a fragile, elderly, combative individual (McDonald and Collins, 2000). Moreover, most existing measures are biased toward factors related to physical abuse and neglect, with less attention paid to factors of psychological and financial abuse or violation of the person's rights.

Intervention Goals

Following efforts by advocates to recognize the basic humanitarian need for assistance, most intervention and prevention efforts in elder abuse, child abuse, and domestic violence began with broadly based services offered within existing social networks. As greater recognition occurred, some communities introduced additional specialized services and resources, such as changes to laws and policies, training of professionals, and establishing abuse registries and telephone hot lines. The next stage of intervention usually involves coordinated, system-integrated approaches to enhance the quality of services already available, which are in place in many North American communities for child and woman abuse, but much less so for elder abuse. Once in place, prevention programs in schools, law enforcement agencies, and similar organizations can begin to promote awareness and deterrence of elder abuse and related forms of domestic violence in the true prevention sense (Wolfe and Jaffe, 2001).

Like child abuse, elder abuse interventions have primarily arisen from either agency- or community-based initiatives. This reflects the mandate of adult protective service agencies and their procedures for responding to abuse and neglect, whereas community-based efforts attempt to integrate or coordinate services found throughout the community in other social service agencies. Typically, intervention protocols include a variety of approaches that include legal, therapeutic, educational, and advocacy complements (Reis and Nahmiash, 1995). Throughout the 1990s some progress was made in terms of initiatives for elder abuse designed for both protection efforts and community services, although no systematic evaluations have been conducted.

Existing approaches to elder abuse intervention focus primarily on three overlapping goals and strategies: (1) legislative, including statutory adult protection service programs, modeled after child abuse initiatives; (2) community services, based on integrated models that attempt to provide coordinated services spanning legal, medical, and psychosocial needs of at-risk seniors, modeled after domestic violence strategies; and (3) education and prevention, including advocacy and empowerment for seniors, derived from the aging network (Anetzberger, 2000). Each of these approaches is discussed below, drawing heavily from child abuse and domestic violence intervention experiences in light of limited knowledge specific to elder abuse. As noted in a recent volume on violence in families (Chalk and King, 1998), major issues especially challenging to effective interventions in the area of elder abuse include the degree of dependence between offenders and victims, limited funding for programming support, and striking a balance between privacy and individual rights.

Legislative Intervention

Over the last 30 years, the legal system's response to most forms of domestic violence has gradually shifted from one in which the maltreatment of family members was tolerated and even condoned to one of almost universal condemnation. This change is reflected in criminal law, tort law, family law, immigration law, and even international human rights law. During the 1970s, for example, a series of international and national conferences on child abuse, woman abuse, and abuse of the elderly resulted in new laws and initiatives at all levels of jurisdictions designed to cope with these concerns in both the United States and Canada. Some of these efforts represented extensions and revisions of existing civil and criminal statutes, while others were attempts at new forms of intervention and services. The end result was that, in one manner or another, new statutes concerning domestic violence in all its forms are now in place throughout North America. However, there are still fewer legal options available to older victims than for other victims of domestic violence (Jaffe et al., 1996).

Adult Protection

All U.S. states and Canadian provinces have enacted special adult protection legislation (McDonald and Collins, 2000). Influenced by child welfare models, such legislation provides legal powers of investigation, intervention, and mandatory reporting. Typically, these methods give extensive powers of investigation to specific agencies, including the authority to apply to the court for provision of services to those found incapable. To assist in implementation of these legal interventions, some communities have developed resource networks consisting of local health, social service, and legal agencies that provide resources to respond to elder abuse and neglect in an integrated and cooperative manner (see Coordinated Community Responses, below). Such networks provide a continuum of services to abused adults, act as a resource for service providers, and offer reliable and consistent service to consumers (McDonald and Collins, 2000).

Adult protection laws relating to the elderly closely resemble the protective services model derived from child abuse legislation, in contrast to the law enforcement model of domestic violence laws. Advocates of adult protection legislation argue that older adults are safeguarded by such means, and attempts can be made to improve their level of functioning while protecting them from harm. Similar to the foster care crisis pursuant to child welfare legislation, however, an overemphasis on adult protection poses the risk of increased placement of seniors in institutions. In the absence of evaluation findings, the value of adult protection legislation is considered below in light of similar measures accompanying child welfare and domestic violence initiatives.

Child Protection

State intervention for children was predicated on the assumption that alternative care by the state (i.e., removing children from abusive or dangerous family environments) was a benevolent intervention when families had failed or violated standards of care. Alternative care was assumed to remove the child from harm and provide a stable and therapeutic environment, as well as to provide a brief period for family rehabilitation. This view has been challenged more recently by the realization that not all interventions are beneficial and, in fact, can do more harm than good in some cases by introducing further victimization and disruption into the child's life (Melton, 1990; Wolfe and Jaffe, 1991). Thus, confusion remains between the needs and rights of children and families.

The traditional response of the juvenile court system that emerged from child welfare legislation was, generally, to maintain or reunify the entire family, including the abuser. This policy became controversial, however, as authorities argued that often the best protection for abused children is to assist their mothers in keeping the abusive father away from both the child and the mother. Some courts now advocate reunification for only the nonviolent family members.

Wald and colleagues (1988) examined whether maltreated children benefit more from foster care or from home care. They found that improved services to families, such as counseling, health care, parent education and support, can help to keep abused and neglected children in their home residences, but not without significant costs. That is, children in both settings showed signs of emotional stress and adjustment difficulties that related to the dilemmas in their respective environments. At home, they had to deal with ongoing family disorganization and conflict, and in foster care settings children had to confront disruption and adapt to a new family system. Therefore, the impact of either placement must be evaluated not only in terms of the children's personal safety, but also in reference to their social, emotional, and intellectual development (a similar argument often arises in the debate concerning protection of elders from abuse). In either home or foster care these children require a high level of services for many years to cope with the trauma they have experienced. In effect, legal interventions for children were intended to provide a safety net for abused children, based on the belief that it is in their best interest to be protected from abuse and neglect. Paradoxically, such protection carries with it certain risks to the child's ongoing development and family relationship.

Domestic Violence Laws

Men who are physically abusive toward their partners and/or children typically come to the attention of domestic violence specialists through either arrest or treatment referral. Unfortunately, studies on the efficacy of both arrest and treatment outcomes with this population are discouraging: Neither arrest nor treatment has been shown to have large effects on men's violent behavior toward their partners. This finding points to the need to intervene before patterns of abusive behavior are developed. Specific legal interventions derived from the domestic violence literature are considered below in terms of their relevance to the elderly and how they might be changed to suit the elderly.

Restraining (Protection) Orders. Restraining orders, an approach that emerged in both U.S. and Canadian legal systems to deal with domestic violence, are intended to "restrain" someone (usually a family or ex-family member) from contact with another family member. All North American courts authorize the use of restraining orders, although jurisdictions may issue them under different conditions (e.g., in some cases a restraining order may be issued simply on the basis of threats, while in others physical abuse must be alleged). They also differ in how the order is enforced and in its duration. Many states also authorize juvenile court judges to issue restraining orders against one or both parents of an abused child, reducing the risk of further harm to the child.

Although few studies offer a definitive conclusion, the overall effect of such orders appears to be beneficial; nonetheless, a restraining order can also increase the risk to the petitioner. Such orders apparently work best in cases where the conditions in the order are clearly specified, where the defendant understands the consequences for violating the order, and where the punishment is strictly enforced if the order is violated (Jaffe et al., 1996).

Criminal Law and Arrest Policies. In the mid-1980s considerable attention was focused on arrest as a possible treatment for domestic violence offenders, prompted by the publication of results from the Minneapolis Domestic

Violence Experiment (Sherman and Berk, 1984; for detailed review see Chalk and King, 1998). However, replications of the Minneapolis experiment largely revealed that arrest has, at best, a small deterrence effect for domestic violence offenses; men's history of assault is, by far, the strongest predictor of future domestic violence offences (Scott and Wolfe, 2000).

Since enactment of the Violence Against Women Act, communities have increased coordination and cooperation among police, prosecutors, victim advocates, the judiciary, and other community institutions related to domestic violence (Sullivan and Allen, 2001). Although controversy over the relative benefits of arrest in domestic violence cases continues, many state and provincial legislatures and local police departments have adopted pro-arrest, warrantless arrest, or mandatory arrest policies in such cases. Some policies have mandated arrest for violations of restraining orders; others do not mandate arrest for spouse abuse or restraining order violations but do require the investigating officer to file a report stating why an arrest was not made. In some jurisdictions, mandatory arrest policies have led to high numbers of battered women being arrested; the current trend is to require officers to determine which party is the primary aggressor, so that victims acting in self-defense are not arrested (Edleson, 1999). Finally, many states and police departments have mandated training programs on domestic violence as part of their initial and ongoing advanced officers' training programs. Increasingly, policies also call for law enforcement to provide a resource card to victims, arrange for medical help, and provide transportation for the victim to a safe place.

Implications

Domestic violence laws, aimed at protecting abused women (and sometimes men) from abusive partners remain controversial and untested in relation to elder abuse. On the one hand, the nature of the dependency relationship between older persons and their caregivers is different from other forms of domestic violence. For example, an older person may depend on a relative for survival in the community, with relatively few alternative residential options. Abused partners sometimes have other options with respect to leaving an abusive relationship and/or having the abuser removed without jeopardizing their own survival. The nature of the dependency relationship, therefore, has important implications for the relevance of domestic violence laws such as restraining orders or criminal law and arrest policies.

On the other hand, approaches to elder abuse that underscore power and control issues (rather than caregiving stress or other contributing factors) remain viable (Harbison, 1999). In this regard, courts may need to protect older persons while considering their best interests in terms of existing family and community supports and living arrangements, including necessary accommodations (e.g., for mobility, hearing, or memory impairments) to improve the experiences of older victims with the court system (Brandl and Meuer, 2000). Although elder abuse laws are viewed by practitioners as more effective when mandatory reporting is included (Bond et al., 1995), opponents argue that mandatory reporting to identify elder abuse must be accompanied by appropriate programs and services (Macolini, 1995).

Recent evaluations of the benefits derived from mandatory child abuse reporting laws that have been in place for four decades provide some direction to this issue. Due to mounting criticisms of the lack of services following child protection investigations and the ensuing family disruption (U.S. Advisory Board on Child Abuse and Neglect, 1993), efforts at reform were initiated in the 1990s. Several states have implemented a dual response system in which only the most serious cases are investigated and less serious cases are referred to community-based services. The states of Florida and Missouri have both conducted major evaluations of these reforms and have found that a dual response system can result in positive changes in child safety, family satisfaction, and community involvement in child protection. Child protective services reforms in both of those states were related to lower rates of re-referral, improved family satisfaction, and increased use of community services (Gordon, 2000).

Community Services

Community services for child abuse and domestic violence have been widely used, and similar approaches to elder abuse and neglect have gained proponents in recent years. Community responses are usually integrated to reduce costs and oversights and involve crisis intervention services (such as hot lines, police involvement in laying charges, protection orders, and emergency and secondary shelters) as well as legal clinics and ongoing support groups. Such methods usually involve educating the public and the abuse victim about their rights as well.

Although this approach has considerable strength, some practitioners caution that some components, such as the use of crisis intervention, are problematic with the elderly because their problems tend to take a longer time to sort out (McDonald and Collins, 2000). Moreover, community services tend to focus primarily on cases of physical abuse and thus may be less geared to the needs of the neglected elderly. Below we consider medical and psychological efforts to address elder abuse, followed by the beginnings of a coordinated community response to elder abuse.

Medical/Psychological

Because few high-risk elderly people are involved in social networks (e.g., school, employment, etc.), opportunities to respond to suspected cases of abuse and neglect are limited to those who come into contact with the family (e.g., physicians, visiting nurses, hospital staff, caseworkers, and others). These professionals have often received training in detecting abused women and children, which suggests that a similar campaign could be implemented to enhance their ability to detect and report suspected cases of elder abuse.

Changes in medical practice related to improved assessment in domestic violence cases include refined standard medical procedures as needed for domestic violence assessment and improved history taking and assessment as needed to complement the medical examination (McDonald and Collins, 2000). These efforts have resulted in physicians, nurses, and ancillary personnel being more skilled in recognizing and reporting relevant cases of woman or child abuse, and providing medical testimony when needed. In many communities physicians and nurses have been instrumental in mobilizing resources, supporting shelters, and volunteering their expertise in a variety of ways.

With the growing acknowledgment of the magnitude of elder abuse, medical practitioners have also developed systems to inform doctors and nurses regarding procedures for examining suspected cases of maltreatment in elderly patients. Kingston and Penhale (1995), for example, provide a list of physical findings and risk factors that are related to physical abuse, sexual abuse, and neglect in elderly patients who come to the attention of emergency room staff. The need for further expansion in this area has been recently documented (Institute of Medicine, 2001).

Although very few psychosocial interventions for elder abuse have been evaluated, two studies warrant discussion. Scogin and colleagues (1992) conducted a controlled treatment study designed to assist abusive caregivers, in which participants received didactic presentations, group discussions, role-playing, and guided practice. They were compared with caregivers who did not receive training, based on measures of general mental health, anger, self-esteem, and degree of burden. Although the program had only a minor impact on anger and self-esteem, caregivers in the treatment program reported reduction in personal costs associated with caregiving. An important finding was that the no-treatment group experienced an increase in symptoms of distress while treatment participants experienced a decrease.

Anetzberger and colleagues (2000) focused their evaluation on an educational curriculum on issues of elder abuse, cross-training initiatives on Alzheimer's disease, and additional materials to aid caregivers in identifying their own risk of abuse and how to access resources. Although the study lacked a control group, benefits were deduced on the basis of positive changes in knowledge, attitudes, and behavior of staff that participated.

Coordinated Community Responses

A number of coordinated programs designed to improve services for the elderly have emerged in the United States and Canada. These programs are characterized by efforts to assess overall needs and then integrate them into a plan that best meets consumer priorities. In most cases, optimal independent living status is the preferred outcome, which is dependent on financial, health, and emotional support. To assist in this effort, many communities have moved toward development of multidisciplinary teams composed of workers from many different community agencies. These teams provide consultation on abuse cases and help coordinate and assist agencies in providing services, especially those that may not be readily available in the community (Wolf, 1992). This approach is modeled after interagency domestic violence task force teams, which serve as the means by which various relevant players (e.g., legal services, child protection, shelters, service providers, and educators) can communicate and solve problems.

A program described by Adele Weiner of Long Island University illustrates a coordinated approach for elderly victims in a large urban area (Weiner, 1991). Her program brought together representatives from several resources, including health care professionals, community leaders, religious groups, and families with elderly members. A series of workshops and consultation/referrals served as the means for training the participants in identifying and preventing elder abuse, and in providing them with information regarding the availability of services. Although not all the project's goals were realized, Weiner's experiences serve as a practical guide to the problems one might encounter in developing such programs, especially in urban communities.

The multiservice program by the San Francisco Consortium for the Prevention of Elder Abuse represents another state-of-the-art approach to dealing with this problem. A team consisting of representatives from the major service entities meets once every month to review and assess elder abuse cases that involve a coordinated combination of needs. Professionals from case management, family counseling, mental health, geriatrics, civil law, law enforcement, financial management, and adult protective services organize an integrated plan for assisting even the most difficult cases. Although the benefits of this and similar programs have not been scientifically evaluated, the advantages to such a systematic approach are evident and may serve as a model for other communities (Goldman Institute on Aging, 2001).

Contributions from Child Abuse and Domestic Violence

Offender Treatment: Child Abuse. Psychosocial interventions with reported maltreating parents developed gradually from an individual-focused pathology model to a more encompassing ecological model, with an evolving emphasis on the importance of the parent-child relationship and its context. Simultaneously, the orientation toward treatment shifted gradually away from a deviance viewpoint and more toward one that accounts for the vast number of stress factors that impinge on the developing parent-child relationship (Wolfe, 1999). This shift toward a more contextual theory of maltreatment places greater emphasis on the importance of promoting parental competence and reducing the burden of stress on families.

Although intervention models have greatly improved and have contributed to encouraging gains in treatment outcomes, the field remains split between promising research findings and the realities of child protection and welfare. Unfortunately, the dominant theme in most services to maltreating families remains that of protection, not treatment (Azar and Wolfe, 1998). This conundrum leaves inadequate services available to the larger number of parents who are at risk of child abuse or neglect and who could benefit the most from early intervention. Nonetheless, important strides have been made in ways to reduce child abuse and neglect among high-risk samples of parents and children. Most relevant to elder abuse intervention is the finding that multileveled programs, that is, programs offering additional services tailored to individual and family needs over time, are worth the additional effort and expense, compared to less intensive services.

Early methods of treatment for physical abuse (e.g., lay counseling, psychotherapy, and provisions of support services) were too narrow in scope to produce changes in the disturbed family interaction patterns that are central to child abuse and neglect. By the late 1970s, national evaluation studies indicated high recidivism rates both during and after treatment (Cohn, 1979; Herrenkohl et al., 1979), which prompted strategies that targeted child-rearing attitudes, skill deficiencies, and anger control. Intervention techniques for the kinds of deficits exhibited by physically abusive families were modified for this population on the basis of well-developed behavioral training methods, such as child management skills training, stress and anger management training, and cognitive restructuring approaches (Wolfe, 1999).

Based on an awareness that child abuse may arise from poor parental preparation and assistance, especially in the early years, intervention strategies for physical abuse have emphasized education, training, and resources for at-risk families and community service providers, as well as direct assistance to caregivers to reduce stress, anger, and similar issues. Evaluations of interventions for child physical abuse and neglect indicate that cognitive-behavioral approaches are the most widely supported methods for assisting maltreating parents (Corcoran, 2000; Hansen et al., 1998). These methods are effective (relative to standard protective-service interventions involving brief counseling and monitoring) in modifying parental behaviors that are most relevant to child maltreatment, such as appropriate child-rearing and self-control skills. Techniques such as relaxation and self-management skills training, cognitive restructuring (viewing child behavior more appropriately), problem-solving training, and stress and anger management training are often combined with structured training in basic child-rearing skills. These methods, either singly or combined, have been successful at teaching coping and problem-solving skills to abusive as well as neglectful parents (Fantuzzo et al., 1986; Kolko, 1996; Wolfe and Wekerle, 1993). Regardless of these advances in treatment, however, the prevailing view for preventing child abuse and neglect is to act earlier rather than later.

Offender Treatment: Woman Abuse. Counseling centers for abusive men are now regarded as an important addition to community services for domestic violence. Offender treatment programs originated in the early 1970s as voluntary programs for men whose partners were seeking the aid of shelter services. In recent years, the criminal justice system has been making increasing use of treatment programs for sentencing men arrested for assaulting their partners. Currently, an average of 80 percent of clients in such programs are referred by probation officers or are attending treatment due to a court mandate (Scott and Wolfe, 2000). Many of these programs use group approaches that encourage participants to take responsibility for their behavior and to find new ways to relate to their partners and to any children involved. The central characteristics of these programs involve accepting responsibility for one's behavior (in contrast to blaming victims), confrontation from other batterers familiar with evasion and denial, challenging attitudes and behaviors that promote male dominance and sexist values, and training in self-control and alternative approaches to dealing with anger, stress, and frustration.

Intervention for abusive men is usually conducted in small groups that emphasize pro-feminist explanations for partner violence and use cognitive-behavioral or psychotherapeutic techniques to bring about change. Although the overall effectiveness of these efforts is still a matter of debate, existing studies endorse their efficacy over alternative models, such as treatment for drug abuse, one-on-one psychotherapy, insight therapy, etc., especially if these alternative approaches do not require the man to accept responsibility for his behavior or if he remains unaccountable for his actions. However, the major limitation of these new programs is that most men refuse to participate unless court-ordered. Moreover, even those who do make an initial inquiry on their own, or are court-mandated, rarely continue to complete the entire program once the crisis has passed or the court's authority has been withdrawn (drop-out rates for batterer treatment programs vary from 20 to 80 percent, depending on how rates are calculated; see Scott and Wolfe, 2000). Even those men who are court-ordered to attend treatment drop out at rates similar to voluntary clients. Moreover, among the few evaluations of batterer intervention programs judged to be methodologically sound, small and generally nonsignificant differences are found in recidivism rates of those who attend intervention and those who do not. Approximately one-third of men participating in various programs re-assault in the year following intervention (32 percent to 39 percent re-assault rates; see Gondolf, 1998).

Coordinated Community Response. The domestic violence movement sparked innovative programs, such as support and advocacy services, which elder abuse efforts have begun to emulate. Importantly, domestic violence intervention models adhere to the belief that victims or potential victims should not be treated as patients, but rather should be empowered through supportive groups, advocacy in the legal system, and awareness of the entire range of options available (Jaffe et al., 1996). Furthermore, advocacy initiatives maintain that the least restrictive and intrusive interventions should be applied to an older person's situation. In practice, advocates advise clients of their rights and alternative services available and can assist in carrying out plans. An important feature of advocacy is the advocate's independence of any formal delivery system, which allows him or her to establish a positive relationship. Studies suggest that when victims have advocates they report less social isolation, are better linked to community services, achieve more goals, and are less likely to suffer abuse (Filinson, 1999). Nonetheless, many older adults may not know how to act on the rights they now understand they have and may not get the assistance they deserve.

A systems-based response to violence against women and children may be of direct benefit to prevention initiatives regarding elder abuse. Each of these issues carries the added complexity of involving not only multiple social service organizations but also other systems such as health care, criminal justice, education, and government, religious, and business organizations. A principal component of such initiatives in domestic violence is a well-developed and coordinated community response, involving community-wide efforts to bring together relevant stakeholders to respond to domestic violence comprehensively. A coordinated community response typically involves a coordinating council, with the goal of enhancing the response by reducing fragmentation and facilitating a shared vision among community members. These councils often consist of representatives from service systems organizations involved in child abuse or woman abuse.

One of the benefits of such coordinating councils is to encourage exchange among persons throughout the community and working in different organizations and settings, as well as developing more highly integrated service delivery systems and enhancing communication (Sullivan and Allen, 2001).

Conclusions and Implications

Although the field of elder abuse clearly lacks scientific evaluations of effective interventions, several implications may be drawn from intervention studies involving child abuse and domestic violence. First, there is evidence to suggest that interventions aimed at assisting caregivers in their important role hold promise for this population. Interventions that have been successfully used with abusive *parents*, in particular, have a clear parallel to elder abuse. Importantly, both forms of abuse emerge in the context of a dependency relationship, whereby the caregiver must learn about and respond appropriately to the needs and demands of the dependent child or adult. Cognitive-behavioral methods addressing misunderstandings about the reasons for a child's behavior, misattributions, and limited knowledge of normal development, for example, have been particularly successful with abusive parents and would likely apply to elder abuse caregivers as well.

In addition, there is converging evidence supporting the utility and acceptance of certain interventions for elder abuse, based largely on clinical reports, uncontrolled studies, and practitioner surveys. Based on professional consensus, Nahmiash and Reis (2000) conclude that the most successful strategies involve concrete services such as nursing care and homemaking assistance, followed by empowerment strategies such as support groups, education, and volunteer buddy/advocates (e.g., Hiatt and Jones, 2000). Moreover, similar to abusive parents discussed above, caregiver abusers require individual supportive counseling to reduce anxiety, stress, and depression, as well as education and training concerning care of the elderly. These valuable clinical impressions and accepted practices from the field point to areas of important intervention priorities and evaluation.

The intervention literature for caregivers of older adults with dementia offers further insights into promising psychosocial interventions. Although these studies do not, for the most part, focus on elder abuse populations, they provide valuable guidance on ways in which caregivers can be helped to minimize their distress and presumably decrease the likelihood of elder abuse. In a recent review, Schulz and colleagues (2001) concluded that caregiver intervention studies show promise of achieving clinically significant outcomes in improving depressive symptoms and reducing anxiety, anger, and hostility, symptoms that have been causally linked to various forms of domestic violence. As in the child abuse literature, intervention methods with nonabusive but stressed adult caregiver populations include a variety of educational and psychotherapeutic interventions such as problem solving, coping skills training, behavior management training, support groups, cognitive-behavioral therapy, and other types of counseling. In general, caregivers of adults with aging impairments are likely to benefit from enhanced knowledge about the disease, the caregiving role, and resources available. Caregivers may also benefit from training in general problem-solving skills and specific anger-management skills related to their role (Schulz et al., 2001).

EDUCATION AND PREVENTION

Similar to child abuse and woman abuse, prevention of elder abuse focuses on educational initiatives, which are believed to be critical elements in any comprehensive approach to domestic violence. These strategies have focused on education of older adults concerning their rights and how to seek help, as well as educating professionals, caregivers, and the general public regarding the nature of elder abuse and its prevention.

Educating the Elderly

Educating older adults provides them with knowledge as to how to protect themselves and their rights, which contributes to feelings of increased control and self-efficacy. Some communities offer support and problem-solving assistance as an adjunct to broader education strategies. For example, Project Care in Montreal incorporates both individual and group support to empower clients (Reis and Nahmiash, 1995). This program involves volunteer "buddies" who meet regularly with abused seniors on a one-to-one basis, in an effort to reduce social isolation and inform seniors of their rights. In addition, the program offers an empowerment group that meets weekly to help victims discuss feelings and brainstorm ways of dealing with specific problems they are encountering. Similar strategies have been used in other cities (Wolf and Pillemer, 1994).

Similar to child sexual abuse prevention initiatives that teach children about safety and protection (Wolfe et al., 1995), education programs for seniors have also attempted to make them active players in the development and day-to-day operation of their services. Seniors can be assisted in reducing abuse in a number of ways, including professional recognition of their contributions, collaboration between seniors and professionals, generating their interest and commitment, ensuring a meaningful experience, brainstorming, using seniors as advisers, and central coordination (ARA Consulting Group, Inc., 1994). Moreover, significant progress has been made to increase professional awareness and involvement through training sessions and seminars on abuse, with the specific aim of examining bias or fears concerning treatment of the elderly among staff and administration (McDonald and Collins, 2000).

Educating Caregivers and the General Public

Because caregivers' stress has been implicated as a risk factor of abuse and neglect of the elderly, education and training programs are seen as a vital aspect in prevention. Available in most communities, such programs offer mutual support, stress reduction, and problem-solving strategies. The underlying assumption is that some social support and education/training works to reduce the likelihood that anger, aggression, and conflict will emerge in the caregiving relationship (Schulz et al., 2001).

Public education campaigns geared toward seniors as well as those in positions to assist have been implemented in recent years. These include a wide variety of pamphlets on the topic of advocacy for resources, lobbying activities, public media, and conferences. Coalitions consisting of service providers have also been established to educate community members about other abuse issues. Moreover, some communities are attempting to develop preventive programs to teach children to respect older adults and create opportunities for intergenerational relationships (Podnieks and Baillie, 1995). Others have taken the lead by offering public educational efforts, such as billboards, TV commercials, and newspaper ads, informing families of the necessity to provide care and support to seniors living at home. Nonprofit corporations or health care facilities that serve a geriatric population typically sponsor these efforts. Although formal evaluation is lacking, these efforts base their support on the success of similar initiatives in the fields of child abuse and domestic violence, described below.

Child Abuse and Domestic Violence Initiatives

Child abuse prevention has been approached through both universal efforts (e.g., educating the general public about its various signs; learning healthy childrearing skills) and more selected and targeted approaches, such as efforts to assist young parents who may or may not be at risk of abuse due to socioeconomic or other factors. An example of selected prevention that may share some common elements with elder abuse prevention is the recent work of David Olds and his colleagues. This program seeks to build on persons' strengths and abilities, rather than their deficits, and as such is a plausible approach to preventing physical abuse, neglect, and related social problems in different age groups. The program itself involves prenatal and postnatal home-visitation services for first-time (under age 19) parents to establish resource linkages and learn about their child's developmental needs. Fifteen years after receiving these services these parents maintained gains over controls on important dimensions: better family planning concerning number and spacing of children, less need for welfare, less child maltreatment, and fewer arrests of their children during adolescence (Olds et al., 1997). Although elder abuse clearly involves a different focus and timing of intervention, any of its components fit with existing knowledge of this issue, such as establishing community linkages, supporting families during stressful periods, teaching basic caregiver skills, and building on strengths of the target adult as well as caregivers and others.

Public awareness campaigns, such as public service announcements and advertisements, have been widely used throughout North America to combat child abuse and domestic violence. These campaigns are usually directed at recognizing the warning signs of such violence, as well as specialized community resources such as shelters for abused women. The Family Violence Prevention Fund (FVPF) in collaboration with the Advertising Council (Klein et al., 1997) developed an illustrative and comprehensive campaign that included a small research component. The campaign involved television ads with the message, "There is no excuse for abuse," and offered local contacts for domestic violence resources. The evaluation involved public opinion data prior to the campaign in 1992 and follow-up data gathered between 1994 and 1996. The findings suggest that Americans at the time perceived domestic violence as an important social issue that required state intervention. Of additional interest is the fact that many Americans excused domestic violence on the basis of alcohol or other circumstances, and they were uncertain and fearful about how to assist or intervene if they knew someone experiencing partner violence.

RECOMMENDATIONS FOR PRACTICE AND RESEARCH

Traditional approaches to child welfare and domestic violence were largely designed for protection rather than assistance, which leaves inadequate services available to a significant number of persons at need and who could benefit from early intervention. With some important exceptions, domestic violence policies related to child, woman, and elder abuse have focused primarily on identification of offenders, which paradoxically reduces the chances for assisting the much larger majority of potentially abusive or inadequate caregivers or partners. That is, if treatment services are tied to an offence and the individual must be identified and labeled, it is understandable that many individuals will perceive them as threatening and undesirable. Moreover, there is often a large gap between what families need in terms of treatment and what is actually delivered in practice. Help should be more easily available to a family or individual before a crisis or tragedy occurs.

Connected to this strategy of earlier family assistance for all forms of domestic violence must be the acknowledgment that intervention after the fact is seldom satisfactory to the individual, the family, or the community. The realities of adult protection, on the one hand, require firm guidelines and legal authority. Individual autonomy and special needs, on the other hand, profit from stability, continuity of caregivers, and a supportive family and community environment. Unfortunately, by the time official attention is drawn to the problem (due to the victims or others' reluctance to seek help, failure of family members or professionals to identify a burgeoning problem, offences that fall below the threshold for official response, etc.), it may be very difficult to reverse some of the patterns that have formed.

To combat the negative connotation associated with treatment and prevention services, policy planners need to study ways to make the available services more attractive to the elderly and those who care for them. As one illustration, prevention and early intervention efforts based on social learning theory have shown considerable promise in addressing the contributing factors related to child abuse; because child and elder abuse share some fundamental features (e.g., a dependent, caregiving relationship), these approaches seem well-suited for elder abuse prevention as well.

· Public Health Models

Emerging changes in public policy, legislation, and service delivery illustrate a commitment to finding ways to reduce the prevalence and harmful effects of all forms of domestic violence. Still, strategies that address the issue at a broader level need to be more fully developed and evaluated. Such strategies must take into account the large number of factors that influence the likelihood of elder abuse, as well as factors that promote proper care and well-being.

Significantly, there are established precedents for addressing complex public health issues facing children and adolescents, such as domestic violence (Wolfe and Jaffe, 2001), substance abuse and peer violence in schools (Cunningham and Henggeler, 2001; Farrell et al., 2001), and personal safety and injury prevention (Tremblay and Peterson, 1999). These approaches, adopted primarily for known health and behavior problems among youth, hold considerable promise for the elderly as well, because they recognize that change occurs through finding positive ways to communicate messages about healthy families and healthy relationships. Alternatives to violence can be activated in each community in a manner that stimulates interest, informs choices, and promotes action to decrease violence and abuse in the lives of children, youth, and families.

Implicit throughout this chapter is the presumption that public health and health promotion approaches to prevention of various forms of domestic violence, including elder abuse and neglect, are promising strategies. Such strategies should not undermine existing efforts at treatment and early intervention but rather would be designed to approach the widespread problem of elder abuse from a broader, more fundamental vantage point. Government fiscal incentives, for example, should be reoriented to emphasize prevention and treatment rather than detection, investigation, and alternative placement. A key health promotion policy issue concerns the need of all families for some degree of support and education (an "enhancement" strategy rather than interception; see Melton and Barry, 1994).

In conjunction with health promotion efforts, program development should focus on providing information for caregivers of the elderly that is easily understood, practical, and accessible to all present and potential populations. In particular, attention should be directed to societal influences that play a role in elder abuse and neglect, especially in circumstances where families are exposed to major effects of poverty, health risks, and environmental conflict. Such a cross-cultural perspective would redirect the focus away from individuals and families and explore societal and cultural conditions that attenuate or exacerbate these problems. In a similar manner, policy planners need to advocate for the establishment of minimum standards of care for their own communities, taking into account the cultural diversity of the community and the imbalance in child-care and elder-care responsibilities on women.

SUMMARY

In sum, the absence of theory-based treatments and outcome research in the area of elder abuse remains striking. Similar to related family violence interventions such as child abuse and women abuse programs, existing elder abuse programs have been largely aimed at individual needs based on victim accounts of abuse and violence, rather than a theory of change based on population based epidemiology (Chalk and King, 1998). This victim response approach has been effective at attracting public attention and resource commitments, but it is inadequate in terms of providing a foundation for measurement and evaluation of long-term outcomes or program effects.

Funding for university-based research efforts is indicated to gather information on ways to address the needs of the elderly, as well as to enhance caregiver(s) functioning enough to ensure safety and proper care. This review points to the conclusion that behavioral and cognitive behavioral approaches show promise as effective means of assisting caregivers and reducing the stresses of caring for an elderly member. Small- and large-scale efforts to validate their effectiveness are needed, as well as work identifying the families or settings for whom these strategies are most useful. Particularly important would be further development of interventions aimed at prevention of elder abuse. Finally, evaluation efforts must investigate the degree to which changes occurred at the community level and the degree to which such efforts may result in changes in the lives of victims and other family members. These levels include individual or family level, the community level, and the state and federal level such as laws and policies regarding response to violence against women and children (Sullivan and Allen, 2001).

REFERENCES

Anetzberger, G.J.
  2000   Caregiving: Primary cause of elder abuse? *Journal of the American Society on Aging* 2:46–51.
ARA Consulting Group, Inc.
  1994   *Older Canadians and the Abuse of Seniors: A Continuum from Participation to Empowerment.* Ottawa, ON: Health Canada.
Azar, S., and D. Wolfe
  1998   Treatment of child abuse and neglect. In: *Treatment of Childhood Disorders,* E.J. Mash and R.A. Barkley, eds. New York: Guilford Press.
Bond, J.B., R.L. Penner, and P. Yellen
  1995   Perceived effectiveness of legislation concerning abuse of the elderly: A survey of professionals in Canada and the United States. *Canadian Journal on Aging* 14(2, Suppl. 2):118–135.
Brandl, B., and T. Meuer
  2000   Domestic abuse in later life. *The Elder Law Journal* 8:297–335.
Chalk, R., and P. King
  1998   Assessing family violence interventions. *American Journal of Preventive Medicine* 14:289–292.
Cohn, A.H.
  1979   Essential elements of successful child abuse and neglect treatment. *Child Abuse and Neglect* 3:491–496.
Corcoran, J.
  2000   Family interventions with child physical abuse and neglect: A critical review. *Children and Youth Services Review* 22:563–591.
Cunningham, P.B., and S.W. Henggeler
  2001   Implementation of an empirically based drug and violence prevention and intervention program in public school settings. *Journal of Clinical Child Psychology* 30:221–232.
Edleson, J.L.
  1999   The overlap between child maltreatment and woman battering. *Violence Against Women* 5:134–154.
Family Violence Prevention Fund
  1998   *Domestic violence advertising campaign tracking survey.* San Francisco: Author.

Fantuzzo, J.W., L. Wray, R. Hall, C. Goins, and S.T. Azar
1986   Parent and social skills training for mentally retarded parents identified as child maltreaters. *American Journal of Mental Deficiency* 91:135–140.
Farrell, A.D., A.L. Meyer, E.M. Kung, and T.N. Sullivan
2001   Development and evaluation of school-based violence prevention programs. *Journal of Clinical Child Psychology* 30:207–220.
Filinson, R
1999   Aging 2000: Consumer empowerment through education. *Educational Gerontology* 25:155–165.
Fluke, J.D., Y.Y. Yuan, and M. Edwards
1999   Recurrence of maltreatment: An application of the National Child Abuse and Neglect Data System (NCANDS). *Child Abuse and Neglect* 23:633–650.
Goldman Institute on Aging
2001   San Francisco Consortium for Elder Abuse Prevention. Available: *www.gioa.org/professional/pro_eap.html.*
Gondolf, E.W.
1998   Do batterer programs work? A 15-month follow-up of multi-site evaluation. *Domestic Violence Report* 3:65–79.
Gordon, A.L.
2000   What works in child protective services reforms. In *What Works in Child Welfare,* M.P. Kluger, G. Alexander, and P.J. Curtis, eds. New York: Child Welfare League of America.
Hansen, D.J., J.E. Warner-Rogers, and D.B. Hecht
1998   Implementing and evaluating an individualized behavioral intervention program for maltreating families. In *Handbook of Child Abuse Research and Treatment,* J. R. Lutzker, ed. New York: Plenum.
Harbison, J.
1999   The changing career of "elder abuse and neglect" as a social problem in Canada: Learning from feminist frameworks? *Journal of Elder Abuse and Neglect* 11:59–80.
Herrenkohl, R.C., E.C Herrenkohl, B.P. Egolf, and M. Seech
1979   The repetition of child abuse: How frequently does it occur? *Child Abuse and Neglect* 3:67–72.
Hiatt, S., and A. Jones
2000   Volunteer services for vulnerable families and at risk elderly. *Child Abuse and Neglect* 24:141–148.
Hollinshead, D., and J. Fluke
2000   What works in safety and risk assessment for child protective services. In *What Works in Child Welfare,* M.P. Kluger, G. Alexander, and P.A. Curtis, eds. New York: Child Welfare League of America.
Hotch, D.
1994   *Identification, Assessment, Care, Referral, and Follow-up of Women Experiencing Domestic Violence Who Come to the Emergency Department for Treatment.* Ottawa, ON: Health Canada, Family Violence Prevention Division.
Institute of Medicine
2001   *Confronting Chronic Neglect: The Education and Training of Health Care Professionals on Family Violence.* F. Cohn, M.E. Salmon, and J.D. Stobo, eds. Washington, DC: National Academy Press.
Jaffe, P., N. Lemon, J. Sandler, and D. Wolfe
1996   *Working Together to End Domestic Violence.* Tampa, FL: Mancorp.

Kingston, P., and B. Penhale
    1995   Elder abuse and neglect: issues in the accident and emergency department. *Accident and Emergency Nursing* 3:122–128.
Klein, E., J. Campbell, E. Soler, and M. Chez
    1997   *Ending Domestic Violence.* Thousand Oaks, CA: Sage Publications.
Kolko, D.J.
    1996   Individual cognitive behavioral treatment and family therapy for physically abused children and their offending parents: A comparison of clinical outcomes. *Child Maltreatment* 1:322–342.
Kozma, A., and M.J. Stones
    1995   Issues in the measurement of elder abuse. In *Abuse and Neglect of Older Canadians: Strategies for Change,* M. J. Maclean, ed. Toronto, ON: Thompson.
Macolini, R.M.
    1995   Elder abuse policy: Considerations in research and legislation. *Behavioral Sciences and the Law* 13(3):349–363.
McDonald, L.
    1996   Abuse and neglect of elders. In *Encyclopedia of Gerontology: Age, Aging, and the Aged,* J.E. Birren, ed. San Diego, CA: Academic Press.
McDonald, L., and A. Collins
    2000   *Abuse and Neglect of Older Adults: A Discussion Paper.* Ottawa. ON: Health Canada.
Melton, G.B.
    1990   Child protection: Making a bad situation worse? *Contemporary Psychology* 35:213–214.
Melton, G.B., and F.D. Barry
    1994   Neighbors helping neighbors: The vision of the U. S. Advisory Board on Child Abuse and Neglect. In *Protecting Children from Abuse and Neglect: Foundations for a New National Strategy,* G.B. Melton, and F.D. Barry, eds.. New York: Guilford Press.
Mulligan, S.
    1990   *A Handbook for the Prevention of Family Violence.* Ottawa, ON: Health and Welfare Canada.
Nahmiash, D., and M. Reis
    2000   Most successful intervention strategies for abused older adults. *Journal of Elder Abuse and Neglect* 12(1).
Olds, D.L., J. Eckenrode, and C. R. Henderson
    1997   Long-term effects of home visitation on maternal life course and child abuse and neglect. *Journal of the American Medical Association* 278:637–643.
Peled, E., P. Jaffe, and J. Edleson
    1995   *Ending the Cycle of Violence.* Thousand Oaks, CA: Sage Publications.
Podnieks, E., and E. Baillie
    1995   Education as the key to the prevention of elder abuse and neglect. In *Abuse and Neglect of Older Canadians: Strategies for change,* M.J. Mclean, ed. Toronto, ON: Thompson.
Reis, M., and D. Nahmiash
    1995   When seniors are abused: An intervention model. *Gerontologist* 35:666–671.
    1998   Validation of the Indicators of Abuse (IOA) screen. *Gerontologist* 38:471–480.
Schulz, R., A. O'Brien, S. Czaja, M. Ory, R. Norris, and L.M. Martire
    2001   *Dementia caregiver intervention research: In search of clinical significance.* Manuscript submitted for publication.

Scogin, F., B. Stephens, J. Bynum, L. Baumhover, C. Beall, and N.P. Grote
  1992   Emotional correlates of caregiving. *Journal of Elder Abuse and Neglect* 4:59–69.
Scott, K.L., and D.A. Wolfe
  2000   What works in the treatment of batterers. In: *What Works in Child Welfare,* M.A. Kluger, G. Alexander, and P A. Curtis, eds. New York: Child Welfare League of America.
Sherman, L.W., and R.A. Berk
  1984   The specific deterrent effects of arrest for domestic assault. *American Sociological Review* 49:261–272.
Sullivan, C.M., and N.E. Allen
  2001   Evaluating coordinated community responses for abused women and their children. In *Domestic Violence in the Lives of Children: The Future of Research, Intervention, and Social Policy,* S.A. Graham-Bermann, and J.L. Edleson, eds. Washington, DC: American Psychological Association.
Tremblay, G.C., and L. Peterson
  1999   Prevention of childhood injury: Clinical and public policy challenges. *Clinical Psychology Review* 19:415–434.
U.S. Advisory Board on Child Abuse and Neglect
  1993   *Neighbors Helping Neighbors: A New National Strategy for the Protection of Children.* Washington, DC: U.S. Government Printing Office.
Wald, M.S., J.M. Carlsmith, P.H. Leiderman, C. Smith, and R.D. French
  1988   *Protecting Abused and Neglected Children.* Stanford, CA: Stanford University Press.
Weiner, A.
  1991   A community-based education model for identification and prevention of elder abuse. *Journal of Gerontological Social Work* 16:107–119.
Wolf, R.S.
  1992   Victimization of the elderly: Elder abuse and neglect. *Reviews in Clinical Gerontology* 2:269-276.
Wolf, R.S., and K. Pillemer
  1994   What's new in elder abuse programming? Four bright ideas. *Gerontologist,* 34:126–129.
Wolfe, D.A.
  1999   *Child Abuse: Implications for Child Development and Psychopathology.* Thousand Oaks, CA: Sage Publications.
Wolfe, D.A., and P. Jaffe
  1991   Child abuse and family violence as determinants of child psychopathology. *Canadian Journal of Behavioural Science* 23:282–299.
  2001   Prevention of domestic violence: Emerging initatives. In: *Domestic Violence in the Lives of Children,* S.A. Graham-Bermann and J.L. Edleson, eds. Washington, DC: American Psychological Association.
Wolfe, D.A., and C. Wekerle
  1993   Treatment strategies for child physical abuse and neglect: A critical progress report. *Clinical Psychology Review* 13:473–500.
Wolfe, D.A., N.D. Reppucci, and S. Hart
  1995   Child abuse prevention: Knowledge and priorities. *Journal of Clinical Child Psychology* 24:5–22.

Index